The Balancing Act

NUTRITION & WEIGHT GUIDE

A No-Gimmick, Step-by-Step Approach That Really Works!

"This may be the most complete and sensible weight loss manual we have seen."
—*The Dallas Morning News*

Georgia G. Kostas, M.P.H., R.D.

Director of Nutrition, Cooper Clinic, Dallas, Texas

FOREWORD by KENNETH H. COOPER, M.D., M.P.H.

PLEASE NOTE

Fitness, diet and health are matters which necessarily vary from
individual to individual. Readers should consult with their own physician
about personal needs before starting any diet program, and especially if
one is on any medication or is already under medical care for illness.

Use of this manual by individuals, health professionals, or organizations
as a teaching tool does not reflect an endorsement by the author or the
Cooper Clinic of the instructor's or the organization's program or practice.

Printed by Quebecor Printing Book Group, Kingsport, Tennessee

---

For inquiries or to order books, write or call:
The Balancing Act Nutrition and Weight Guide
P.O. Box 671281
Dallas, TX 75367-8281
(214) 239-7223

For additional copies, refer to the order form in the back of this manual.

ISBN Number   0-9635969-1-8

This Book

STOP DIETING! LOSE WEIGHT! GET FIT! FEEL GREAT!

Written in a "user-friendly," step-by-step workbook format, **The Balancing Act Nutrition and Weight Guide,** *provides you with the strategies for healthy eating and weight loss that REALLY WORK! This book will direct, organize, and expedite your route to health, fitness, and permanent weight loss. You'll learn the same eating, exercise, and lifestyle habits used to help individuals lose weight successfully at the renowned Cooper Clinic. By designing your own eating plan and exercise routine, your personal success will be assured.*

With this book, you will:

- Reduce your appetite and increase your control over eating

- "Rev up" your metabolism and burn more body fat

- Develop habits that free you from "up and down" weight cycles

- Learn how to include your favorite foods - *even french fries, ice cream, and chocolate*

- Be able to make the best-informed choices at restaurants of all types

- Learn to judge a food by its label

- Improve your nutritional health and fitness

As a result, you'll feel and look your best and experience a greater zest for life and a sense of well-being. **You'll** *be the one "in charge" of your weight and health, and enjoy the freedom of having discovered the best "Balancing Act" for you!*

Dedication

To those who continually strive for healthy lifestyles and weight management through a balanced sensible approach.

Acknowledgments

First and foremost, I wish to acknowledge with gratitude, Dr. Kenneth Cooper and the Cooper Clinic physicians who provided the incentive, the environment and the philosophy in which a balanced weight control program could be established. This manual reflects the clinic's balanced approach to health and well-being and emphasis on preventive medicine, education and personal responsibility for one's health.

*Secondly, I wish to thank Kim Rojohn, R.D., my dear friend and Cooper Clinic colleague who helped author this book in its original form, **The Balancing Act**. Kim's creativity, compassion and expertise in nutrition counseling combined with her personal commitment to fitness and weight management made this manual's first edition an enjoyable team effort.*

A special thank you to all my patients, colleagues, and friends who contributed ideas and successful strategies described in this book. You helped fill these pages with "real" strategies from "real" people!

Thanks to Lisa Rose and Cindy Morrison for their outstanding professional typesetting and layout work. (Lisa even lost 5 lbs. and gave up caffeine while working on this book!) Thank you to Jay Weesner, cover designer and graphic artist; Bruce Peschel, book illustrator; and Floyd Black, Tom Demopulos, and Sondra Carey, R.D., consultants. My sincere appreciation to the Cooper Clinic nutrition staff, Kathy Miller, M.S., R.D., Patty Kirk, R.D., Karen Angevine, R.D., and Veronica Coronado, who helped with nutrition revisions.

To each of you, thank you for your input, contributions, and enthusiastic support.

FOREWORD

*The concept of "wellness" is sweeping the country due to the great interest expressed by the consumer. Initially, I felt "wellness" was secondary to an aerobic exercise program. In fact, I have been guilty of saying that "exercise overcomes many, if not all, of the deleterious effects of diet." Over the past few years, it has been brought to my attention on many occasions that people have followed exercise guidelines exactly, ignored the other component parts of wellness including proper weight and diet, and have died suddenly at relatively early ages from heart disease. This is why I emphasize aerobics as only a part of a total wellness program and state that it is "not enough by itself." I expanded upon that concept in my book, **The Aerobics Program For Total Well-Being**.*

*Georgia Kostas, M.P.H., R.D., Director of Nutrition at the Cooper Clinic, has been involved in the nutritional recommendations in all of my publications since 1980. Her knowledge and expertise in this area is quite evident in her contribution to **The Aerobics Program For Total Well-Being**. She then combined her talents and knowledge of nutrition with Kim Rojohn, a former member of The Cooper Clinic nutrition staff, and prepared an outstanding nutritional manual, **The Balancing Act**. Now she has updated and enhanced this manual as **The Balancing Act Nutrition and Weight Guide**. In this book, the various components of a wellness program are emphasized focusing primarily on diet. Nonetheless, the recommended exercise programs are sound, and in conjunction with proper nutrition, should be of considerable value in helping the reader to achieve optimum health through proper exercise and diet.*

This book provides practical and interesting information which should be of great value in balancing your wellness program. Remember, too, moderation is the key to long-term success.

May your efforts to follow the nutritional and exercise recommendations in this book be successful, enabling you to enjoy a long, healthy and productive life . . . to the fullest.

Kenneth H. Cooper, M.D., M.P.H
Founder and Chairman, Cooper Clinic

About the Authors

Georgia Kostas, M.P.H., R.D., *teaches you winning strategies for weight loss and optimal health. Since founding the Cooper Clinic's Nutrition Program in 1979, she has designed nutrition programs for over 15,000 individuals. Dedicated to helping individuals achieve their health and fitness goals, she is a nutrition consultant to numerous organizations and corporations and to professional athletes. A registered and licensed dietitian, she has authored the nutrition chapters in recent books by Dr. Kenneth H. Cooper —* **The Aerobics Program for Total Well-Being** *(1984),* **Controlling Cholesterol** *(1987), and* **Hypertension** *(1990). Her areas of specialty include preventive and cardiovascular medicine, weight control, physical fitness, sports nutrition, and media communications. As a frequent speaker to professional, corporate, and public groups, she has presented seminars in Brazil, Germany, Spain, Japan, Austria and Poland and a satellite broadcast for the American Dietetic Association. She has served as a consultant to McDonald's "Healthy Growing Up" curriculum, American Airlines, the U.S. Army in Europe, and Mike Ditka's "Straight from the Heart" health video, and is on Gatorade's Speakers Bureau, teaching sports nutrition to coaches and athletic trainers, and professional athletes. Ms. Kostas serves as the American Dietetic Association's Liaison to the President's Council on Physical Fitness and Sports and is a media spokesperson for the American Heart Association. She has co-authored the nutrition information series* **Nutrition Tips***, and designed* **The Cooper Clinic Nutrition and Exercise Evaluation System***, a computerized dietary analysis software package. Her B.A. in Biology is from Rice University, her M.P.H. in Nutrition from Tulane University and residency at Ochsner Hospital. She was "Recognized Young Dietitian of the Year" from Texas in 1981, and received the American Dietetic Association's Sports and Cardiovascular Nutrition National Achievement Award in 1990. She maintains a healthy, active lifestyle.*

Kimberly Rojohn, R.D., *who co-authored this book's first edition, is the former Assistant Director of Nutrition at the Cooper Clinic and Cooper Aerobics Center in Dallas, Texas. As an athlete, marathoner and triathlete, she is an expert in nutrition and fitness counseling and understands the unique role of both in weight control. As a clinical nutritionist and registered dietitian, she often lectures on nutrition. She developed the first "Nutrition for Heart Health" program component of the Cooper Aerobics Center's Cardiac Rehabilitation Exercise Program, and co-authored the* **Nutrition Tips** *series of 13 informative pamphlets for consumers. Her B.A. in Dietetics is from Indiana University of Pennsylvania and her internship was at Baylor University Medical Center in Dallas.*

© 1993, *The Balancing Act Nutrition and Weight Guide*, G. Kostas, M.P.H., R.D., Dallas, Texas

To The Reader

Dear Friends,

Thanks to your positive response to the first edition of *The Balancing Act*, we've decided to publish this second edition called *The Balancing Act Nutrition and Weight Guide*. The new title reflects the fact that this book can be used both as a **nutrition guide** and a **weight loss guide**. This latest edition offers you the most current information on nutrition and winning strategies for managing your weight and optimizing your health and fitness.

In addition, this unique book provides you with *FIVE NEW EATING PLAN OPTIONS* so YOU can choose the one that best fits your lifestyle. Even those of you with busy, on-the-go lifestyles will at last find a plan that works for you!

Our readers report that they have appreciated this "no gimmick", practical approach, and the opportunity to design their own personalized eating and exercise plans. With a wealth of practical nutrition information at your fingertips, you too will be able to make better informed decisions about your diet and health. As a result, you'll reap the benefits of a healthy lifestyle — the ability to take control of your weight, eat well, feel fit and energetic, and enjoy a greater sense of well-being.

Here's to your new discoveries, enjoyment, and successes as you follow the principles and steps outlined in the following pages. *START NOW!* Get fit, eat wisely, and enjoy the satisfaction that comes from leading a healthy, active, productive life!

To your best health and fitness,

Georgia Kostas, M.P.H., R.D.
Director of Nutrition, Cooper Clinic

The Cooper Aerobics Center

The internationally known **Cooper Aerobics Center** provides the most up-to-date preventive medicine expertise in the world. This complete preventive medicine facility was founded in 1971 by Dr. Kenneth H. Cooper, M.D., M.P.H. The center, with its five components the Cooper Clinic, the Cooper Fitness Center, Cooper Institute for Aerobics Research, Guest Lodge and Cooper Wellness Program is located in Dallas, Texas and is staffed by professionals in medicine, nutrition, fitness, exercise physiology, epidemiology and health education.

The **Cooper Clinic** is a cardiovascular and preventive medicine clinic providing comprehensive medical evaluations, coronary risk factor appraisals, and individualized diet, exercise, and lifestyle guidelines. Physicians, nutritionists, and fitness consultants staff the clinic.

The **Cooper Fitness Center** is a total fitness complex where members may participate in medically prescribed and supervised exercise programs.

The **Cooper Institute for Aerobics Research** is a non-profit public corporation dedicated to advancing research and education regarding diet, exercise, living habits and health.

The **Aerobics Center Guest Lodge** offers lovely accommodations for Aerobics Center visitors, clinic patients and In-Residence program participants.

The **Cooper Wellness Programs** offer multiple live-in programs that teach healthy lifestyles through education and first-hand experience.

All divisions are dedicated to the philosophy that proper diet, regular exercise and emotional well-being are the cornerstones of preventive medicine.

TABLE OF CONTENTS

SECTION VIII: HABITS - INNER PSYCHE AND STRESS MANAGEMENT NUTRITION - GROCERY SHOPPING / LABELS 185

INNER PSYCHE AND STRESS MANAGEMENT

GROCERY SHOPPING

SECTION IX: HABIT - BUILDING SUPPORT - NUTRITION - MORE FOOD FACTS 197

BUILDING SUPPORT

FOOD FACTS

SECTION X: TIPS TO CONTINUE ONWARD 215

MAINTAIN YOUR NEW LIFESTYLE...*utilize:*...............................217

APPENDICES

INTRODUCTION

DESIGNING YOUR BALANCING ACT FOR YOUR BEST HEALTH AND WEIGHT

- Do you want to arrange your closet by SEASON and not by SIZE?

- Do you want to eat a fudge brownie, enjoy a cool ice cream cone on a hot summer day, eat Mexican food or a hamburger and still be healthy and lose weight?

- **YOU CAN!** *The Balancing Act Nutrition and Weight Guide* shows you how.

Gone are the days when deprivation and starvation were associated with weight loss. We now have proof that "diets don't work" in the long run; nor do powders, pills, shakes, bars, pre-packaged meals, or gimmicky diets. These methods may result in short-term weight loss, but with time, the weight usually returns. Often, the "post-diet" weight is greater than before the diet began and afterwards, even harder to lose! This is because the body's composition changes with weight re-gain (more fat, less muscle), which slows down metabolism (your body's rate of calorie-burning). Re-gained weight is often re-distributed around the "middle", which increases one's risk of heart problems, high blood pressure, and diabetes.

Very low-calorie, "quick-fixes", **do not work**! Eating too few calories can actually lead to bingeing, uncontrolled eating, muscle loss, and a slowed-down metabolism.

Fortunately, you really can eat foods you enjoy — even **brownies, ice cream**, and **burgers** — and still lose weight. You simply need: (1) a practical system for food selection, balancing high-fat foods with low-fat foods; and (2) a sensible fitness routine that "revs" up your metabolism so you can burn more body fat, even at rest.

Fifteen years of diet counseling over 15,000 individuals has taught me that the key to successful weight loss is a "no gimmick" approach that puts you in charge. You choose what you eat and where - at home or on-the-town. No special foods are required. *The Balancing Act Nutrition and Weight Guide* outlines strategies that have been used successfully by Cooper Clinic patients and class participants.

People who are most successful in losing weight:

1. *Enjoy eating a healthy mix of all foods*, balancing low-fat, high-fiber foods with higher-fat choices, and developing strategies for eating favorite foods in reasonable amounts.
2. *Exercise moderately and consistently* to boost metabolism, decrease appetite and burn more body fat.
3. *Practice "I'm-in-charge", sensible eating habits and the lifestyle* that promotes one's chosen weight.
4. *Shift thinking to "lifestyle" (not "dieting") and "lifetime" (not "quick-fix").* This shift away from the "on again - off again" dieting mentality *sets you free* and enables you to maintain a more productive life focus.
5. Work toward *moderation, balance, and variety* with food choices and exercise.

---

6. *Set realistic goals*. Since you didn't gain overnight, you can't expect to lose overnight.

7. *Have a meaningful purpose* for losing the weight and keeping it off, lifelong.

8. *Write down* a daily description of food consumed and daily exercise. Records build awareness and motivate action. (One woman was amazed to discover she was eating thousands of calories while cooking, preparing and clearing her family's plates!)

The "80-20 rule" is good news to many. It means if you make healthy choices 80% of the time, you can eat "fun foods" 20% of the time and still stay healthy and achieve your weight goals. For example, go ahead and enjoy that brownie, with its 250 calories and 10 grams of fat. You can still lose weight. How? By using fat-free salad dressing on your salad and skipping the croutons. Or, hold the extra tablespoon of butter on your baked potato, and have a refreshing glass of water instead of a 12 oz. regular soda. Either way, by making these simple trade-offs, you can enjoy the brownie, guilt-free. Chances are, you won't miss the croutons, fat-laden dressing, butter, or soda. You've simply traded the calories and fat.

Can you eat fast foods and burgers? Of course, with the "80-20 rule," and a little "balancing act", here's how:

Example One				
BREAKFAST	**LUNCH**	**DINNER**	**TOTALS**	**OPTIONS**
1 fruit	hamburger (1/4 lb)	Chinese stir-fry		
1 cup cereal	small fries	dinner or low-fat		Omit fries;
1 cup skim milk	1 fruit	frozen dinner		
	1 diet drink	1 fruit		TOTALS =
300 Calories	700 Calories	350 Calories	**1350 Calories**	1030 Calories,
0 Fat	36 Grams Fat	8 Grams Fat	**44 Grams Fat**	28 Grams Fat
Example Two				
BREAKFAST	**LUNCH**	**DINNER**	**TOTALS**	**OPTIONS**
1 bagel	fast food grilled	2 slices cheese pizza		
1 banana	chicken sandwich	huge salad with		Omit fries;
8 oz. fat-free fruit	(no mayonnaise)	oil-free dressing		
yogurt	small fries (or candy bar)	4 oz. fat-free frozen		
	diet drink or water	yogurt		TOTALS =
350 Calories	550 Calories	500 Calories	**1400 Calories**	1180 Calories,
0 Fat	20 Grams Fat	17 Grams Fat	**37 Grams Fat**	25 Grams Fat

Add a brisk 2 mile walk (30 minutes) and burn 200 calories. You'll net 1150 calories the first day (Example One), and 1200 calories the second day (Example Two). Anyone can lose weight this way!

One gentleman, who lost 120 pounds in one year following our recommended system, said "I couldn't have lost weight without this book...I set up my program just as I would a business. Taking certain steps daily led to success."

With this book and its 10 sections of informative tips and strategies, you will discover the ultimate keys to your best health and weight — developing the lifestyle and skills for your own **"Balancing Act"**! Ready to begin? Read on!

HOW TO USE THIS MANUAL

USE THIS BOOK AS YOUR PERSONAL DAILY COUNSELOR, "COACH", AND GUIDE.

1. **BEGIN** by scanning the Table of Contents. **CHOOSE** the section(s) of the book and topics that most affect your lifestyle, food choices, and weight. Read these sections first.

    For example:
    - You skip breakfast because you rush out the door each morning with no time to eat.
    - **Turn to** page 86 for *"Quick and Easy Breakfast Ideas."*

    -OR-
    - You hear that "fat makes you fat," but you don't see fat on your dinner plate. Where is it hidden and what can you do about it? What meats are O.K. to eat?
    - **Turn to:** — *"Trim Fat — Save Calories"* (Page 100)
        - *"Fat Gram Counter"* (Page 108)
        - *"Be Calorie-Wise and Fat-Smart"* (Page 93)
        - *"Meats"* in the Food Groups Section (Page 59)
        - *"Fats"* in the Food Groups Section (Page 67)
        - *"Cooking Tips"* (Page 127)

    -OR-
    - You eat out frequently and can't figure out your best choices.
    - **Read** *"Eating Out"* sections (page 167) and *"Meals Out - Comparisons"* (page 175)

2. **DESIGN YOUR OWN ACTION PLAN** — in Section I. Select an **EATING PLAN** (Section II) and **EXERCISE PLAN** (Sections I and VII) suited for your lifestyle. Read the entire book to learn strategies that enable you to utilize your plan successfully. Progress through the book in your preferred sequence of sections.

3. **READ** one section of the manual each week and concentrate only on that section. Take two weeks on a particular section , if necessary. Identify the most workable strategies for you in each section, and try them!

    EMPHASIZE WEEKLY:
    - one positive eating **HABIT**
    - one new **FOOD** or nutrition goal
    - one step forward with your **EXERCISE** plan

4. **KEEP RECORDS.** Records increase your awareness and promote your desired behavior changes.

RECORD:

- Daily eating on your **FOOD RECORDS**
- Daily exercise on your **EXERCISE LOG**
- Weekly weight on your **WEIGHT CHART** or **GRAPH**
- Weekly achievements on your **LADDER TO SUCCESS**
- Monthly progress checks on your **END-OF-MONTH PROGRESS CHART**

These records are in Appendix A.

5. **REWARD YOURSELF**: Plan rewards for each notable achievement — big or small. Rewards reinforce your successes.

6. **SOLICIT SUPPORT**: Include family, friends, conducive environments and activities. Think positive thoughts, attitudes and feelings.

7. **REVIEW DAILY**:

- Assess yesterday's successes to repeat and anticipate problems to prevent today. Learn from yesterday. Live for today!
- Commit yourself.
- Expect success.
- Enjoy a rewarding day.

8. **YOU'LL FIND RESULTS YOU CAN ANTICIPATE** — the best "balancing act" for you! You'll enjoy easier decision-making, healthier eating, the right exercise, easier weight control, less guilt, and a sense of personal control over your well-being, energy, and looks. More good news follows. Read on!

I. PROGRAM OVERVIEW: LIFESTYLE CHOICES

HABITS AND LIFESTYLE FOCUS

1. Make a COMMITMENT. Get a MIND SET! BEGIN!
2. What's ahead? Discover two key *Hints for a Healthier You* (6).
3. Become familiar with *Optimal Nutrition* (8), *Basic Guidelines for Weight Control* (11), how to *Strike a Balance* (12) for healthy weight loss.
4. Understand how *Body Composition* affects metabolism and how to change your body to change yiour weight (14).
5. Is your exercise adequate? (15)
6. Which of your eating habits promote or prevent over-eating? (16-17)
7. Identify your past weight loss and eating patterns (18-20).

NUTRITION FOCUS

1. Test your nutritional IQ with the *Quiz* (21).
2. Learn why most diets don't work (22-25) and what to look for in a food plan (26).
3. *Calculate Your Calorie Needs* for weight loss (27-29).
4. To encourage new habits, enjoy some *Pleasure Activities* (30).
5. Name your game plan. Record *My Action Plan* (31-32).

EXERCISE FOCUS

1. Review the examples on pages 15 and 29.
2. Start exercising! Begin with 3 days of exercise this week. Every little bit helps.

RECORDS

1. Records are the tools for your success. Begin keeping food and exercise records daily (33-35).
2. Chart your weight and list your achievements on the *Ladder to Success* (36) at the end of the week.
3. Keep in mind the *Success Tips* (37) that will keep you going!

GOALS

HABIT:	3 meals per day
FOOD:	remove all "problem foods" at home
EXERCISE:	30 minutes per session, 3 days this week
RECORDS:	food, exercise, weight

HINTS FOR A HEALTHIER YOU

The **Balancing Act Nutrition and Weight Guide** shows you how to eat right, exercise successfully, and create the lifestyle habits that promote a permanent, healthy weight. As a result, you'll look and feel your best. But, first there are a couple of points to grasp as you prepare to become a healthier you.

1. GIVE UP THE BELIEF IN A "QUICK-FIX".

Later in this section, you will read more about the pitfalls of "miracle diets" that entice Americans to spend 13 billion dollars each year pursuing leanness and youthfulness. These quick-fix diet programs don't work long term because they do not produce lasting solutions. Beyond the negative physiological impact of repeatedly losing and regaining weight, the psychological impact can be devastating. Start now to avoid the disappointment and frustration that can be so demoralizing!

WHY MOST QUICK-FIX DIETS FAIL

1. New behaviors, healthy eating habits, good food choices and smart "trade-off" eating cannot be learned if you are relying on fad diets, special products, etc. "Food replacements" are not serious food "trade-offs", nor are they "habit replacements".

2. Standardized programs become boring and too rigid to follow long-term. By choosing your own personalized, varied eating plan, you'll enjoy your meals and "stay with the program" for lifetime success.

3. Your metabolism slows down. Fast weight loss means muscle loss. When you lose weight more slowly and exercise, however, your body can begin to burn more body fat, retain muscle, boost your metabolism, speed weight loss, and keep the weight off.

4. Medical complications can arise from some diets and /or from repeated weight gain/loss "seesawing". (See "Dieting" page 22).

REMEMBER: There is no "MIRACLE CURE" to melt fat away!

A HEALTHY WEIGHT = eating right + exercise + sensible lifestyle habits!

---

2. COMMIT YOURSELF TO UN-LEARNING OLD BEHAVIORS AND RE-LEARNING NEW ONES.

Eating is one of our most complex behaviors. Eating behaviors are deeply entrenched and learned through a lifetime of family, ethnic, cultural and religious customs. Fortunately, just as we learn how to eat, we can *re-learn* to eat. New behaviors enable us to attain and maintain a desired weight. To get started, don a fresh attitude, an open mindedness and a commitment to change.

WHAT EXPERIENCES AND ATTITUDES INFLUENCE YOUR EATING HABITS?

1. "Clean your plates. Children in far-off lands are starving."
2. "Eat your vegetables and clean your plate before you can have dessert."
3. "A fat child is a healthy child."
4. Food may be served as rewards. Food may be equated with love.
5. Food is associated with social life.

WHAT ADVERTISING INFLUENCES YOUR EATING BEHAVIOR?

- discount coupons, mailers
- all-you-can-eat promotions
- tantalizing magazine and newspaper ads
- colorful billboard adds
- enticing food packaging

Learning new eating behaviors and how to make informed food decisions is a gradual process that becomes ingrained over time. Repeated behaviors becomes "habit". Make your habits work for you...not against you. Create habits that work!

Small, permanent lifestyle changes are better than large, temporary ones.
Small, permanent weight losses are better than large, temporary ones.

ARE YOU READY TO BECOME MORE ENERGETIC, VIBRANT, PRODUCTIVE, AND STRESS RESISTANT? Start with good nutrition, summarized on the following two pages. **Become informed!**

GUIDELINES FOR OPTIMAL NUTRITION

For your best health and easiest weight loss or weight control, here's what to eat and why:

1. BALANCE YOUR CALORIE INTAKE WITH EXERCISE TO ATTAIN AND MAINTAIN YOUR DESIRED BODY WEIGHT. Over-eating or under-exercising upsets your caloric balance. Extra pounds result.

2. BALANCE YOUR INTAKE OF PROTEIN, COMPLEX CARBOHYDRATES AND FAT FOR WELL-BALANCED MEALS. COMBINE P-C-F AT EACH MEAL...to satisfy your appetite, reduce hunger for hours, and give you lasting energy between meals.

NUTRIENT	% OF CALORIES	EAT DAILY
PROTEIN	10 - 20 %	4-6 ounces fish, poultry, lean meat, dried peas or beans + 2-3 cups skim or low-fat milk or yogurt
COMPLEX CARBOHYDRATE	50 - 70 %	5 - 8 fruit and vegetables, at least 2 raw, plus 5 - 8 starches, at least 2 wholegrain
FAT	15 - 30 %	3 - 8 teaspoons added fats (margarine, oil, dressing) Eat only baked, broiled foods — not fried
WATER		4 glasses (1 quart) minimum plus 1 quart other fluids

3. CHOOSE A WIDE FOOD VARIETY AT EACH MEAL TO MAXIMIZE NUTRIENT VARIETY. Select a protein source, grain/starch, vegetable, and/or fruit. Color variety also makes a meal more appealing and psychologically satisfying.

4. CHOOSE FRESH, WHOLESOME, UNPROCESSED FOODS...fresh fruit and vegetables, wholewheat bread and cereals, etc. These contain more nutrients and fiber, and less sugar and salt.

5. ESTABLISH CONSISTENT EATING PATTERNS, i.e., 3 MEALS A DAY. This promotes sound nutrition, reduces stress, increases energy, prevents over-eating and puts you in control of your appetite and eating. Do not skip meals...particularly breakfast. Eat every 5-6 hours to keep your blood sugar normal, regulate appetite, and reduce between meal snacking.

6. CHOOSE MORE COMPLEX CARBOHYDRATES ("plant foods"), at least 3-4 per meal, for vitamins, minerals, energy, fiber, water and few calories. Eat fresh fruits and vegetables, wholegrained and enriched cereals (bread, cereals, rice, pasta, grits, oatmeal, cracked wheat, bran), potatoes, corn, peas, beans, lentils, popcorn, pretzels. These foods should make up at least half of your daily calories.

7. CHOOSE MORE DIETARY FIBER (at least 8 fiber foods daily) for good digestion, prevention of digestive problems, colon cancer, and regulation of blood sugar and cholesterol levels. Fiber in foods helps you feel more full so that you eat less per meal. Fiber is in: bran, wholegrains, fruits and vegetables (including peels and seeds), nuts, seeds, popcorn, beans, peas, brown rice, oatmeal, potatoes, corn.

8. CHOOSE FEWER FOODS HIGH IN FAT. These include: fried foods, butter, margarine, mayonnaise, oils, sauces, salad dressings, nuts, avocado, granola, party crackers and dips, chips and dips, fast foods, convenience foods, commercial pastries, high-fat meat (bacon, sausage, cold cuts, hot dogs, marbled beef, lamb, pork), high-fat dairy products (whole milk, sour or sweet cream, cheese, ice cream). Since fats contain twice the calories per gram as carbohydrates and proteins, fats concentrate a lot of calories into a small amount of food. **One tablespoon of fat** (oil, margarine, mayonnaise, peanut butter, butter, etc.) **contains 100 calories!**

9. EAT UNSATURATED FATS IN PLACE OF SATURATED FATS WHENEVER POSSIBLE. *Saturated fats* are usually *animal fats*, found in dairy and meat products, but sometimes are vegetable fats, as in chocolate, coconut, palm oils, and "hydrogenated" (hardened) fats in baked goods. *Polyunsaturated fats* are primarily from *vegetable sources,* and found in vegetable oils, tub margarines and unhydrogenated peanut butter; and also in fish. Use safflower, corn, sunflower, soybean and cottonseed oils and margarines. *Monounsaturated fats* are in olives, peanuts, olive oil, peanut oil, canola oil, avocados, and some nuts.

10. EAT LESS PROTEIN...just 4 to 6 ounces per day of fish, poultry and lean meat. Most protein-rich foods contain fat and cholesterol. Eat more fish, poultry and veal (10+ meals per week) in place of beef, lamb, pork and cheese (4 meals per week).

11. EAT LESS CHOLESTEROL...less than 300 mg a day. Limit these: egg yolks, organ meats, crawfish, meat and meat products (sausage, cold cuts, bacon, etc.), dairy products (whole milk, sour or sweet cream, cheese, ice cream, butter), and fried foods.

12. EAT LESS SUGAR...limit sweets to 1 - 3 weekly. Sugar is in: table sugar, honey, jam, jelly, soft drinks, desserts, candy, cookies, cakes, pastries, processed foods and beverages, sweetened juices and fruit, sugar-coated cereals, peanut butter containing sugar. Most desserts are rich in sugar, fat, and calories.

13. LIMIT SODIUM...to less than 4000 mg daily. Sources: salt, pickles, olives, luncheon meats, hot dogs, ham, bacon, sausage, cheeses, processed foods, fast foods, snack foods (chips, crackers, pretzels), canned soups and vegetables, sauces (chili, barbecue, soy, steak), pizza, commercial bakery products.

14. LIMIT CAFFEINE (a stimulant) to 200 mg daily, as found in 2 cups of coffee. Caffeine is in: coffee, tea, cola drinks, chocolate.

15. LIMIT ALCOHOL as your doctor directs; and at most, 1 to 2 drinks per day. A "drink" is 1 1/2 ounces liquor, 4 ounces wine, 1 light beer, 8 ounces regular beer. Each contains 100 calories. Also, alcohol sabotages your weight loss efforts by slowing down your burning of fat stores.

16. DRINK AT LEAST 8 GLASSES OF FLUIDS DAILY, 4 OF WHICH ARE WATER. Sources: water, juice, milk, other beverages. Fluids are filling, helping you eat fewer high-fat foods. Fluids also prevent mistaking hunger for thirst.

17. ENJOY YOUR MEALS! EAT SLOWLY IN A RELAXED ENVIRONMENT. This aids digestion and weight control and makes meals more satisfying, which reduces over-eating. How you eat is almost as important as what you eat. Find ways to deal with stress effectively, without food or alcohol. Slow down and enjoy each bite of a good meal.

18. ADJUST YOUR FOOD INTAKE ACCORDING TO YOUR SPECIAL NEEDS (such as hypertension, high cholesterol levels, diabetes, etc.).

19. ENJOY THE PLEASURE OF EATING HEALTHY FOODS THAT TASTE GOOD.

WHAT'S ON YOUR PLATE?

Healthy, balanced meals are 15-30% fat, 50-60% complex carbohydrate, and 10-20% protein, as described on page 8.

On your dinner plate, this means eating: **3/4ths plant foods (complex carbohydrates)** such as 1/2 cup carrots, 1/2 cup green beans, 1/2 cup rice; and **1/4th protein** (3 oz. of fish, chicken, lean meat).

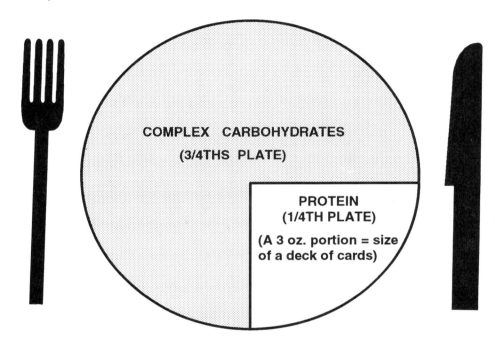

Translated into "grams", this means a daily recommended intake of:

CALORIES	FAT (gms)	COMPLEX CARBOHYDRATES (gms)	PROTEIN (gms)
1000	15-30	125-150	25-50
1200	18-40	150-180	30-60
1500	22-50	190-225	40-75
2000	30-60	250-300	60-100

You need not get this technical with numbers! Use the plate as your guide.

Note: 1 gram complex carbohydrate contains 4 calories
1 gram protein contains 4 calories
1 gram fat contains 9 calories

BASIC GUIDELINES FOR WEIGHT CONTROL

1. Refuse second HELPINGS, except vegetables.

2. Eat smaller PORTIONS of most foods.

3. Double your intake of fresh VEGETABLES and FRUIT, especially raw.

4. Choose CRUNCHY foods...apples, salads, popcorn, toast, vegetables.

5. Eat less PROTEIN: just 4 to 6 ounces per day of meat, fish, poultry, veal!

6. Reduce ALCOHOL consumption.

7. Reduce SWEETS (candy, soft drinks, desserts, sweet rolls, sugar, etc.)

8. Reduce FATS (margarine, mayonnaise, salad dressings, sauces, fatty meats, fast foods, fried foods). Buy lower-fat and fat-free options.

9. Avoid SNACKS, unless pre-planned and healthy.

10. Drink at least 4 glasses (1 quart) of WATER daily, and 4 glasses of other fluids (or water).

11. EXERCISE more.

12. REMEMBER: 3500 calories = 1 pound fat ... Therefore, use the chart below to determine how much to decrease your calorie intake and increase your calorie expenditure to lose 1 to 2 pounds a week.

CALORIES Food + Exercise	CALORIES Save Daily	CALORIES Saved Weekly	LOSE Weekly
↓ 250 + ↑ 250 = ↓ 750 + ↑ 250 =	500 1000	3500 7000	1 pound 2 pounds

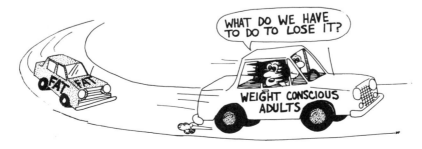

STRIKE A BALANCE!

1. **LOSE GRADUALLY**
   A gradual weight loss of 1/2 to 2 pounds per week is best to:
   - maintain nutritionally balanced meals
   - lose body fat — not muscle
   - produce big results
   - maintain your weight loss

2. **SUPPLEMENTS**
   If your eating program includes less than 1200 calories per day, take a multiple vitamin and mineral supplement to be sure you are getting the essential nutrients each day. Do not go below 1000 calories per day!

3. **3500 CALORIES = 1 POUND**
   - To lose **1 pound** per week, decrease your daily calories by 500;
     500 x 7 days per week = 3500 calories
   - To lose **2 pounds** per week, decrease your daily calories by 1000;
     1000 x 7 days per week = 7000 calories

A SIMPLE APPROACH:	Calories omitted per day
↓ 8-ounce meat portion to 4 ounce	280
↓ salad dressing to 1 tablespoon (not 3 tablespoons)	200
Have a crunchy apple snack instead of 1/2 cup peanuts	270
Exercise: Walk 36 minutes per day (2-1/2 miles per day)	250
TOTAL CALORIES SAVED:	1000!

   IN 7 DAYS LOSE 2 POUNDS!

4. **ADD UP THOSE CALORIES**
   - An extra 100 calories, such as a large apple, 20 peanuts or 1 tablespoon margarine, each day adds up to 36,500 calories in 1 year. That's 10 EXTRA POUNDS!!!
   - Walk 30 minutes daily, using 210 calories per day, and burn 76,650 calories. That's 22 pounds lost a year!!!

5. **A REGULAR INDIVIDUAL EXERCISE PROGRAM HELPS! EXERCISE:**
   - Burns calories and helps maintain weight loss
   - Promotes fat-burning and decreases body fat
   - Speeds metabolism (calorie-burning)
   - Improves physical fitness and muscle tone
   - Increases cardiopulmonary health
   - Suppresses appetite
   - Minimizes stress
   - Maximizes energy
   - Enhances mental health
   - Enhances emotional well-being

6. **ESTABLISH EATING AND EXERCISE HABITS THAT PROMOTE LIFELONG WEIGHT CONTROL.**

THE RIGHT BALANCE

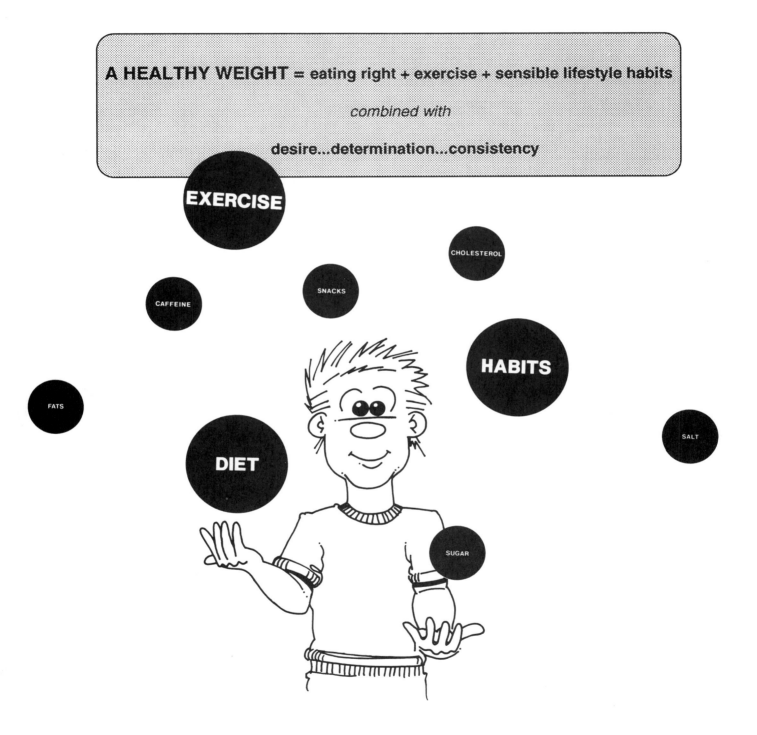

A HEALTHY WEIGHT = eating right + exercise + sensible lifestyle habits

combined with

desire...determination...consistency

EXERCISE

CHOLESTEROL

CAFFEINE

SNACKS

HABITS

FATS

SALT

DIET

SUGAR

EAT RIGHT! GET FIT! LOSE WEIGHT! FEEL GREAT!

BODY COMPOSITION

You must change your body composition to change your weight for life! Focus on body composition as your primary weight objective. The more muscle you have, the more permanent is your weight loss. Muscle speeds metabolism (calories you burn daily), so that you burn more body fat and leave it off.

Your **TOTAL WEIGHT** is comprised of 2 basic components:

TOTAL WEIGHT = FAT + LEAN BODY MASS (muscle, bone, water)

You cannot maintain or gain muscle without **EXERCISE!!!**

- Each year, as part of the aging process, we lose muscle and gain fat.
- This process slows your metabolism and consequently, you gain body fat and weight.
- The only way to prevent or reverse this process is to **EXERCISE!**
- Exercise helps you "keep the muscle; lose the fat".

If you lose weight without exercise, you lose approximately 50 percent lean tissue and 50 percent fat. To lose almost 100 percent fat, exercise and cut back on fat calories!

BODY COMPOSITION AND METABOLISM:

You can be the same height and weight and have different body compositions at different times in life, and therefore, have different calorie needs. The more muscle you have, the more you can eat to maintain weight because your metabolism is higher.

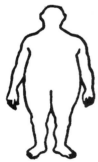

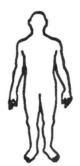

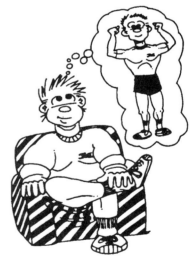

200 Pounds
150 pounds lean body mass
50 pounds fat (25%)
needs **2000 calories** per day
(200 lbs x 10 calories per lb)

200 Pounds
175 pounds lean body mass
25 pounds fat (12.5%)
needs **3000 calories** per day
(200 lbs x 15 calories per lb)

COOPER CLINIC PERCENT BODY FAT RECOMMENDATIONS

Your most appropriate percent body fat and weight are based on your age, health status, fitness level, body build, and other individual factors. Check with your physician or dietitian for the most appropriate body fat for you. General guidelines are as follows:

MEN:	10-20%	(AVG: <20%)	
WOMEN:	18-27%	(AVG: <24%)	

Let your body fat goal determine your corresponding weight goal.

YOUR EXERCISE

HOW ACTIVE ARE YOU? HOW MUCH ACTIVITY DO YOU NEED FOR WEIGHT LOSS?

You can improve your body composition, fitness, fat-burning, and metabolic rate if you exercise regularly and strive to live an active lifestyle.

YOU WILL LOSE 1 POUND WEEKLY IF YOU:

- expend 250 calories/day (by walking approximately 2.75 miles in 42 minutes or by jogging 2.5 miles in 25 minutes), and
- omit 250 food calories/day.

A REGULAR AEROBIC EXERCISE PROGRAM:

- complements your eating program and provides lasting fitness and weight loss results.
- burns calories - if you walk 30 minutes daily (180 calories/day), you burn 65,700 calories/year = **18 pounds!**
- burns fat stores and promotes faster fat-burning.
- prevents "creeping" weight gain.

YOUR EXERCISE:

The American College of Sports Medicine recommends:
- aerobic exercise 30-45 minutes, 4-5 times a week to lose body fat and burn 200-300 calories a day.
- strength training (i.e., weights) 20-30 minutes, 2-3 times a week to build muscle.

THIS COMBINATION BUILDS MUSCLE AND BURNS FAT.

Gradually, work up to burning approximately 250 calories a day with this much exercise:

Activity	Calories Per Hour	Time Needed to Burn 250 Calories
Walking 4 mph (15 min per mile)	350	42 min.
Tennis (doubles	400	37 min.
Aerobic Dance	400	37 min.
Downhill Skiing	400	37 min.
Skating (moderate)	475	32 min.
Swimming, crawl (45 yd/min.)	550	28 min.
Jogging 5 mph (12 min. per mile)	550	28 min.
Biking 13 mph	550	28 min.
Stair-Climbing (machine)	550	28 min.
Jogging 6 mph (10 min. per mile)	680	23 min.
Jogging 7 mph (8.5 min. per mile)	780	20 min.
Handball, Squash	815	19 min.

NOTE: *These figures are for a 150 pound person. If you weigh more, you'll burn more calories in the same time; if you weigh less, you'll burn fewer calories.*

See Appendix C for calories burned from various exercises at various body weights. See Chapter IV to develop your own best exercise and fitness program and to learn more about exercise.

OUR KEY MESSAGE: MOVE DAILY!

HABIT ASSESSMENT

IDENTIFY YOUR EATING HABITS:

Complete the **"ASSESSMENT OF EATING HABITS"** to identify key habits that contribute to your over-eating. These are chief factors that affect eating behavior.

Be honest and circle the habits that you need to modify. Be aware and work toward new ways of eating.

ASSESSMENT OF EATING HABITS

FACTOR	EATING BEHAVIOR - DO YOU:	YES	NO
Meal Time	1. Eat at regular meal times daily?		
	2. Eat in a relatively consistent pattern day to day?		
	3. Eat 3 meals a day?		
	4. Skip meals?		
	5. Snack between meals?		
Length	6. Eat rapidly? (Less than 20 minutes a meal)		
Place	7. Eat in more than one room at home?		
	8. Eat in more than one place in your kitchen?		
	9. Eat standing up or lying down oftentimes?		
	10. Eat while involved in other activities (i.e., reading, writing, watching TV, working)?		
Social Environment	11. Eat more food when alone? If "yes," why?		
	12. Eat more with others? If "yes," why?		
Mood	13. Eat under stress?		
	14. Eat in response to moods? Which moods?		
Amount	15. Take second helpings?		
	16. Ever leave an "unclean" plate?		
	17. Add more "extras" — butter, jam, salad dressing gravies, sauces?		
Type of Food	18. Frequently (daily) eat high-calorie foods (fried foods, creamy foods, desserts, soft drinks, alcohol)?		
	19. Frequently (daily) eat low-calorie foods (fresh fruits and vegetables)?		
	20. Drink 6-8 glasses of fluid daily?		

A "yes" answer to any of these questions: 4 through 15, 17, 18, and a "no" answer to any of these questions: 1, 2, 3, 16, 19, 20, means you must re-train these behaviors for successful weight loss.

 © 1993, *The Balancing Act Nutrition and Weight Guide*, G. Kostas, M.P.H., R.D., Dallas, Texas

HABITS

You must change your habits to change your weight...your eating habits, exercise patterns, and your way of thinking about food, moods, and physical activity. This means making a few lifestyle changes...for life! Focus on one to two key habits per week.

The following habits will help you control your eating and lose weight. Focus on one to two habits a week, until all these habits are yours.

GUIDELINES

1. **EAT 3 MEALS AT REGULAR MEAL TIMES DAILY.** Do not skip meals and change your eating patterns daily. Skipped meals lead to over-eating or bingeing. Feel more energetic and speed your metabolism by eating every 5-6 hours. This also reduces appetite.

2. **EAT SLOWLY** taking at least 20 minutes for meals, 10 minutes for snacks. You will feel more satisfied with smaller food quantities and eat less than those who eat fast. It takes 20 minutes for the brain to sense the stomach's signal: "I'm full!"

3. **CHOOSE ONE SPECIFIC LOCATION TO EAT; MAKE EATING A SINGULAR ACTIVITY.** Beware of unconscious eating — in front of the TV, at the movies, while reading or studying, driving, cooking or standing. **EAT SITTING ONLY. ENJOY EATING!** When you are involved in an activity while eating, you can be distracted from really tasting or enjoying your food; consequently it is easy to over-eat, frequently unconsciously. Savor each bite. Taste and chew slowly.

4. **BE AWARE OF THE SOCIAL INFLUENCES THAT AFFECT YOUR EATING BEHAVIOR.** Avoid or be cautious in situations that encourage your over-eating. Choose low-fat, low-calorie foods. Don't stand next to the food table, etc.

5. **PLAN AHEAD**...this promotes quality food choices and eating strategies for restaurants, parties, weekends, etc. With the right foods present, meals and snacks are healthier. Plan daily. Avoid restaurants (i.e., buffets) where it's easy to over-indulge.

6. **KEEP FOOD OUT OF SIGHT.** Make problematic foods inconvenient or unavailable. Keep low-calorie foods convenient. Keep raw vegetables and fruit in front of refrigerator. Serve food from the stove — not in bowls on the table.

7. **CONTROL EMOTIONAL EATING.** Don't reach for food to make you content or relaxed. Food is not the answer. Those who use activity rather than mood-triggered eating find a quick, surer means of mood resolution.

8. **ADD PLEASURE** to your life in ways other than with food. Reward yourself.

9. Put yourself in situations that **SUPPORT YOUR EFFORTS AT CONTROLLED EATING.** Don't let week "dieters" weaken you! You are not on a "diet!"

10. Learn to **CONTROL BOTH THE TYPE OF FOOD** as well as the **QUANTITY OF FOOD.**

HOW TO CHANGE HABITS:
- Be alert to your eating patterns - what, where, when, why you eat.
- Keep records daily - to be aware constantly.
- Take small steps in a consistent direction. Practice, practice, practice!

YOUR BACKGROUND

Do you understand how your past eating and "dieting" habits have affected you up to now?
To prevent repeating past patterns, complete this form. What have you learned?

WEIGHT HISTORY

1. What do you consider a good weight for yourself? _____ Current weight?_____

2. What is the most you have weighed? _____ at what age?_____

3. What is the least you have weighed? _____ at what age?_____

4. Have you lost or gained weight recently? _____ How much? _____

5. Is your spouse overweight? _____ Children?_____ Parents?_____

6. Are you overweight right now? _____

7. How long have you been overweight? _____

RELATED FACTORS

8. What do you see as the reason(s) for you being overweight or over-eating?

_____eat the wrong type of food	___depression	___job
_____eat too much (large portions)	___emotions	___fats (fried foods)
_____drink too much (alcohol)	___anger	___sugar
_____lack of exercise	___boredom	___fast foods
_____snacks	___nervousness	___soft drinks
_____travel or eating out often	___stress	___desserts
_____habits	___fatigue	___meat
_____socializing	___quit smoking	___other: _____
_____watching T.V., sports, movies	___relaxation	

9. Are you dissatisfied with the way you look at this weight? _____

10. Why do you want to lose weight?

_____appearance	___improve physical fitness
_____pressure from family/friends	___health
_____feel better	___physician/nutritionist
_____other: _____	

11. How do others influence your weight loss goals? Give their names.

INFLUENCE	NAMES	HOW
Positive	_____	_____
Negative	_____	_____
None	_____	_____
Other	_____	_____

  © 1993, *The Balancing Act Nutrition and Weight Guide*, G. Kostas, M.P.H., R.D., Dallas, Texas

DIETING HISTORY

12. List diets and/or weight loss plans you have followed in the past.

TYPES	SHORT-TERM RESULTS	LONG-TERM RESULTS
1._____	_____	_____
2._____	_____	_____
3._____	_____	_____
4._____	_____	_____

Which worked best? _____Why?_____

13. What do you wish to achieve now? _____

14. Is it more difficult for you to lose weight or maintain weight? _____

EATING AND EXERCISE PATTERNS

15. List any food allergies or intolerances. _____

16. List vitamin/mineral/dietary supplements with the amounts you take.

_____   _____

_____   _____

17. How many meals a day do you eat? _____Skip?_____

18. How many times a day do you snack? _____On what?_____

19. Where do you eat your meals (M) and snacks (S)?Example: __M__kitchen,__S__den

_____kitchen _____dining room _____TV room

_____den _____bedroom _____other:_____

20. How many meals do you eat out each week? _____Where?

____restaurant____fast food____deli____cafeteria____other:_____

21. Who prepares your meals at home? _____

22. What is your eating pace? ___fast ___slow ___moderate

23. List foods in which you overindulge (your problem foods): _____

_____

24. Do you exercise? _____If yes, describe below.

	SAMPLE	FILL IN	FILL IN
Form of exercise (jog, swim, stationary bike, etc.)	Walk		
Length of workout (minutes)	40 minutes		
Distance per workout	2 miles		
Number of workouts per week	4		

25. Do you smoke? _____ If yes, how many (cigarettes) do you smoke daily? _____

26. Do you drink alcohol? _____ Amt. daily: ____ beer _____ liquor _____ wine

YOUR HEALTH

27. Present medical conditions:

    _____ heart disease   ____ liver disease   ___ ulcer
    _____ diabetes   ____ kidney disease   ___ gastrointestinal problem
    _____ high blood pressure ____ cancer (type)   ___ hiatal hernia
    _____ overweight   ____ elevated cholesterol   ___ diverticulosis
    _____ gallbladder disease ____ elevated triglycerides   ___ diverticulitis
    _____ other _____

28. Rate your health: ___ excellent   ___ good   ___ fair ___ poor

29. Do you feel this is a good time for you to begin your eating and exercise program? Have you checked with your doctor and received his O.K.?   _____

30. If your overeating is linked to moods, emotions, or unknown causes have you worked with a professional counselor to help with this aspect of over-eating? _____ We recommend counseling when habits are difficult to change and compulsive over-eating and weight and food preoccupation continue.

31. Please describe a day's eating with comments about variations you may have. PLEASE BE ACCURATE AND SPECIFIC!

SAMPLE		
BREAKFAST	8 oz. orange juice 1 egg, scrambled in 1 tsp. margarine	2 wholewheat toast with 2 tsp. margarine + 1 Tbsp. jam 1 cup coffee + 1 Tbsp. cream
BREAKFAST		
LUNCH		
DINNER		
SNACKS		

What did you learn about your eating style and habits? _____

QUIZ

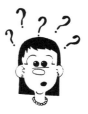

TEST YOUR NUTRITIONAL I.Q.: ANSWER TRUE OR FALSE

1. A "high protein diet" is a reduction diet. _____
2. Quick reducing diets are the best way to reduce and maintain a desired weight. _____
3. On a reducing diet, omitting all carbohydrates from your food intake
   will be beneficial. _____
4. You don't need diet foods to diet. _____
5. Grapefruit causes weight loss. _____
6. Low calorie diets are expensive. _____
7. Meal skipping is a good way to lose weight. _____
8. Diet pills can be habit forming. _____
9. Cider vinegar in a glass of water, taken at each meal,
   makes it possible for the body to burn fat. _____
10. Toasting bread decreases the calories. _____
11. Fats give more than twice as many calories as carbohydrates. _____
12. Cellulite is nothing more than body fat. _____
13. Carbohydrates are more fattening than protein. _____
14. Margarine contains fewer calories than butter. _____
15. Pork causes heart disease. _____
16. "Diet ice cream" has no calories. _____
17. Optimum health requires "health foods." _____
18. Vitamins take the place of food. _____
19. If a small amount of vitamins are good, larger quantities will be better. _____
20. Vitamin E has specific curative or age retarding properties
    and gives specific sexual powers. _____
21. "Natural" vitamins are better than "synthetic" vitamins. _____
22. "Organically grown food" is better than food grown with synthetic fertilizers. _____

Answers:

1.) F 2.) F 3.) F 4.) T 5.) F 6.) T 7.) F 8.) T 9.) F 10.) F 11.) T
12.) T 13.) F 14.) F 15.) F 16.) F 17.) F 18.) F 19.) F 20.) F 21.) F 22.) F

DIETING

The federal government has issued U.S. Dietary Guidelines that recommend eating sensibly and moderately, cutting back calories, and exercising to lose weight safely. Weight loss results from eating less and/or exercising, over time! DIETS (as temporary programs) DON'T WORK! Lifestyle eating and exercise patterns DO WORK.

The DESPERATE DIETER turns to the abundance of books with misinformation and gimmicks that promise magic, quick weight loss. "Dieting" schemes come and go, and there is one to suit every taste, budget, and misconception:

Hollywood Eighteen Day Diet	The Egg Diet
Banana Diet	All Meat Diet
Crenshaw Super Beauty Diet	Never Say Diet
Easy No-Flab Diet	Dallas Diet
Three-Day Prune Diet	Doctor's Diet
"Spring Shape-Up"	Beverly Hills Diet
No-Aging Diet	Liquid Diets

The Amazing Diet Secret of a Desperate Housewife

...and many, many more!!!

BE AWARE

- These diets do not teach controlled eating or sensible meal planning.
- They are poor preparation for a lifetime of eating ahead!
- They can be dangerous because they often restrict or eliminate foods that supply essential nutrients for good health and nutritionally balanced meals.
- A BALANCED DIET is one that provides protein, carbohydrates, fats, vitamins, and minerals for sound nutritional health.
- An UNBALANCED DIET is one that drastically departs from this by overemphasizing one food group or single nutrient at the expense of others.

HOW MANY POUNDS

HAVE YOU LOST

IN A LIFETIME?

_____

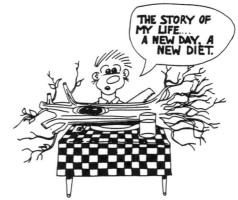

LET'S LOOK AT A FEW "POPULAR" DIETS

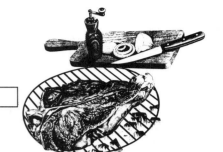

1. **LOW CARBOHYDRATE, HIGH PROTEIN DIETS (HIGH-FAT)**

   A. Dr. Atkins Diet, Scarsdale Diet, Stillman Diet, etc.

   B. **Rules**:
      - Eat all you want, any time, of the foods that have no carbohydrates (steak, fish, chicken, eggs, cheese, spareribs, lobster Newburg, etc.)
      - Limit amounts of carbohydrate foods such as salad greens, certain vegetables, fruits.
      - Avoid sugar and starches (potatoes, bread).

   C. **Claims**:
      - Atkins — A no carbohydrate diet stimulates a fat-mobilizing hormone which helps to burn body fat!
      - Stillman — Protein molecules are so large that extra energy is required to digest them!

   D. **Criticisms**:
      - You decrease body fat through exercise and reduced calorie intake.
      - Energy (fat) does not just "disappear."
      - Not a balanced diet that provides all needed nutrients.
      - High in saturated fats and cholesterol.
      - Does little or nothing to alter overall eating behavior for long term weight maintenance.
      - Too rigid and monotonous to follow over a long period.
      - Results in abnormal fat breakdown due to inadequate carbohydrates.
      - Ketosis occurs when there is not enough carbohydrate to meet caloric needs. The waste products from fats are called ketones.
      - The state of ketosis is unhealthy and if continued over a long period of time may damage the liver and kidneys.
      - Side effects of ketosis: temporary dizziness, headache, weakness, diarrhea, nausea, low blood pressure, dehydration, fatigue, sleeplessness.

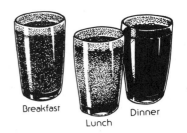

Breakfast Lunch Dinner

2. LIQUID DIETS

A. Liquid Protein Diet, Protein Supplements, Liquid Meals, The Last Chance Diet

B. **Rules**:

Daily doses of "liquid nutrition," "liquid protein," and limited carbohydrates.

C. **Claims**:

Offer "quick weight loss" with freedom from having to choose, plan and manage food intake.

D. **Criticisms**:

- These diets do nothing to alter eating habits permanently; "normal" eating is resumed, weight is regained.

- Serious health hazards may result form prolonged use: irregular heart beat and heart damage, kidney and liver damage, diarrhea, low blood volume, dehydration, nausea, hair loss, nervous disorders, abdominal cramps, death.

3. HIGH CARBOHYDRATE DIETS

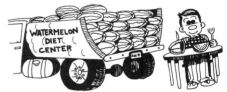

A. Rockerfeller, Watermelon, Quick Inches-Off

B. **Rules**:

- High complex carbohydrates, reduced sugar, saturated fat, protein.

C. **Criticisms**:

- A balanced vegetarian diet has advantages but an unbalanced high carbohydrate diet can be dangerous, leading to protein and Vitamin B12 deficiency. (Vegetable proteins must be combined properly to obtain sufficient protein for health.)

4. FADS

A. Grapefruit, Rice, Banana, Ice Cream, Hamburger Diets, etc.

B. **Rules**:

- One or a few foods are permitted which are said to have magical properties (i.e., "grapefruit contains enzymes which help increase the fat burning process" — eat 1/2 grapefruit at the start of every meal.)

C. **Claims**:

- Easy to remember, no calorie counting.

D. **Criticisms**:

- There are no special foods that "melt" fat away or make foods less fattening.
- A limited diet results in vitamin and mineral deficiency, and is too boring to follow.

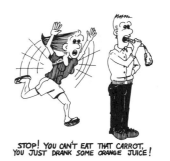

STOP! YOU CAN'T EAT THAT CARROT,
YOU JUST DRANK SOME ORANGE JUICE!

5. HIGH FIBER, COMBINATION DIETS

A. Beverly Hills Diet, Fit for Life, etc.

B. **Rules**:

- Combine foods properly to allow the enzymes in foods and those in your body to effectively digest food and make it less fattening. As new foods are introduced, in the Beverly Hills diet, you may eat as much as you want as long as you eat foods separately. (for example, fruit should be eaten alone or it gets "trapped" by other foods in your stomach.)

- Beverly Hills Diet: First 11 days — fruit only; second week — vegetables and breads introduced; third week — lobster; fourth week — regimen of bran.

- Fit for Life Diet: Only fruit can be consumed in the morning; milk and milk products cannot be consumed; certain foods cannot be eaten together.

C. **Claims**:

- When certain foods are combined your body cannot digest them and they turn to fat.
- Combine foods properly for most efficient digestion.

D. **Criticisms**:

- There is no magic combination of foods to make them less fattening. Undigested food is eliminated from the body, not stored as fat. All foods are digested as soon as they pass through the digestive system.

- Single food diets can lead to serious illnesses and death. Large quantities of fruit may lead to severe diarrhea with water loss, causing potassium deficiency and an irregular heat beat. Fever, muscle weakness, rapid pulse, and fatal drop in blood pressure may develop.

6. OTHER ATTEMPTED METHODS FOR WEIGHT CONTROL

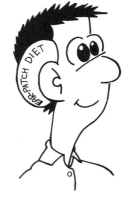

acupuncture	intestinal bypass surgery
hypnosis	gastric stapling
"fat farms"	starvation
diet pills	semi-starvation
jaw wiring	ear patches

CHOOSING A FOOD PLAN FOR WEIGHT LOSS

1. **A HEALTHY FOOD PLAN FOR WEIGHT LOSS** should contain:

    *   A balanced variety of food on a daily basis.

    *   Ample calories (1000-1500/day) to prevent muscle loss and a slower metabolism.

    *   Less than 30 percent fat calories, (meaning 20-50 fat grams daily).

    *   50 to 70 percent complex carbohydrate calories to energize you and to prevent muscle loss. This means at least 10 fruit, vegetables, starches daily.

    *   Sufficient vitamins and minerals for health.

    *   Re-education toward new eating habits for life-long weight maintenance.

2. **HOW TO RATE A WEIGHT LOSS DIET:**

    *   <u>Is the diet based on sound principles of nutrition?</u> Is it well balanced nutritionally? Does it eliminate one or more of the basic six food groups? Or, does it claim that one food or food group will promote weight loss? Be careful. A well balanced diet includes foods from all six food groups ★ and is safe.

    *   <u>Is the diet based on a "secret" no one has discovered?</u> Does it promote extremely rapid weight loss of more than three pounds per week? Are unlimited amounts of food promised? If the answer is *yes*, remember there are no miracles for losing weight and keeping it off!

    *   <u>Could you eat like this for the rest of your life?</u> Does the diet allow for individual preferences, practice and taste? Rigid diets that tell you what and when to eat and give no nutritional information are doomed to fail.

    *   <u>Is the author credible?</u> Check degrees and work experience. Distinguish between "nutritionist" and R.D. (registered dietitian), "doctor" or M.D. The national credentialed professionals are known as "R.D.'s" and "M.D.'s".

    *   <u>Has the author supported "success" claims?</u> Was the diet tested on a sufficient number of overweight people and the results objectively compared to the results of a similar group of people following another weight-reducing diet? Were the results published? If the answer is *no*, consider the claims to be questionable. Congressional rulings in 1992 require that any claims be substantiated with published research.

    ★*Basic six food groups: Milk, Meat/Protein, Fruit, Vegetable, Grains/Starches, Fats.*

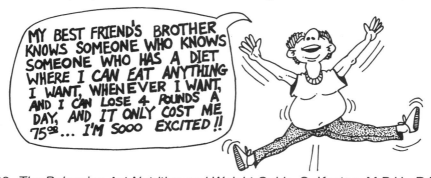

© 1993, *The Balancing Act Nutrition and Weight Guide*, G. Kostas, M.P.H., R.D., Dallas, Texas

CALCULATE YOUR CALORIE NEEDS

You must eat sensibly to control your weight and promote your best health. Always eat at least 1000-1200 calories a day (women) or 1200-1500 calories a day (men) for healthy weight loss. You'll be more likely to lose body fat, feel energetic, and not slow your metabolism. Moreover, you won't "starve" and binge. And you'll be able to stay with these eating principles for life.

WHAT SHOULD YOU EAT TO STAY HEALTHY AND STILL LOSE WEIGHT?

1. **A VARIETY OF FOODS** to meet your body needs for energy and approximately 50 nutrients (protein, fat, carbohydrate, vitamins, minerals). There is no magical food that supplies all these nutrients. Therefore, eat a mixture of vegetables, fruit, starches, protein foods and limited fat.

2. **A MODERATE AMOUNT OF FOOD** to keep you going - not excess amounts of foods that will lead to excess weight, or too little, which slows metabolism.

3. **THE P-C-F (p**rotein, **c**arbohydrate, **f**at) **BALANCE** at each meal, 3 meals a day. This helps to maximize energy, minimize stress and limit "empty-calorie" snacks, by stabilizing your blood sugar. See Section II for details.

4. **SMALLER SERVINGS of CALORIE-DENSE FOODS** - foods with fat, sugar, alcohol, meat products, and cheese.

WHAT SHOULD YOU WEIGH?

- The more accurate method of determining your **TARGET WEIGHT** is by body composition - using **SKINFOLD MEASUREMENTS** and /or **UNDERWATER WEIGHING**. Your **TARGET WEIGHT** is calculated from your percentage of body fat versus lean tissue (muscle). Generally, the percentage of body fat for **MEN** should not exceed 19 percent and for **WOMEN**, 23 percent. A reliable health or fitness facility in your area can measure your body fat. Consult with a health professional to identify your healthiest weight and body fat.

- Or, refer to Appendix C for a Height / Weight Chart of suggested weights.

- Or, calculate your **TARGET WEIGHT** with this simple formula:

  women: 100 + (inches over 5 ft. X 5 lbs.) = **TARGET WEIGHT**

  men: 106 + (inches over 5 ft. X 6 lbs.) = **TARGET WEIGHT**

  Add or subtract 10% for a large or small frame, respectively.

  For example, if you are a 5' 6" woman:

    100 + (6" X 5) = 100 + 30 = 130 = **TARGET WEIGHT**

  (handwritten: 105)

- **My target weight is:** _105_

HOW DO YOU LOSE WEIGHT?
  1) eat fewer calories   2) expend more calories   3) do both

---

HOW MANY CALORIES CAN YOU EAT TO LOSE WEIGHT?

1. **CALCULATE YOUR BASELINE CALORIE NEEDS AT YOUR CURRENT WEIGHT:**
   CURRENT WEIGHT in pounds X 12 calories per pound = **BASELINE CALORIES PER DAY**
   For example: 130 pounds X 12 calories per pound = **1560 calories per day**
   Note: Most people need 10-15 calories per pound:

Ages 20-30:	weight X 13-15
Ages 30-40:	weight X 12
Ages 40-50:	weight X 11
Ages 50 +:	weight X 10

   My Baseline Calorie Needs are:

   _____1248_____

2. **CHOOSE HOW TO LOSE WEIGHT:**
   Since 3500 calories = 1 pound body weight,
   - Omit 1000 Calories per day to lose 2 pounds per week
   - Omit 500 Calories per day to lose 1 pound per week
   - Omit 250 Calories per day to lose 1/2 pound per week. If with exercise alone:
     — Walk 1 mile briskly in 15 minutes to burn approximately 100 calories.
     — Walk 2 1/2 miles in 37 minutes or jog it in 25 minutes to burn 250 calories.
   - Combine diet and exercise for maximum results!

3. **CALCULATE YOUR EXERCISE CALORIES BURNED:**
   - Use the Exercise Chart on the following page or Appendix C to calculate the calories you expend weekly.
   - Determine the calories you burn daily (an average):

Minutes of exercise each week	X	Calories burned per minute	÷ 7 days in a week	=	AVERAGE CALORIES BURNED DAILY

   Example One: **Your Usual Exercise -**
   Walk 5 times a week X 40 minutes (2 miles) each time = 200 minutes weekly
   200 minutes weekly X 5 calories per minute = 1000 calories weekly
   1000 calories a week ÷ 7 days in a week = **140 average calories burned daily**

   Example Two: **Extra Exercise -**
   - Strive to burn 200-300 calories/day for optimal weight loss.
   - Here's How:
     Walk 5 times a week X 60 minutes (2 1/2 miles) each time = 300 minutes weekly
     300 minutes weekly X 5 calories per minute = 1500 calories weekly
     300 calories a week ÷ 7 days in a week = **215 average calories burned daily**
   - If you walk/run 15 miles weekly, as Dr. Cooper recommends for cardiovascular health, you'll burn 200-300 calories per day.

   - **Calories I burn daily:** _____

EXERCISE CALORIES

This chart shows approximate exercise energy expenditure*. To compute more specifically by rate of calories burned per pound of body weight, see Appendix C.

5 Calories Per Minute	7 Calories Per Minute	10 Calories Per Minute
walking 3 mph	walking 4.5 mph	stationary jogging
cycling 5-1/2 mph	cycling 9.5 mph	cycling 12 mph
volleyball	stationary cycling	jogging 6 mph
table tennis	tennis singles	skipping rope
dancing slow step	dancing fast step	calisthenics (heavy0
domestic work	swimming 30 yd/minute	swimming 45 yd/minute
golf (no cart)	skiing (water)	snow skiing
bowling	badminton (singles)	paddleball
light gardening	heavy gardening	squash, handball
	skating (ice, roller)	climbing stairs
	horseback riding (trot)	(up and down, approx. 35 steps per minute)

* for a 150 pound person. (Add or subtract 10% of calories for each 10 pounds you are above or below 150 pounds.)

4. CALCULATE CALORIE NEEDS TO LOSE WEIGHT:
- Here are 3 ways to omit 500 calories a day to lose 1 pound a week:

  1. Adjust **FOOD** Only:
Baseline Calories =	1560
Subtract 500 Calories	- 500
Eat daily: =	**1060 Calories**

  2. Add your **USUAL EXERCISE** to Baseline Calories: +140 Calories
Eat daily: =	**1200 Calories**
-or-	Baseline Calories = 1060 Calories

  3. Add **EXTRA EXERCISE** to Baseline Calories: +215 Calories
     Eat daily: = **1275 Calories**

- We recommend this last method because you can eat more; and 215 calories of exercise daily promotes a leaner body composition and speeds metabolism and fat-burning...all keys to optimal success!
- If you wish to lose faster (1 1/2 to 2 lbs a week), add more exercise and/or decrease calories consumed. Never eat less than 1000 calories per day (women) or 1200 calories per day (men).

5. WHAT CALORIE INTAKE MAINTAINS YOUR TARGET WEIGHT?

Baseline Calorie Needs + Exercise Calories Burned = CALORIE REQUIREMENTS

6. NOW SET YOUR GOALS
1. My current weight: ~~120~~ 104   My target weight: ~~105~~ 100   *15 pounds*
2. My current baseline calorie needs daily: ~~1200~~ 1248
3. Minus calories I will omit daily to lose _____ lbs/wk: _____
4. Plus exercise calories (average) I will burn daily: _____
5. Calories I will eat daily to lose weight: _____
6. I will reach my TARGET WEIGHT in _____ weeks.

PLEASURE ACTIVITIES LIST

REWARD YOURSELF:

. . . Enjoy rewards when you

- exercise regularly
- practice new eating habits
- follow your meal plan
- lose 5 pounds, 10 pounds, etc.

and...

Use these ideas to reduce

- stress
- boredom
- loneliness
- anger
- anxiety
- nervousness
- moodiness

REWARDED BEHAVIORS
TEND TO BE
REPEATED BEHAVIORS.

YOU DESERVE
REWARDS AND TREATS!!!

BUT

NEVER USE FOOD
AS A REWARD!

MARK THE ACTIVITIES YOU DO TO REWARD YOURSELF.

Activity	none	a little	much	very much
1. Watching Television				
2. Listening to Radio/Records				
3. Playing Cards				
4. Doing Crossword Puzzles				
5. Reading Books, Magazines				
6. Dancing				
7. Sleeping Late				
8. Shopping				
9. Buying New Clothes				
10. Buying Kitchen Appliances				
11. Buying Records				
12. Buying Books/Magazines				
13. Telephoning a Friend				
14. Calling a Friend Long Distance				
15. Visiting Friends				
16. Taking a Relaxing Bath or Shower				
17. Attending Sporting Events				
18. Attending Movies				
19. Attending Plays or Concerts				
20. Playing Recreational Sports (golf, bowling, etc.)				
21. Aerobic Exercise (walk, jog, bike, tennis)				
22. Participating in Team Sports				
23. Participating in Organizations				
24. "Pamper" self (manicure, facial, pedicure, massage, hair style)				
25. Personal Time				
26. Camping				
27. Traveling				
28. Hiking				
29. Gardening				
30. Hobbies (painting, drawing, needlework, carpentry)				
31. Other items that you enjoy:				

MY ACTION PLAN

I AM COMMITTING MYSELF TO THESE SPECIFIC HEALTH GOALS:

- I will LOSE _____ pounds in _____ weeks.

- I will EAT _____ calories per day for ____ weeks.

- I will burn an average of _____ calories per day and will EXERCISE _____ times a week for _____ weeks.

- I will MODIFY these eating BEHAVIORS:

  _____   _____

  _____   _____

  _____   _____

- I will enjoy these REWARDS _____ when _____

  _____   _____

  _____   _____

I WILL UTILIZE THESE STRATEGIES: *NO (Healthy low cal sweets)*

1. I WILL DECREASE MY **CALORIE** INTAKE IN THESE WAYS:
   ____ a. Decrease alcohol, soft drinks, sweets, junk food, _____.
   ____ b. Control portions by skipping seconds, serving smaller first portions, or
   _____.
   ____ c. Eat more nutritious, high fiber foods: fruit, vegetables, wholegrains.
   ____ d. Eat less "extras": sauces, toppings, butter, dressing.
   ____ e. Eat less fat. How: _____.
   ____ f. Other: _____.

2. I WILL INCREASE MY CALORIES BURNED THROUGH **EXERCISE** AND WORK TO BUILD LEAN BODY MASS.

   Determine calories as calculated on pages 28-29 or Appendix C.)

ACTIVITY	CALORIES PER MINUTE	X	MINUTES PER WEEK	=	CALORIES PER WEEK
_____	_____		_____		_____
_____	_____		_____		_____
_____	_____		_____		_____
_____	_____		_____		_____
			TOTAL	=	_____ calories per day

3. I WILL DEVELOP THESE **LIFESTYLE** SKILLS:

   ____ a. Plan meals in advance

   ____ b. Consistently practice my new eating habits.

   ____ c. Take charge of my environment. How: _____

   ____ d. Involve myself in activities that build my self-esteem: _____

   ____ e. Build and utilize an effective support team.

   My key supports are _____, _____, _____.

   ____ f. Respond to stress without food. How: _____

   ____ g. Other:_____

   Signed _____

   Support Person _____

   Date _____

RECORDS

1. **WRITE DOWN YOUR EATING HABITS:**

   Studies show that people who keep food and exercise records daily are more successful with changing eating patterns and losing weight.

   Keep accurate food records each day. RECORD EVERYTHING you eat and drink, even if you overeat. It is best to do the food record right before or right after you eat. Include the TIME you eat, how LONG it takes to eat, the exact PLACE, with WHOM, MOOD or ACTIVITY WHILE EATING, the AMOUNT, and HOW THE FOOD IS PREPARED. Then choose to list fat grams, calories, food groups — which ones best fit your goals?

FOOD RECORDS

NAME *Mary Smith*

DATE *Monday, October 1*

DAILY TOTAL
_____ MILK _____
_____ VEG_____
_____ FRUIT ___II_____
_____ BREAD __I____
_____ MEAT___I____
_____ FAT _HHL I____

Write **ONE** food on each line.

Time/ Min. Eating	Place/ With Whom	Mood/Activity	Amount	Food — How Prepared	Food Group or Calories	Fat Grams
7:15 am	kitchen table	nervous	8 oz.	orange juice	2 Fruit	0
			1	egg, scrambled	1 Meat	5
10 min.	alone		2 tsp.	margarine (egg, toast)	2 Fat	10
			1 slice	wholewheat toast	1 Bread	1
			2 strips	bacon	2 Fats	10
			1 cup	coffee	Free	0
			2 tbsp	cream	2 Fat	10

Your **FOOD RECORD** forms are in Appendix A. Use them daily!

2. CHART AND GRAPH YOUR WEIGHT:

Post your weight record in a prominent place and record your weight weekly. Weigh at the same time and day each week, using the same scale. Day to day fluctuations in weight (as shown below) are typical due to fluid shifts, activity level, etc. Look for an overall downward trend. NOTE: It is normal to gain **water** weight when losing body **fat**. Expect a **weight gain** (from water) on the scales at some point, even when you are doing everything consistently to lose! Hang in there! The water will go away with time.

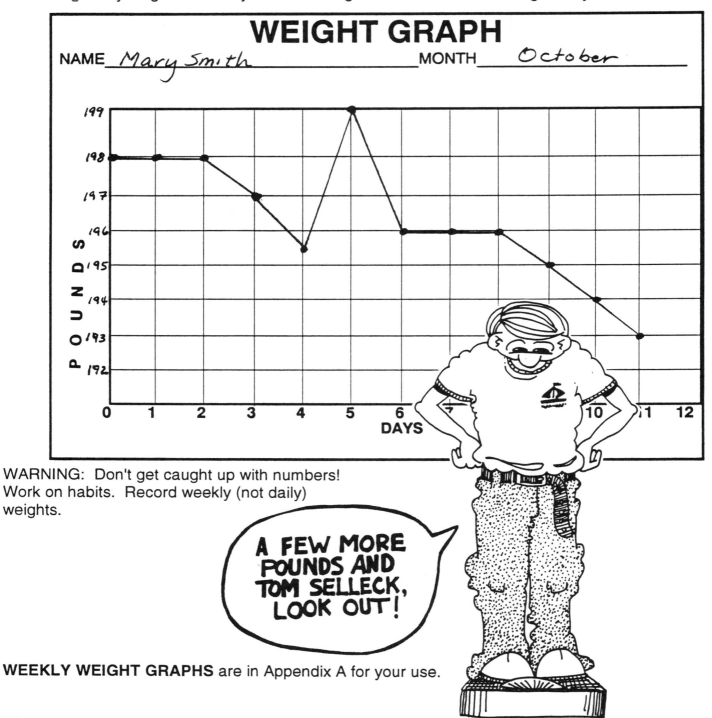

WARNING: Don't get caught up with numbers! Work on habits. Record weekly (not daily) weights.

WEEKLY WEIGHT GRAPHS are in Appendix A for your use.

3. **RECORD YOUR EXERCISE:**

Post your **EXERCISE LOG** to remind yourself to exercise 5 days a week.

EXERCISE LOG							
Sunday	Monday	Tuesday	Wednesday	Thursday	Friday	Saturday	**Weekly Totals**
	① Walk 2 miles (40 min.)	② Beginner Aerobic Dance class (60 min.)	③ Walk 2 miles (40 min.)		④ Stationary Bike 5 miles (30 min.)	⑤ Pleasure Bike Ride (60 min.)	Walk — 4 miles Dance — 1 hr. St. Bike — 30 min. Outdoor bike 60 min.

Your **EXERCISE LOGS** are in Appendix A.

4. **CLIMB THE LADDER TO SUCCESS**

List your weekly achievements at the end of each week.

LADDER TO SUCCESS

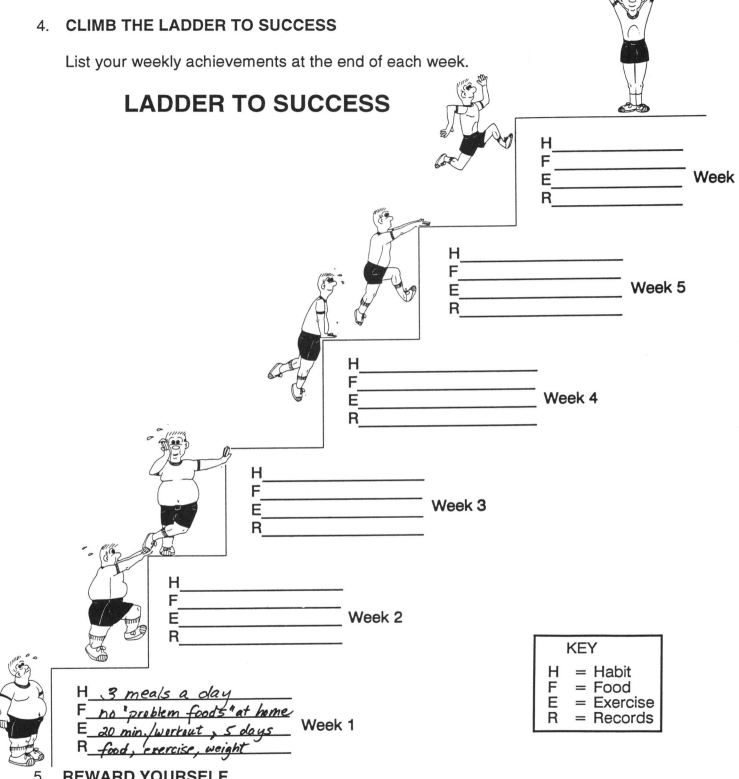

H _____
F _____
E _____ Week (
R _____

H _____
F _____
E _____ Week 5
R _____

H _____
F _____
E _____ Week 4
R _____

H _____
F _____
E _____ Week 3
R _____

H _____
F _____
E _____ Week 2
R _____

	KEY	
H	=	Habit
F	=	Food
E	=	Exercise
R	=	Records

H *3 meals a day*
F *no "problem foods" at home*
E *20 min./workout, 5 days* Week 1
R *food, exercise, weight*

5. **REWARD YOURSELF**

Use list on Page (30) for ideas.
See Appendix A for **LADDER TO SUCCESS** forms and **END-OF-MONTH PROGRESS CHECKS**.

SUCCESS TIPS

THINK POSITIVE!

1. *BE COMMITTED* — *to a new lifestyle of health and fitness.*

2. *TAKE CHARGE* — *assert yourself and your program.*

3. *BE RESPONSIBLE* — *for nutritious meals and regular exercise.*

4. *DEVELOP A PLAN* — *stick with it daily.*

5. *BE POSITIVE AND ENTHUSIASTIC about your new endeavor.*

6. *BELIEVE IN YOUR GOALS and in YOURSELF.*

7. *EXPECT SUCCESS.*

8. *REWARD yourself.*

9. *ENJOY AND SAVOR THE RESULTS* — *feeling better, looking better, more vitality.*

> TAKE CHARGE OF YOUR EATING BEHAVIORS - Be aware of your habits.
> BE PATIENT - It takes practice to learn new habits and maintain them.
> BECOME SENSITIVE TO YOUR FEELINGS THAT HINDER WEIGHT LOSS.
> LEARN TO EAT FOR YOUR BODY'S NEEDS AND NOT FOR EMOTIONAL COMFORT.

LIFETIME SUCCESS

1. *Set your own **"ground rules"** for weight loss and maintenance. Design your own eating plan, based on "low-fat, high-fiber" eating. Include foods you enjoy and know realistically you'll eat.*

2. ***Exercise** 3-5 times per week...an active life is absolutely essential to keep metabolism up and pounds off.*

3. *Keep food and exercise **logs**. They boost your awareness and help you make progress.*

4. *Surround yourself with **support** — individuals, groups, places, events that motivate and reinforce the good habits and lifestyle you wish to continue.*

5. *Stay **accountable** — join a group, see a qualified nutritionist (registered dietitian) periodically, weigh-in at your doctor's office, weigh yourself at home weekly.*

6. *Keep in mind your **personal incentives** to lose weight and keep it off.*

7. *Never think of yourself as "dieting". **Focus** on "healthy eating"!*

8. *If you have an "off" day, **get back "on track"** the next meal! The longer you delay, the harder it is to resume new habits.*

II
DESIGN YOUR EATING PLAN

*The upcoming pages will introduce you to **five ways** you can tailor an eating plan to fit your lifestyle and personality. Choose the best approach for you.*

NUTRITION FOCUS

1. Read Chapter 2; then return to page 50 to select your favorite eating plan. Note the five proposed options are all "variations on a theme". The **best option** is the one you can follow most readily.
2. As you review the general "Eating Plan Basics" (45), especially notice how the P-C-F concept (45-48) works to control your appetite and maximize your energy.
3. Understand how you benefit from focusing first on fats (49).
4. See how you can "Design your own eating plan" based on five key approaches (50-51).
5. Get acquainted with Options I and II (52-53).
6. Notice how P-C-F and fat priorities are integrated in the "Food Group" eating plan system (53).
   a. Select "Your Healthy Eating Plan" from the Daily Eating Plans (58) and record it on page 57, if you choose to use this food group approach. Note the two sample menus (59).
   b. See how easily food groups can convert to calories (73) and how to eat the most food for the same 100 calories (60)!
   c. Know how much you eat with these tips on identifying portion sizes (61).
   d. Acquaint yourself with "food groups", portion sizes, and "hidden fats" (62-74).
7. Enjoy Option IV: Two Weeks of Sample Menus (using food groups) at your chosen calorie level of 1000, 1200, or 1500 calories (75-87).
8. Try Option V: Mix & Match Meals, based on fat grams and calories. Notice how easy the quick-fix meals are to prepare (88-94).
9. Now return to page 50 and select the eating plan option that fits you best. If you choose the Food Group system, be sure to record your DAILY EATING PLAN on page 57.
10. Get ready to put your successful "game plan" of strategies into action!

HABIT FOCUS

Plan and eat 3 meals a day with P-C-F balance.

EXERCISE FOCUS

Keep exercising!

RECORDS

Continue your food, exercise, weight records daily.

GOALS

HABIT:	spend 20 minutes per meal, plan meals in advance
FOOD:	practice the P-C-F balance; measure portions
EXERCISE:	incorporate more activity into your daily routine
RECORDS:	food, exercise, weight

EATING PLAN BASICS

UNDERSTANDING A FEW EATING PLAN BASICS WILL HELP YOU DESIGN YOUR **DAILY EATING PLAN**. As described in the previous section, no matter which approach to weight loss you choose, a successful **HEALTH AND WEIGHT** program must include:

- your specific eating plan, tailored to fit you
- your fat-burning exercise program
- your behavior strategies (positive eating habits)
- your lifetime commitment to total well-being.

YOUR EATING PLAN will include:

- a variety of foods for optimal nutrition
- low-fat, high-fiber foods
- the right combination of 3 nutrient groups:

  50-70% **Complex Carbohydrates (C)**
  10-20% **Protein (P)**
  15-30% **Fat (F)**

- **P-C-F** Balance at each meal to maximize energy, reduce stress, control appetite, and promote a sense of well-being

FOODS THAT MAKE UP THIS TOTAL BALANCE:

NUTRIENT GROUPS	COMPLEX CARBOHYDRATES (C)	PROTEIN (P)	FAT (F)
SIX FOOD GROUPS	• Fruits • Vegetables • Starches/Breads (bread, cereal, pasta, rice, corn)	• Milk/Milk Products • Meat/Substitutes (poultry, fish, meat, eggs, cheese, dried beans and peas)	• Fats (margarine, oils, dressings, nuts, peanut butter, etc.)

YOUR GOALS

- Lose 1/2-2 pounds per week. (Women, aim for 1/2-1 lb. a week; men aim for 1-2 lbs. a week). Faster weight loss usually results in muscle and water loss, plus a slowdown of your metabolism.

- Eat healthy foods and nutritionally balanced, P-C-F meals. Choose foods you enjoy. Select high-fiber, low-fat foods.

- Exercise regularly to:
  - Lose body fat - not muscle and water.
  - Build lean body mass (muscle) and burn fat.
  - Prevent a slowdown of your metabolic rate.

- Eat sufficient calories to boost energy, control appetite, and prevent fatigue. Never eat fewer than 1000 calories a day. It may lead to bingeing as well as a metabolic slowdown.

- Maintain your weight loss and good habits for life.

THE P-C-F PRINCIPLE

Choose **P-C-F** meals as part of any eating program to benefit in numerous ways: to boost your energy, reduce stress, feel your best, control over-eating, and lose weight.

1. **WHAT SHOULD YOU EAT?**

   - Combine foods with **protein (P), carbohydrate (C),** and **fat (F)** at meals for the **P-C-F balance**. The result: better nutrition and appetite control.
   - **Carbohydrate** meals (fruits, starches, vegetables) give short-term energy; hunger may return within 1-3 hours.
   - Add **protein** (skim milk or meat products, eggs, beans and peas) to delay hunger and promote energy for 3-5 hours.
   - Add a little **fat** (margarine, mayonnaise, etc.) to delay hunger for 5-6 hours.

2. **WHEN SHOULD YOU EAT? TO MAXIMIZE ENERGY AND MINIMIZE STRESS:**

   - "Re-fuel" at regular intervals throughout the day.
   - Eat three meals a day, and planned snacks, if needed.
   - Space meals 4-6 hours apart.
   - Keep a **P-C-F balance** at each meal.

3. **PLAN MEALS WITH THE P-C-F- BALANCE OF FOODS:**

The **P-C-F** (protein-carbohydrate-fat) **BALANCE** at each meal, 3 meals a day will help you lose weight by moderating your blood sugar levels and appetite. As a result:

   - you won't be as hungry and battling food cravings
   - you'll be more energetic and alert all day long
   - you'll enjoy a greater sense of well-being and more enthusiasm
   - you'll experience less stress and fewer emotional "ups and downs"
   - you'll be able to skip "empty calorie" between-meal snacks
   - you'll make better food choices (who can make good decisions when your blood sugar is low?)
   - plus you'll be eating balanced meals for your best health

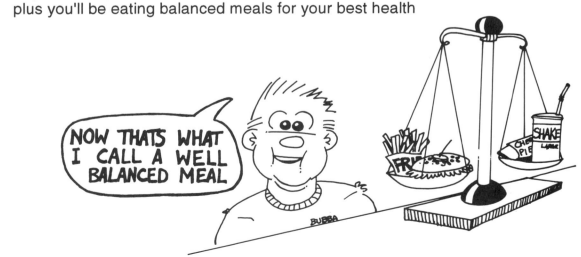

P-C-F BALANCE

This is how the P-C-F Principle works to moderate blood sugar levels and appetite:

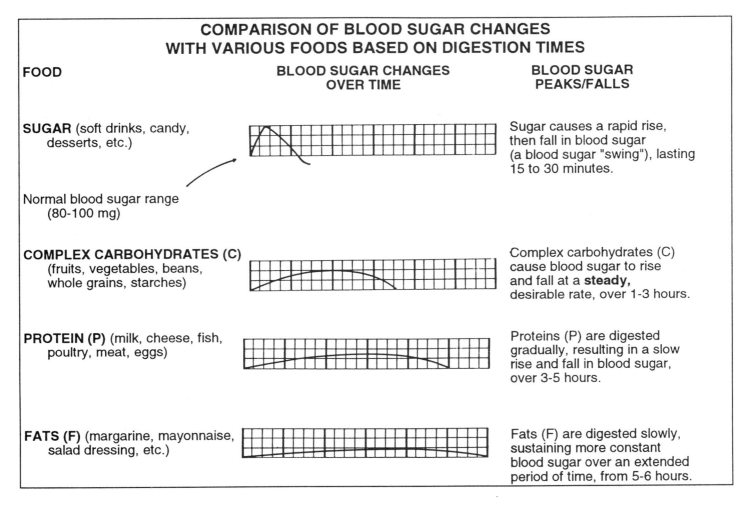

COMPARISON OF BLOOD SUGAR CHANGES WITH VARIOUS FOODS BASED ON DIGESTION TIMES

FOOD	BLOOD SUGAR CHANGES OVER TIME	BLOOD SUGAR PEAKS/FALLS
SUGAR (soft drinks, candy, desserts, etc.)		Sugar causes a rapid rise, then fall in blood sugar (a blood sugar "swing"), lasting 15 to 30 minutes.
Normal blood sugar range (80-100 mg)		
COMPLEX CARBOHYDRATES (C) (fruits, vegetables, beans, whole grains, starches)		Complex carbohydrates (C) cause blood sugar to rise and fall at a **steady,** desirable rate, over 1-3 hours.
PROTEIN (P) (milk, cheese, fish, poultry, meat, eggs)		Proteins (P) are digested gradually, resulting in a slow rise and fall in blood sugar, over 3-5 hours.
FATS (F) (margarine, mayonnaise, salad dressing, etc.)		Fats (F) are digested slowly, sustaining more constant blood sugar over an extended period of time, from 5-6 hours.

EAT THIS WAY FOR OPTIMAL BLOOD SUGAR CONTROL!

- Eat a **P-C-F COMBINATION** every time you eat (Example: turkey, bread, fruit, mayonnaise)
- Eat every 4-6 hours
- Eat an afternoon snack (if needed) to keep blood sugar levels stable
- This pattern of eating regulates blood sugar levels (and appetite) all day

7:00 a.m.   Breakfast   12:00 p.m.   Lunch   6:00 p.m.   Supper

REMEMBER: Exercise 1-3 hours after eating while blood sugar levels are high enough to meet energy demands.

SAMPLE P-C-F MEALS

These healthy meals fit into any eating program.

Note:	P = protein	C = complex carbohydrate	F = fat (in grams)	Cal = calories
	tbsp = tablespoon	tsp = teaspoon	oz = ounce	tr = trace

QUICK AND EASY BREAKFAST IDEAS

	Cal.	Fat		Cal.	Fat
2 Tbsp raisins (C)	60	0	1 banana (C)	120	0
2/3 cup bran flakes (C)	80	tr	2 slices wholewheat bread (C)	160	tr
1 cup skim milk (P,C)	90	tr	1 Tbsp peanut butter (P,F)	100	8
TOTALS	230	tr	TOTALS	380	8

QUICK AND EASY BROWN-BAG LUNCHES

	Cal.	Fat		Cal.	Fat
2 slices wholewheat bread (C)	160	tr	1/2 cup low-fat cottage cheese (P,F)	80	2
2 oz. chicken, turkey, or			1/3 cup pineapple chunks (C)	60	0
lean beef (P,F)	100	2	3/4 cup strawberries (C)	30	0
1 tsp mayonnaise (F)	45	5	1/2 banana, sliced (C)	60	0
lettuce, tomato slices	10	0	Topping: 3 Tbsp Grapenuts (C)	80	tr
1 small orange (C)	60	0			
38 stick pretzels (C)	80	tr			
TOTALS	455	7	TOTALS	310	2

QUICK AND EASY SUPPER IDEAS

	Cal.	Fat		Cal.	Fat
Oriental Stir-fry:			3 oz. baked chicken (no skin) (P,F)	150	3
3 oz. chicken or turkey (P,F)	150	3	seasoned with 2 Tbsp reduced-		
2 cups vetetables (C)	100	0	calorie Italian dressing (F)	45	2
cooked in 1 tsp oil (F)	45	5	1/2 cup steamed spinach (C)	25	0
2/3 cup brown or wild rice (C)	160	2	1/2 cup steamed carrots (C)	25	0
1/2 cup fruit salad (C)	60	0	1/2 cup noodles (C)	80	tr
			1 fruit (C)	60	0
TOTALS	530	10	TOTALS	385	5

More quick and easy breakfast, lunch, and supper P-C-F meals are on pages 86-91. Use these sample meals to "mix-and-match" for your desired calorie and fat intake.

 © 1993, *The Balancing Act Nutrition and Weight Guide*, G. Kostas, M.P.H., R.D., Dallas, Texas

FOCUS FIRST ON FATS

LOW-FAT EATING IS ESSENTIAL TO ANY EFFECTIVE, HEALTHY EATING PROGRAM.

FAT CALORIES
Fat calories seem to promote weight gain more readily than other calorie sources. Fat calories also contribute to body fat, raise cholesterol levels, and increase one's risk of cancer, heart disease, and diabetes. If you want to stay healthy, feel fit, lose weight, and keep the weight off, **focus first on fats.**

HOW MUCH FAT SHOULD YOU EAT?
Although most Americans eat 100-150 grams of fat daily, most nutrition experts agree that we should consume only 20-30 grams of fat per 1000 calories. This means:

WOMEN:	20-30 grams to lose weight
	30-60 grams to maintain weight
MEN:	30-60 grams to lose weight
	50-75 grams to maintain weight

These figures translate into eating 20-30% of your calories from fat.

The following table specifies how much fat (in grams) to eat by calorie intake:

	FAT GRAMS		
CALORIES	**20% FAT**	**25% FAT**	**30% FAT**
1000	20	25	30
1200	25	30	40
1500	30	40	50
1800	35	45	60
2000	40	50	65
2200	45	55	70
2500	50	65	80

HOW DO YOU STAY WITHIN THIS FAT LIMIT?
You can count fat grams or simply use this daily guide:

DAILY FOOD TO EAT	FAT GRAMS
4-6 oz. lean meat, fish, poultry	4-18
3-6 tsp. (1-2 Tablespoons) fats/oils	15-30
4-8 starches/breads/cereals	0-8
3+ fruit	0
3+ vegetables	0
2-3 skim milk products	0
TOTAL	**20-55**

Appendix C and a condensed Fat Gram Counter (p. 108) lists fat grams in foods. **Read food labels for fat information also.**

WARNING:DO NOT OMIT FAT COMPLETELY! Fat-free eating may lead to constant hunger and over-eating. A little fat provides "staying power," giving longer-term energy and less hunger.

HOW TO DESIGN-YOUR-OWN EATING PLAN

NOW THAT YOU'VE LEARNED THE BASIC COMPONENTS OF HEALTHY EATING, IT'S TIME TO DESIGN YOUR OWN EATING PLAN! We will introduce you to five effective ways to pattern your daily meals and food calories to enjoy optimal nutrition and lose or manage weight. You may select one of the following five options, whichever best fits your personality, lifestyle, and preferences.

I.   THE "KEEP IT SIMPLE PLEASE" PLAN — "LOW-FAT, HIGH-FIBER EATING" (p. 48).
Based on the United States Department of Agriculture's new Pyramid guide for healthy eating, you simply emphasize high-fiber foods (fruit, vegetables, wholegrains, peas, beans, starches) and limit fats (such as margarine and oils) and keep protein-rich foods moderate.

II.   THE FAT GRAM PLAN (p. 49)
Using a fat-gram counter, you tally the amount of fat you eat daily. By keeping your fat intake at about 20-30 grams daily for women, and 30-60 grams daily for men, you automatically cut calories and lose weight quickly and effectively.

III.   THE FOOD GROUPS PLAN (p. 50)
Instead of counting fat grams or calories, you simply eat a set number of servings daily from each of six food categories (or "food groups") … fruit, vegetables, bread/starches, meat/fish/poultry, milk, and fats (margarine, oil, etc.). You'll lose weight while enjoying the maximum flexibility plus structure in meal planning.

IV.   2-WEEK MENU PLAN — BASED ON FOOD GROUPS (p. 71-83)
If you want to start out with the least decisions and get quick results, follow 2 weeks of **Sample Menus** at 1000, 1200, or 1500 calorie levels. All menus are low-fat and high-fiber, and utilize food groups for meal planning. This structured approach is for the person who "can't wait to get started" and/or tends to over-eat without boundaries. Eventually, you want to progress to making the right food decisions on your own. Use these menus as a start-up guide, taking note of portions and the mix of food choices per meal. Note the emphasis on plant foods, and smaller protein and fat servings. After 2-4 weeks, "spice up your life" with more food variety and meal flexibility by choosing a less structured approach. Re-read the remaining four eating plan systems described in this section and select the program that best fits your personality and eating needs.

V.   MIX-AND-MATCH MEALS PLAN — BASED ON FAT GRAMS (p. 85-91)
This plan works well for busy persons wanting to eat-on-the-run and figure out at-a-glance what to eat. A quick and easy system, based on fat grams and calories, this system offers structure, flexibility, convenience, and planned meal ideas. Combine any P-C-F breakfast, lunch and dinner meals listed on pages (85-91). You'll automatically eat healthy, nutritionally balanced meals and 1000-1500 calories (average 1200 calories) daily with 20-30 grams of fat. Out of 20 breakfast choices, 20 lunch and 20 dinner choices, you'll enjoy plenty of options and pre-planned quick-fix meal ideas. For meals out, review the "Meals Out" meal options in Section VII and the Fast Food options in Appendix C. Balance the week. If you are "over" one day and "under" the next, you'll still lose weight.

All of these plans for weight loss are based on these sound principles:
- **regularly spaced meals** • **P-C-F balanced meals**
- **low-fat, high fiber foods** • **food variety for optimal nutrition**

More specifically, all eating plans recommend:

Women:	Eat 1000-1200 calories, 20-30 grams fat, 20-30 grams fiber daily
Men:	Eat 1500-1800 calories, 30-60 grams fat, 20-30 grams fiber daily

Research by Judith Stern, D.Sc. at the University of California at Davis indicates that 66% of those most successful with long-term weight loss are those who design their own eating programs and set up their own "ground rules" based on healthy eating principles. The next step is to select your "game plan" for successful weight loss from the options proposed.

IT'S TIME TO ACT!

Now that you've read the five basic eating plans, which one will you put into action? Select your favorite approach and become better acquainted with it by reading the pages recommended. Then begin! As you read other book sections, you'll discover new facts, behaviors, and "tricks of the trade" that will help you be successful.

OOPS! . . . WHAT IF YOU "BLOW IT"??

Don't let one meal out of 21 weekly destroy your frame of mind and enthusiasm! Even 3 meals "off" shouldn't throw you off balance. Make up the extra calories and fat by eating 2-4 extra "all-vegetable" or "fat-free" meals that week. It will all balance out. "All-vegetable" plates cut 250-500 calories per meal. Get back on track and keep moving! Don't waste time, morale, and energy looking back. Remember: it's the week's balance of meals that counts — not necessarily a single meal!

BEYOND DIET

HABITS

Along with any of these healthy eating approaches, eating **habits** are key to lifelong weight success. Learning to plan and eat three meals daily, to choose low-fat snacks, eat slowly, and establish other healthy habits requires repeated practice. Repeated patterns become habits. Once new habits are established, they reinforce the eating styles that enable healthy weight control without as much conscious effort. The sooner you get started, the better.

EXERCISE

Along with healthy eating habits, you must exercise! Remember, burn 200-300 calories aerobically, 4-5 times a week to burn sufficient fat calories and body fat. Add two or three 20-30 minute sessions of resistance or strength training weekly to build muscle (lean body mass), which speeds metabolism. five days a week of exercise will increase fitness; three days a week will maintain fitness.

If your busy schedule prevents exercise now and then, look for ways to increase daily activity by taking stairs, longer walking routes to meetings, offices, your car, etc., and walk long hotel and airport corridors. Simply, **KEEP MOVING!**

LIFELONG WEIGHT MAINTENANCE

The above behaviors will help you lose weight and keep it off. In addition, become familiar with the size meals that enable you to enjoy your desired weight for life!

JUST DO IT!

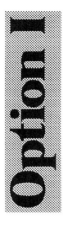

OPTION I

THE "KEEP IT SIMPLE PLEASE" PLAN:
"LOW-FAT, HIGH-FIBER" EATING

This plan is the most flexible and least structured.

For fiber, eat 10 or more "complex carbohydrates" (plant foods) daily, choosing at least 3 fruit, 3 vegetables, and 4 starches (cereal, wholewheat bread, pasta, rice, corn, peas, potatoes) daily. Keep all portions at 1/2 cup, or 1 fruit, 1 vegetable, 1 slice bread or roll. These foods are virtually fat-free and provide 20+ grams of fiber, the minimum needed daily. Eating this way provides at least 50% of your calories from complex carbohydrates. To increase fiber further, eat more bran cereals and beans, and always eat wholewheat bread.

For low-fat protein sources, eat 4-6 oz. lean meat/fish/poultry daily and 2 glasses skim milk. You may choose up to 3-6 teaspoons (= 1-2 tablespoons) of oils/fats daily. Automatically, you'll be limiting your fat intake to 20-30 grams per 1000 calories. For example:

WOMEN		
Choose	**Fat (gm)**	**Fiber (gm)**
5 oz. lean meat, fish, poultry =	5-10	0
2-3 teaspoons oils/fats =	10-15	0
4-5 starches =	0-5	10+
2-3 fruit, 3 vegetables, 2 cups skim milk =	0	10+
TOTALS: 1000-1200 calories	**20-30**	**20+**
MEN		
Choose	**Fat (gm)**	**Fiber (gm)**
6 oz. lean meat, fish, poultry =	6-12	0
4-6 teaspoons oils/fat =	20-30	0
6-8 starches =	0-8	14+
3-4 fruit, 3 vegetables, 2 cups skim milk =	0	16+
TOTALS: 1500-1800 calories	**32-50**	**30+**

Emphasize large vegetable servings to consume the most food volume and fiber (to feel "full") for the least fat and calories.

OPTION II

THE FAT-GRAM PLAN

With this approach, cut fat, not calories, to lose weight. Many individuals lose weight readily when fat calories (not total calories) are reduced.

To count fat grams, use the foods lists in **Appendix C** and on **pages 89-90** and/or food packages which list fat grams.

This system works well, especially for men. Calories are still important, however. A quart of orange juice contains 500 calories, 0 fat. Too many of even the best of calories can lead to weight gain. So, focus on fats first, keep calories reasonable, and vary food choices from all food groups.

As with other approaches, here are your goals:

> **WOMEN:** 20-30 grams of fat daily
> **MEN:** 30-60 grams of fat daily

This plan is perfect for label-readers. Some days, you can even eat that chocolate bar for 15 grams fat as part of your day's total fat intake! For a woman, 15 grams represents 50% of your daily 30-gram target. This leaves you with 15 grams of fat for your 3 meals . . . a challenge, but you can do it ... occasionally! For meal ideas, use the breakfast, lunch and supper ideas (p. 55) and dining out ideas (p. 179-182). This is self-education at its best.

HOW TO EAT FAVORITE FAT-RICH FOODS

Note the fat content in your favorite foods (see Sections III, IV, and Appendix C). When you eat higher-fat foods, cut back on dressings, margarines, mayonnaise, and other fats/oils. For example, if you choose a Snickers bar or danish roll or slice of apple pie (each contain 15 grams of fat), omit 1 tablespoon of vegetable oil or 2 tablespoons of salad dressing (each contain approximately 15 grams fat). Even though fat is "swapped" or "traded out" in this example, calories and quality nutrients are not equally traded. Now and then, that's O.K. You will still lose weight and be healthy.

CONSIDER THIS SAMPLE EATING PLAN:

DAILY EATING PLAN FOR 1200 CALORIES, 20-40 GRAMS FAT		
Food Groups	**Calories**	**Fat grams**
3 fruit	180	0
3 vegetables	75	0
5 starches/breads	400	0-10
2 skim milk	180	0
5 oz. protein foods	275	5-15
2 tsp fat/oils	90	10
TOTALS	**1200**	**15-35**

OPTION III
THE FOOD GROUPS PLAN

If you want structure, flexibility, and simplicity, use the FOOD GROUPS EATING PLAN system. The **FOOD GROUPING** system is based on the principle that all foods can be divided into six groups according to their nutrient content. By selecting a specific number of servings from each of these groups daily, you can enjoy optimal nutrition and automatically consume the right amount of fiber, fat, and calories. **You never count calories or fat grams!** Simply count food groups at your desired calorie intake.

FOOD GROUPS:

This chart shows the average nutrient content in each Food Group serving.

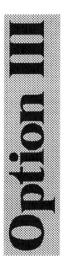

FOOD GROUP	SERVING SIZE	CALORIES	FAT (gm)	CARBOHYDRATE (gm)	PROTEIN (gm)
Milk (skim)	1 cup	90	trace	12	8
Meat/Subst.	1 ounce	55	0-3	0	7
Starch/Bread	1/2 cup; 1 slice	80	0-2	15	3
Fruit	1 whole; 1/2 cup	60	0	15	0
Vegetable	1/2 cup	25	0	5	2
Fat	1 tsp	45	5	0	0

DAILY MEAL PLANS:

To determine how many food group servings to eat, choose your calorie intake and turn to page 54 to select your favorite **DAILY EATING PLAN** of food groups. Then plan meals that include these foods. Refer to page 55 for two days of sample menus, and enjoy the two weeks of sample menus at the end of this chapter.

NOTICE HOW SIMPLE FOOD GROUP EATING PLANS CAN BE:

SAMPLE 1200-CALORIE EATING PLAN:				
You select:		**You automatically consume:**		
Amount	Food Group	Calories	Fat (gm)	Fiber (gm)
3	fruit	180	0	6+
3	vegetables	75	0	6+
5	starches	400	0-10	10+
2 cups	skim milk	180	0	0
5 oz.	lean meat	275	5-15	0
2 tsp	fats	90	10	0
TOTALS:		**1200**	**15-35**	**22+**

NOTE: Just like Plans I and II, this plan also provides 1200 calories, 20-30 grams fat, 20+ grams fiber.

GUIDELINES:

- Each food per group contains about the same number of calories, and grams of protein, carbohydrate, and fats. Therefore, you can vary foods within a group and not alter calorie intake. For example, if your plan calls for you to eat one vegetable, you may select a carrot or a tomato or green beans, and consume approximately the same calories.

- Do not swap foods from different groups. For example, if your plan calls for a vegetable, don't swap cheese for a vegetable.

- Familiarize yourself with foods included in each **Food Group** (p. 56).

- Be consistent with your caloric intake for continued weight loss or maintenance. If you eat more one day, cut back the next. Think of your week, and daily *averages*. If you are low on vegetables one day, eat more the next.

- Eat the same foods as other family members except in different amounts. There's no need to cook separate meals!

- Eat 1,000-1,500 calories daily, and 2-6 servings (teaspoons, usually) of fats daily for weight loss. See your nutritionist or physician for special needs. See page 54 for your DAILY EATING PLAN options.

PORTION CONTROL AIDS:

- Food weighing scale to measure the weight of meat and cheese

- Standard measuring cups and spoons (teaspoons and tablespoons) to measure liquids and other foods

- Measuring and weight equivalents:

1 ounce = 28 grams	4 tablespoons = 1/4 cup
1 pound = 16 ounces (oz.)	1 pint = 2 cups
1 cup = 8 ounces = 16 Tbsp	2 pints = 4 cups = 1 quart
1 tablespoon = 3 teaspoons	4 quarts = 1 gallon
2 tablespoons = 1 fluid ounce	

REFER TO FOODS IN FOOD GROUPS ON PAGE 56!

YOUR HEALTHY EATING PLAN

DESIGN YOUR OWN EATING PLAN!

Remember: you will count **food servings** — not calories — daily for balanced nutrition, easy meal planning and calorie and fat control.

Follow these steps:

1. Choose your appropriate calorie intake for weight loss. (*See pages 27-28 if you need help.*)

2. Using this chart below, note the number of servings you can eat daily from each food group at your calorie level.

3. Record the "totals" of servings from each group in the far right column of your Eating Plan chart (p. 53).

4. Distribute the servings into 3 meals, recording them on your chart, so that now you have a meal plan for each meal. Follow as an example this 1200-calorie eating and meal plan on the right.

MY DAILY EATING PLAN

1200 CALORIES   **25** FAT (GRAMS)

	B'fast	Snack	Lunch	Snack	Dinner	Snack	Totals
Milk	1			1			2
Meat			2oz.		3oz		5oz.
Starches	1		2		1	1	5
Fruit	1		1	1			3
Vegetables			1		2		3
Fats			1		1		2
Extras							
CALORIES	230		400	150	340	80	1200
FAT GRAMS	0		10–15	0	10–15	0	20–30

YOUR EATING PLAN

CALORIES AND FAT	10-20% PROTEIN	15-30% FAT	50-70% CARBOHYDRATE
1000 cal. 20 gm fat	4 oz. Meat/sub 2 cups skim Milk	2 tsp Fat	2 Fruit 4 Starches 3 Vegetables
1200 cal. 25 gm fat	5 oz. Meat/sub 2 cups skim Milk	2 tsp Fat	3 Fruit 5 Starches 3 Vegetables
1500 cal. 40 gm fat	6 oz. meat/sub 2 cups skim Milk	4 tsp Fat	3 Fruit 7 Starches 3 Vegetables
1800 cal. 55 gm fat	7 oz. Meat/sub 2 cups skim Milk	6 tsp Fat	3 Fruit 9 Starches 3 Vegetables
2000 cal. 60 gm fat	7 oz. Meat/sub 2 cups skim Milk	6 tsp Fat	5 Fruit 10 Starches 3 Vegetables

- Familiarize yourself with the Food Groups (p. 56-68).

- If you eat less than 1200 calories daily, Take a multiple vitamin/mineral with 100% of the R.D.A.'s. If you cannot drink milk, add 400-600 milligrams calcium supplement.

- Drink at least 2 quarts of fluids daily, half of which is water.

- For more variety of food plans at your calorie level, select from any of the additional **Daily Eating Plans** on page 54.

MY DAILY EATING PLAN

	CALORIES				FAT (GRAMS)		
	B'fast	Snack	Lunch	Snack	Dinner	Snack	Totals
Milk							
Meat							
Starches							
Fruit							
Vegetables							
Fats							
Extras							
CALORIES							
FAT GRAMS							

DAILY EATING PLANS

SELECT YOUR OWN CALORIC LEVEL AND FOOD DISTRIBUTION — **YOUR DAILY EATING PLAN.**

CIRCLE YOUR CHOICE

All plans have 15-30% fat calories, 10-20% protein calories, 50-70% carbohydrate calories.

Total Daily Calories	Skim Milk (8 oz.)	Vegetables (1 or 1/2 Cup)	Fruit (1 serving)	Starches (1 serving)	Meat (1 ounce)	Fats (1 teaspoon)
1000	0	3	4	5	4	2
	0	4	3	5	4	2
	* 2	3	2	4	4	2
	2	3	3	4	3	2
	2	4	2	4	3	3
	2	3	3	3	4	2
1200	0	4	5	5	5	3
	0	3	4	6	5	3
	0	3	4	5	6	4
	2	4	3	5	4	3
	* 2	3	3	5	5	2
	2	3	5	4	5	3
1400	0	3	4	8	5	4
	0	4	4	7	5	5
	0	4	5	6	6	4
	2	3	3	6	5	5
	2	3	3	7	5	3
	2	4	4	6	4	4
1500	0	3	5	8	6	4
	0	4	4	8	6	4
	* 2	3	3	7	6	4
	2	4	3	6	6	5
	2	3	4	6	5	6
	2	4	4	6	5	5
1800	0	4	7	8	7	6
	0	3	6	9	7	6
	2	4	5	8	7	5
	2	4	4	8	7	6
	2	3	5	8	7	5
	2	3	5	8	6	6
2000	0	4	5	11	7	7
	0	4	6	11	7	6
	2	4	5	9	7	7
	2	4	6	9	7	6
2400	0	4	8	13	7	9
	2	4	6	13	7	7
	2	4	7	12	7	8
	3	4	5	12	7	9

WOMEN: Select 1000-1200 calorie plans for weight loss; 1300-1800 for weight maintenance.
MEN: Select 1500-2000 calorie plans for weight loss; 2000-2400 for weight maintenance.

NOTE: The "no-milk" plans are for those who cannot drink milk. For calcium, drink calcium-fortified orange juice and a calcium supplement as directed by your physician or dietitian.

* The two-week sample menus are based on these plans at the end of this section (Option IV).

 © 1993, *The Balancing Act Nutrition and Weight Guide*, G. Kostas, M.P.H., R.D., Dallas, Texas

TWO SAMPLE MENUS FOR 1200-CALORIE LEVEL

TOTALS each day: 2 cups Milk, 5 oz. Meat/substitute, 5 Starches, 3 Fruit, 3 Vegetables, 2 Fats

Breakfast	Day #1	Day #2
1 Fruit	1/2 cup unsweetened orange juice	1/4 cantaloupe
1 Starch	1 slice wholewheat toast with	1/2 English wholewheat muffin
Free	1 tsp jam	1 Tbsp apple butter
1 Meat	1 egg	1/4 cup low-fat cottage cheese or Eggbeaters
1 Milk	1 cup skim milk	1 cup skim milk
0 Fat		
Beverages	water	water

Lunch

	Day #1	Day #2
2 Meat	1/2 cup water-packed tuna	2 ounces turkey
2 Starch	2 slices wholewheat bread	2 slices wholewheat bread
1 Fat	1 Tbsp reduced-calorie mayonnaise	1 tsp mayonniase or 1 Tbsp reduced-calorie mayonnaise
Free	pickle, lettuce slices	lettuce, tomato slice, mustard
1 Vegetable	1 tomato, sliced in wedges	1 raw carrot, in sticks
1 Fruit	1 apple	1 pear
0 Milk	0	0
Beverages	water	water

Supper

	Day #1	Day #2
2 Meat	2 ounces broiled, skinless chicken	2 ounces broiled fish w/lemon
1 Starch	1 small baked potato with	1 small ear corn
1 Fat	1 tsp margarine or 1 Tbsp reduced-calorie margarine	2 Tbsp reduced-calorie dressing (about 20 calories/Tbsp) on
2 Vegetables	1/2 cup carrots, steamed	tossed salad w/1 tomato
	1/2 cup green beans, steamed	1/2 cup broccoli, steamed, with
Free	tossed salad of "free" vegetables and 1 Tbsp fat-free dressing	lemon and "butter" sprinkles
1 Fruit	1 1/4 cup strawberries	1/2 cup mixed fruit cup
0 Milk	0	0
Beverage	water	water

Snacks

	Day #1	Day #2
1 Milk	1 cup skim milk	1 cup sugar-free hot cocoa
1 Starch	3 cups air-popped popcorn	3 graham cracker squares

SEE SAMPLE 2-WEEK MENUS PAGE 71-83.

SEE FOOD GROUPS (PAGES 56-68)

FOOD GROUP CALORIE AND FAT CONVERSION

Here's a quick way to know your calorie and fat intake daily, based on food groups:

FOOD GROUP (1 serving)	CALORIES	FAT (gms)
1 Milk (skim)	90	0
1 Meat or substitute	55	0-3
1 Starch	80	0-2
1 Fruit	60	0
1 Vegetable	25	0
1 Fat	45	5

Total your day's food group intake and calculate calories and fat grams consumed.

Example:

DAILY TOTAL		CALORIES	FAT (gms)
1 Milk (skim)	= 1 x 90	90	0
6 ounces Meat	= 6 x 55	330	12
5 Starch	= 5 x 80	400	5
3 Fruit	= 3 x 60	180	0
4 Vegetable	= 4 x 25	100	0
3 Fat	= 3 x 45	135	15
DAY'S TOTAL		**1235**	**32**

100-CALORIE FOOD EQUIVALENTS

2 cups vegetables (non-starchy)
1 medium fruit
1 small potato (4 inches long)
4 cups popcorn (without butter)
1/2 cup starch (potato, rice, pasta, etc.)
1/2 cup beans (lentils, pinto, garbanzo, etc.)
1 1/2 slices bread
1 1/2 cups (1 bowl) soup at home; 1 cup at restaurants
1 ounce cheese or 2 ounces low-fat cheese
1 ounce high-fat meat (prime rib, brisket, etc.)
1 1/2 ounces lean meat (flank, filet, tenderloin)
2 ounces fish or poultry
1 cup skim milk or yogurt
1/2 cup low-fat cottage cheese, tuna, crab, salmon
1 tablespoon salad dressing
2 pats (2 teaspoons) margarine, oil, mayonnaise

GO FOR VOLUME!

TIPS FOR IDENTIFYING FOOD PORTIONS

Meat, Poultry, Fish (cooked)

3 ounces	=	size of palm of a lady's hand (don't count fingers!)
	=	amount in a sandwich
	=	amount in a "quarter pounder" (cooked)
	=	half chicken breast (3 inches across)
6 ounces	=	restaurant split chicken breasts (6 inches across)
	=	common luncheon or cafeteria portion
8 ounces	=	common evening restaurant portion

Cheese

1 cunce	=	1 slice on sandwich or hamburger
	=	1 inch cube or 1 wedge airplane serving
1/2 cup	=	1 scoop cottage cheese

Salads

1 cup	=	dinner salad
2-4 cups	=	salad bar

Vegetables

1/2 cup	=	cafeteria or restaurant portion
	=	coleslaw or beans at a barbecue restaurant

Potato

1 small (3 oz)	=	80 calories	=	3 inches long = 1/2 cup
1 medium (6 oz)	=	160 calories	=	5 inches long
1 large (8 oz)	=	200 calories	=	6 inches long
1 huge (9 oz)	=	250 calories	=	6+ inches long = meal-in-one potato

Fruit

1 medium (3 inches across) fruit	=	60 calories
1 large fruit (apple, banana, pear)	=	120 calories

Fats

1 teaspoon margarine/butter	=	45 calories	= 1 pat
1 tablespoon mayonnaise	=	100 calories	= typical amount on sandwiches
2 tablespoons dressing	=	160 calories	= typical amount on a dinner salad
			= 1 small ladle (restaurant)
			= 1/2 large ladle (restaurant)

Ice Cream

1/2 cup (1 scoop)	= 4 ounces

Beverages

6 ounces	= typical juice portion
8 ounces	= common milk portion
4 ounces	= small glass of wine
12 ounces	= a can of beer or soft drink
1 1/2 ounces	= 1 jigger per alcoholic drink

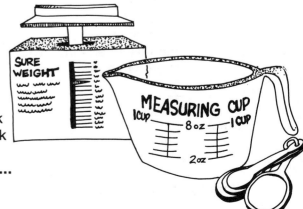

...Every Bite Counts...

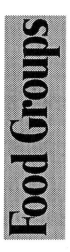

FOOD GROUPS

FROM OPTION III

Milk

Key nutrients: calcium, phosphorous, high-quality protein
Amount needed: 2-3 servings per day (for adults)

One serving contains 90 calories (8 grams protein, 12 grams carbohydrate, 0 fat)

🍴 CHOOSE

	One Serving
Milk (non-fat, skim, 1/2%, 1%)	1 cup
evaporated skim	1/2 cup
powdered (dry), nonfat..	1/4 cup
buttermilk, skim or low-fat	1 cup
low-fat (2%)..	3/4 cup
Yogurt	
from skim milk, plain, unflavored	1 cup
from low-fat milk, plain, unflavored	3/4 cup
from nonfat milk, flavored, sugar-free	1 cup
Low-calorie hot cocoa or milkshake (nonfat, sugar-free)	
(i.e., Alba, Swiss Miss Lite, Diet Carnation, etc.)	1 cup

---

✋ LIMIT

Whole milk products:
   chocolate
   condensed
   dried
   evaporated
Buttermilk (made from whole milk)
Flavored milk drink mixes

Instant breakfast drinks
Flavored yogurts
Hot cocoa mixes
Eggnog
Ice cream
Custard
Pudding

Note: 1 cup milk/yogurt = 300 mg calcium
1 cup orange juice with calcium = 300 mg calcium
We need 800-1500 mg calcium daily.

More Options: Occasionally, it's okay to substitute 1/2 cup fat-free frozen yogurt, 1/2 cup fat-free cottage cheese, or 1/2 cup fat-free pudding for 1 cup milk serving.

58 © 1993, *The Balancing Act Nutrition and Weight Guide*, G. Kostas, M.P.H., R.D., Dallas, Texas

Meat

Key nutrients: *protein, iron, zinc, Vitamin B12, B-complex vitamins, phosphorous*
Amount needed: *4-6 ounces per day*

Per 1 oz. Meat						
	Cal.	**Fat (gm)**			**Cal.**	**Fat (gm)**
Fish	40	0-1		Low-fat cheese	35-50	2-3
Poultry (no skin)	50	1		Reduced-fat cheese	50-80	3-5
Poultry (w/skin)	60	2		1/4 cup beans	50	0
Lean meat	60	3		Average	55	0-3

One serving (1 ounce, usually) contains 55 calories
(7 grams protein, 0-3 grams fat)

🍴 CHOOSE 10+ MEALS PER WEEK:

One Serving

Poultry:	Chicken, turkey, Cornish hen, ground poultry (all without skin)	1 oz
Fish:	Any kind (fresh or frozen)	1 oz
	Water-packed canned tuna or salmon	1/4 cup
	Crab, lobster, clams, scallops, shrimp (fresh or canned in water)	2 oz
	Oysters	6 medium
	Shrimp (limit to 2 oz per day)	2 oz (10 large)
	Sardines, canned and drained	2 medium
Veal:	Any cut except veal cutlets (ground or cubed)	1 oz
Venison:	Lean cuts	1 oz

Cold Cuts: *(3 grams of fat or less per ounce)*
     Poultry, lean beef, ham, Canadian bacon ....1 oz

Low-Fat or Nonfat Cheese: *(3 grams of fat or less per ounce)*
     Low-fat cottage cheese, Laughing Cow (reduced-calorie), farmer's,
     Skim ricotta, Borden Lite Line, Weight Watcher's slices, etc............1 oz (1/4 c or 3 Tbsp)

Other: Egg substitutes (cholesterol-free) ....1/4 cup
           Egg whites 3
           Dried beans, peas or lentils, cooked   ....1/4 cup
           (count 2/3 cup beans = 1 meat + 1 starch; 1 cup beans = 1 meat + 2 starches)

♦ LIMIT TO 4 MEALS PER WEEK:

LEAN AND WELL-TRIMMED MEATS (12-16 oz. total per week)

Lean Beef Cuts: *(per 3 oz, these cuts contain less than 200 calories and less than 10 grams fat)*
     Steak: tenderloin, sirloin, T-bone, porterhouse, round, flank............1 oz
     Roasts, stews: sirloin tip, eye of round, arm.....................1 oz
     Cooked and rinsed ground round or sirloin (10% fat)...................1 oz

Lean Lamb Cuts: leg, chops, loin, shoulder.............................1 oz
Lean Pork & Ham: center cut steaks, loin chops, smoked ham, tenderloin .... 1 oz
Reduced-Fat Cheese: *(3-5 grams of fat per ounce)*
     Part-skim mozzarella, Neufchatel, Kraft Natural Light Reduced-Fat cheeses
     (Cheddar, Swiss, Monterey Jack, etc.), Parmesan ....1 oz (1/4 c or 3 Tbsp)

LIMIT

THESE CHOLESTEROL-RICH FOODS:

Eggs (with yolks):... 1-3 per week
Organ Meat (Liver, heart, brains, kidney, tongue, pate): .... 3 oz. per month

THESE FOODS HIGH IN TOTAL FAT, SATURATED FAT AND CHOLESTEROL:
       (Count 1 oz. as 1 meat + 1 fat = 100 calories, 8-10 gms fat)

Poultry:	Domestic duck, goose
Fish:	Fish roe (caviar) or fried
Meats:	Fried, with gravies, sauces, breading, casseroles
	High fat meats: brisket, corned beef, ground beef or pork or lamb, club or rib steaks, rib roasts, spare ribs, deviled ham, sausage, cold cuts, hot dogs, luncheon meats, meatloaf
Cheese:	All (Cheddar, American, Swiss, blue, etc.). Select only low-fat and reduced-fat cheeses.

Note: Cured and canned meats and cheese are high in sodium.

WAYS TO TRIM MEAT FAT

1.   Eat approximately 4-6 ounces of meat, fish or poultry daily to trim fat, cholesterol, calories. Limit beef, lamb, pork to 12-16 ounces per week.

2.   Choose only lean cuts of meat (see list page 61). Avoid cuts where fat is visible or known to be "hidden" throughout the meat (i.e., brisket, rib roast, prime rib). Look for lean meat cuts labeled as "loin" (tenderloin, top sirloin, sirloin tips) or "round" (round roast, eye of round, top round). These cuts contain less than 10 grams of fat per 3 oz. portion.

3.   Trim all visible fat; remove skin from poultry before cooking.

4.   Bake, broil, or grill meats; do not add fats (as in sautéing, frying, adding sauces, gravies, cheeses, breading, etc.). Cook with non-stick sprays.

5.   Roast and bake meats with a rack to allow excess fat to drain off meat.

6.   Prepare eggs fat-free by poaching, boiling, scrambling or cooking in non-stick pans or with non-stick sprays.

7.   Remove fat from meat drippings: refrigerate drippings so that the cold fat will rise to the top and harden. Skim off or use a "gravy skimmer" which separates fat from hot drippings.

8.   Weigh meat after cooking and without bone. A 3-ounce serving of cooked meat equals approximately 1/4 pound (4 ounces) of raw meat.

9.   Rinse cooked ground beef in a sieve under hot water to rinse away fat. Then add beef to skillet, add tomato sauce, etc.

    © 1993, *The Balancing Act Nutrition and Weight Guide*, G. Kostas, M.P.H., R.D., Dallas, Texas

TYPICAL PORTIONS

Meat, Poultry, Fish

3 ounces	=	size of palm of lady's hand (don't count fingers!)
	=	amount in a sandwich
	=	amount in a "quarter pounder" (cooked)
	=	chicken breast half (3 inches across)
6 ounces	=	restaurant chicken breast (6 inches across)
	=	common luncheon or cafeteria portion
8 ounces	=	common evening restaurant portion

Cheese

1 ounce	=	1 slice on sandwich or hamburger
	=	1 inch cube of 1 wedge airplane serving
	=	3 Tbsp grated (1/4 cup)
1/2 cup	=	1 scoop cottage cheese (2 oz.)

3-Ounce Portions

1 pork or veal chop, 3/4 inch thick

2 rib lamb chops or 1 shoulder chop

1 leg-and-thigh or 1/2 breast of a 3-pound chicken

1 meat patty, 3 inches x 3/4 inches

2 thin slices roast meat, each 3 inches x 3 inches x 1/4 inch

3 medium size pieces of stew meat

1 small beef filet or 1/2 small sirloin tip

1 fish filet, 3 inches x 3 inches x 1/2 inch

3/4 cup tuna, salmon, crab, cottage cheese

15 large shrimp

3 boiled crabs or 18 oysters

1/2 Rock Cornish hen

Starches

Key nutrients: B-vitamins, iron, fiber, energy, potassium
Amount needed: at least 4 servings per day
Choose: wholegrains; high-fiber, unprocessed foods

One serving contains 80 calories
(3 grams of protein, 15 grams of carbohydrate, 0-2 grams of fat)

🍴 CHOOSE

One Serving

Bread and substitutes:

Bread, any type (1 oz)	1 slice
Bread, reduced-calorie (40 calories per slice)	2 slices
Bread crumbs	3 Tbsp
Bagel, small	1/2 (1 oz)
Croutons (lowfat)	1 cup
English muffin	1/2
Hamburger or hot dog bun	1/2
Pancake (4 in. across)	1
Pita or pocket bread (6 in. across)	1/2
Rice cakes	2
Mini rice cakes	6
Roll, plain	1
Tortilla (6 in. diameter, made without lard)	1
Waffle, fat-free (Eggo or Special K)	1
Submarine or hoagie roll (6 inches long)	1/2

Cereals, Grains and Pasta:

Bran cereals, concentrated (i.e., All-Bran or Muselix)	1/3 cup
Bran cereals, flaked (i.e., Bran Flakes, Fiber One)	1/2 cup
Cheerios or Kashi	1 cup
Dry cereal, flaked (i.e. Corn Flakes)	3/4 cup
Dry cereal, puffed (i.e., puffed rice or wheat)	1-1/2 cup
Grape Nuts or low-fat granola	3 Tbsp
Shredded Wheat (1 biscuit)	1/2 cup
Cooked cereal (oatmeal, grits, etc.)	1/2 cup
Noodles, spaghetti (cooked)	1/2 cup
Rice, white or brown; couscous (cooked)	1/3 cup
Unprocessed bran	1/2 cup
Wheat germ, buckwheat	3 Tbsp

Starchy Vegetables:

Corn	1/2 cup
Corn-on-cob (6 in. long)	1
Lima beans	1/2 cup
Mixed vegetables (corn, peas, carrots, lima beans)	1/2 cup
Peas, green (canned or frozen)	1/2 cup
Plantain[3]	1/2 cup
Potato, white[1] or sweet[3], baked (3 oz)	1 small
Potato, mashed	1/2 cup
Pumpkin[3]	3/4 cup
Winter squash (acorn or butternut)[3]	1 cup
Yam[3]	1/3 cup

Dried Beans, Peas and Lentils (cooked):

Baked beans, no pork	1/4 cup
Chickpeas, garbanzo beans	1/4 cup
Beans, peas, lentils, cooked	1/3 cup

(1 cup = 2 starches + 1 meat) (2/3 cup = 1 starch + 1 meat)

[1] high in Vitamin C   [2] high in Vitamin A   [3] high in Vitamins A & C

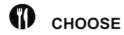

CHOOSE

Crackers and Snacks: One Serving

Animal 8
Bread sticks (4 in. x 1/2 in.) 2
Gingersnaps or Chocolate Snaps 3
Graham (2-1/2 in. square) 3
Matzoh..3/4 oz.
Melba rounds...7
Melba toast..5
Oyster (1/2 cup) 24
Popcorn (air-popped, no fat added) ....3 cups
Popcorn, microwave light (2 or less grams of fat) ....3 cups
Pretzels (stick) (3/4 oz.)......................................38
Pretzels (small 3-ring tiny twist) (3/4 oz.) 12
Rye Krisp (2 inch x 3-1/2 in.) 4
Saltines (2 in. square) 6
Whole grain crackers (i.e., Harvest Crisp).............6
Whole-wheat crackers, no fat added(crisp breads, i.e. Finn,
    Kavli, Wasa) (3/4 oz.). ....2-4 slices

Miscellaneous:

Catsup, chili sauce or BBQ sauce.........................1/4 cup
Spaghetti sauce, meatless ....1/2 cup
Tomato sauce...1 cup
Cornmeal, cornstarch, flour ....3 Tbsp
Cornflake crumbs and bread crumbs ....3 Tbsp

Soups:

Broth or tomato-based (i.e., vegetable, chicken
    noodle - homemade or canned) ....1 cup
Lentil or bean soup
    (count as 1 starch + 1 meat + 1 vegetable).......1 cup

✋ LIMIT STARCHES PREPARED WITH FAT (3 servings or less per week)

                                                                 One Serving

Count as 1 starch/bread, + 1 fat:

Biscuit (2-1/2 in. across).....................................1
Movie popcorn (unbuttered) or Microwave popcorn ....3 cups
Boboli .... 1/2 individual or 1/4 large
Chow mein noodles..1/2 cup
Corn bread (2 in. cube) (2 oz.) 1
Crackers, specialty (i.e., Ritz, Triscuits) 6
Cream soup, condensed ....4 oz.
Doughnut, cake ....1 small
French fried potatoes (2 in. to 3-1/2 in. long) 10
Granola..1/4 cup
Muffin, plain, homemade ....1 small
Stuffing, bread (prepared) ....1/4 cup
Taco shells (6 in. across) 2
Tortilla chips, Restaurant style (1 oz.) 7
Waffle (4-1/2 in. square) 1

Count as 1 starch/bread + 2 fats:

Corn chips, small (1 oz.).......................................34 small
    dipsize (1 oz.) 13
Croissant, large 1/2
Doughnut, yeast or glazed 1
Muffin, commercial 1
Potato chips (1 oz.) 15
Sweet Roll or Danish, small..................................1

Label Tip: Choose breads, cereals, crackers and snacks that have 2 or less grams of fat per serving.

Sodium Tip: Salt-free or low-sodium crackers, pretzels, canned goods (beans, soups, tomato-based sauces) are
                available. Commercially prepared baked goods and snack foods are usually high in sodium.

Fruit

Key nutrients: Vitamin C, Vitamin A, fiber, multiple vitamins and minerals
Amount needed: at least 2 servings per day

One serving contains 60 calories
(15 grams of carbohydrates, 0 protein, 0 fat)

🍴 CHOOSE

Fresh, frozen, canned fruit or fruit juice without sugar or syrup:

Apple (3 in. diameter)...	1 (4 oz.)
Applesauce, unsweetened..	1/2 cup
Apricots[3], fresh	4
dried[3]	7 halves
Banana (9 inches long)	1/2 (2 oz.)
Berries:	
Blackberries	3/4 cup
Blueberries..	3/4 cup
Boysenberries..	3/4 cup
Raspberries...	1 cup
Strawberries[1]	1 1/4 cup
Cherries	12 large
Dates..	2
Figs, fresh or dried (2 inches across)	2
Fruit cocktail, unsweetened	1/2 cup
Grapefruit[1]...	1/2
sections..	3/4 cup
Grapes	1 cup
Kiwi	1
Mango[3]	1/2
Melon:	
Cantaloupe[3] (5 inches across)	1/3
Honeydew[1]	1/8
Watermelon[2]...	1 1/4 cups
Melon Balls[3]	1 cup
Nectarine..	1
Orange[1]	1
Orange or mandarin sections[1]	3/4 cup
Papaya[3]..	1 cup
Peach, fresh[2] (3/4 cup)...	1
canned, unsweetened...	2 halves (1/2 cup)
Pear, fresh	1 small (4 oz.)
canned, unsweetened...	2 halves (1/2 cup)
Pineapple, fresh..	1/3 cup
canned, unsweetened...	3/4 cup
Plums[1]..	3 medium
Prunes[2], dried..	3 medium
Raisins	2 Tbsp
Tangerine[3]	2 medium

---

[1]high in Vitamin C   [2]high in Vitamin A   [3]high in Vitamin A and Vitamin C

Juices

Cranberry juice[1], low-calorie	1 1/4 cup
Apple juice/cider	1/2 cup
Grapefruit juice[1]	1/2 cup
Orange juice[1]	1/2 cup
Pineapple juice[1]	1/2 cup
Cranberry juice[1], regular, sweetened	1/3 cup
Grape juice	1/3 cup
Nectar	1/3 cup
Prune juice	1/3 cup

[1] *high in Vitamin C*   [2] *high in Vitamin A*   [3] *high in Vitamin A and Vitamin C*

 LIMIT

All sweetened frozen juice or canned fruit in syrup, commercial fruit fillings.

Tips:

1. Try to get the most fruit for your calories:
   Eat 1 cup cantaloupe (1/3 melon)   =   60 calories
   vs. 2 tablespoons raisins   =   60 calories
   or 1/3 cup grape juice   =   60 calories

2. Fresh, frozen and dried fruits have about 2 grams of fiber per serving.

3. To boost calcium, drink calcium-fortified orange juice (8 oz. juice = 2 fruit) which contains the same amount of calcium as in 8 oz. milk, which is 300 mg. calcium.

4. Key nutrients in fruit — Vitamins A and C and fiber — protect against cancer.

Vegetables

Key nutrients: *Vitamin A, Vitamin C, fiber, potassium, folacin, B_6, iron, magnesium*
Amount needed: *at least 3 servings per day (1 1/2 cups)*
Choose: *fresh or frozen vegetables, raw, baked, broiled, steamed, or boiled*
Serving Size: *1/2 cup cooked or 1 cup raw*

One serving (1/2 cup) contains 25 calories
(2 grams protein, 5 grams carbohydrate, 0 grams fat)

 CHOOSE

Artichoke (1/2 medium)	Okra
Asparagus[2]	Onions
Bean sprouts	Pea-pods
Beets	Rhubarb
Broccoli[3]	Rutabaga
Brussels sprouts[3]	Sauerkraut
Cabbage[1], cooked	Spinach[3], cooked
Carrots[2]	String beans, green or yellow
Cauliflower[1]	Summer squash[2]
Eggplant	Tomatoes[3]
Green beans	Tomato juice[3]
Green pepper[3]	Turnips
Greens, all types[3]	Vegetable juice[3]
Kohlrabi	Water chestnuts
Mushrooms, cooked	Zucchini, cooked

Eat these raw vegetables in any quantity:

Cabbage[1]	Lettuce, all types
Celery	Mushrooms
Chicory[3]	Parsley[3]
Chinese Cabbage	Pickles, dill or sour
Cucumbers	Radishes[1]
Endive[2]	Spinach
Escarole[2]	Watercress[3]
Green onions	Zucchini[1]

[1] *high in Vitamin C*   [2] *high in Vitamin A*   [3] *high in Vitamin A and Vitamin C*

 LIMIT

Creamed, buttered, or fried vegetables
Vegetables with gravies, sauces, marinades, cheese
Vegetables seasoned with bacon fat, salt pork, ham hocks or sausage
Vegetables canned with added salt

Note:
1. Starchy vegetables (i.e., peas, potatoes, corn) are listed with Starches/Breads.
2. Vegetables may contain up to 3 grams of dietary fiber per serving.
3. Choose fresh or frozen to avoid added salt.
4. Vegetable juices, pickles, and sauerkraut are high in salt.

Fats

Key nutrients: *fat soluble Vitamins A, D, E, K; essential fatty acids*
Amount needed: *2-8 portions per day (maximum)*
NOTE: *Fats are concentrated sources of calories - measure these!*

One serving contains 45 calories (5 grams of fat)

 CHOOSE

One Serving

Unsaturated Fats:

Oils* (except coconut, palm)	1 tsp
Margarine, soft tub, stick, or liquid**	1 tsp
Reduced-calorie**	1 Tbsp
Mayonnaise	1 tsp
Reduced-calorie	1 Tbsp
Fat-free	4 Tbsp
Salad dressing (all varieties)	1 Tbsp
Reduced-calorie (all varieties)	2 Tbsp
Nuts, Seeds, and Peanut Butter:	
Almonds, unsalted, dry roasted	6 whole
Peanuts, unsalted	10 large
Peanut butter	1/2 Tbsp
Pecans or walnuts, unsalted	2 whole
Nuts, unsalted (i.e., cashews)	1 Tbsp
Seeds (i.e., sunflower, sesame), unsalted	1 Tbsp
Avocado (medium)	1/8
Olives (large)	5
Coffee whitener, liquid	2 Tbsp
powder	4 tsp

*   Monounsaturated fats - canola, olive and peanut
     Polyunsaturated fats - safflower, sunflower, corn, soybean and cottonseed
** Avoid saturated fats - coconut, palm, "hydrogenated" (hardened) fats. Choose margarine with "liquid oil" as the first
     listed (predominant) ingredient on the label, and "hydrogenated" near end of list.

 LIMIT

Saturated Fats:

Butter	1 tsp
Bacon	1 slice
Coconut, shredded	2 Tbsp
Commercial dips	2 Tbsp
Cream, light, coffee, table	2 Tbsp
Heavy, whipping	1 Tbsp
Cream cheese	1 Tbsp
Light	1-1/2 Tbsp
Gravy	1 Tbsp
Salt pork	1/4 ounce
Sour cream	2 Tbsp
Imitation whipped topping, aerosol	5 Tbsp
Frozen	3 Tbsp

**Avoid commercially prepared foods with coconut or palm oil, lard, cocoa butter and hydrogenated fats,
i.e., shortening.**

Label Tip: Any fat-free dressing, mayonnaise, sour cream or cream cheese not exceeding 20 calories is considered a
              "free" serving.

Sodium Tip: Commercial dressings, olives, salted nuts and seeds, bacon, commercial chips, snack foods and salt pork are
              high in sodium. If you need to limit salt, look for low-sodium alternatives.

Cooking Tips: See page 98 for ways to reduce fats in cooking.

Note: **See Appendix C and pages 138-141 for more details on Fat grams in foods.**

HOW TO ESTIMATE HIDDEN FATS

When eating away from home, such as in restaurants or at parties, it may be difficult to determine the amount of fat added during cooking. These "hidden" fats may not be visible, but they do add fat calories. The following guidelines will assist you in counting hidden fats. When you tally food groups consumed daily, don't forget to include these easily forgotten fats!

Meats, Fish, Poultry

basted	1 oz.	=	1 meat + 1/2 fat
breaded and fried	1 oz.	=	1 meat + 1 fat
marinated	1 oz.	=	1 meat + 1/2 fat, if based with marinade during cooking
sautéed, pan fried, or stir-fried	1 oz.	=	1 meat + 1/2 fat

Vegetables

breaded and fried	1/2 cup	=	1 vegetable or starch + 1-2 fat
seasoned with margarine, oil or other fat	1/2 cup	=	1 vegetable or starch + 1/2-1 fat
stir fried	1/2 cup	=	1 vegetable or starch + 1/2 fat
French fries (small order)	20	=	2 starch + 2 fat

Eggs

fried	1 egg	=	1 meat + 1 fat
scrambled	1 egg	=	1 meat + 1 fat

Salads

meat or tuna salad	1/2 cup	=	2 meat + 2 fat
potato or macaroni salad	1/2 cup	=	1 starch + 2 fat
slaw or fruit salad	1/2 cup	=	1 vegetable or fruit + 2 fat
tossed salad with dressing	1 cup	=	1 vegetable + 2 fat

Sauces

gravy	2 Tbsp	=	1 fat
tartar sauce	2 tsp	=	1 fat
unknown "special" sauce	2 Tbsp	=	1 fat
white sauce	2 Tbsp	=	1 fat

   © 1993, *The Balancing Act Nutrition and Weight Guide*, G. Kostas, M.P.H., R.D., Dallas, Texas

Extras

Here's how to include calorie-containing "extra's" beyond your regular eating plan:

If you eat:	Limit extras to:
1000-1200 calories per day:	1-2 per week
1500+ calories per day:	3 per week

Try to choose foods that do not exceed 150 calories and 5 grams of fat per serving.

Some ideas:

	Cal.	Fat
COOKIES		
Snackwell's Cinnamon Graham Cookies (9), Devil's Food Cake (1)	60	0
Snackwell's Chocolate Chip Cookies (6), Oatmeal Raisin Cookies (1)	60	1
Nabisco Devil's Food Cake (1)	70	1
Health Valley Fat-free cookies - oatmeal raisin (3), apricot (3), etc.	75	0
Entenmann's Fat-free cookies - oatmeal raisin, etc. (1)	80	0
Animal crackers (10), vanilla wafers (5), chocolate snaps (4), ginger snaps (3), grahamy bears (5)	80	3
Homemade cookies - oatmeal (1), sugar (1), chocolate chip (1), etc.	80	3
Chocolate creme-filled (2) or Lovin' Lite brownie (1/24th of mix)	100	3
Fig newtons (2)	120	2
Health Valley fat-free granola bar (1) or fat-free muffin (1)	140	0
DESSERTS/SWEETS		
Angel food cake (1/24th of cake); Entenmann's fat-free cakes (1 oz.)	80	0
Regular gelatin (1/2 cup) or sugar-free pudding (1/2 cup)	80	0
Fat-free pudding snacks (1/2 cup)	100	0
Popsicle twin pop (1 bar), frozen fruit bar, frozen pudding bar	80	0
Fruit ice (1/2 cup), nonfat frozen yogurt (1/2 cup)	80	0
Ice milk (1/2 cup) or low-fat frozen yogurt (1/2 cup)	100	3
Sorbet (1/2 cup)	120	0
Sherbet (1/2 cup)	135	2
CONDIMENTS		
Apple butter (1 Tbsp)	15	0
Sugar, jam, jelly, marmalade, honey, molasses, maple syrup (1 Tbsp)	55	0
Low-calorie jelly or maple syrup (1 Tbsp)	8-35	0
Chocolate syrup (1 Tbsp)	50	0
Low-calorie fudge topping (1 Tbsp)	35	0
BEVERAGES		
Water, club soda, sugar-free tonic water	0	0
Tonic water (6 ounces)	7	0
Wine, dry (3 ounces)	70	0
Liquor (1 ounce, 80 Proof)	70	0
Lite beer (12 ounces)	70-100	0
Regular beer (12 ounces)	150	0
Dessert wine, sherry (3 ounces)	120	0
Port wine (3 ounces)	140	0
Soft drinks, punch (12 ounces)	150	0

Freebies

You can eat a few "extra's" for "free"! These items have only a few calories (less than 20 per serving), are fat-free, and may contain a little sugar. A few of these foods have specified portions listed because large amounts will add too many calories. Enjoy!

water, regular or bottled
carbonated water
sugar-free soft drinks
sugar-free tonic water
club soda
sugar-free drink mixes (lemonade, Kool-Aid)
coffee, tea, Postum
cocoa powder, unsweetened (1 Tbsp)
*barbecue sauce (1 Tbsp)
*catsup (1 Tbsp)
*chili sauce (1 Tbsp)
Pizza sauce (2 Tbsp)
Picante sauce (salsa)
hot pepper sauce, Tabasco sauce
*taco (hot) sauce
tomato paste/puree (1 Tbsp)
*Worcestershire sauce
*soy sauce
steak sauce (A-1, etc.)
vinegar, all flavors

baking powder, baking soda
*bouillon, consommé without fat
*broth
chives
cranberries, unsweetened
rhubarb, unsweetened
lemon, lime
gelatin, sugar-free (1/2 cup)
jam, jelly, regular or sugar-free (1 tsp)
apple butter (1 Tbsp)
pancake syrup, sugar-free (1 Tbsp)
sugar substitutes
whipped toppings (2 Tbsp)
herbs and spices, all types
*mustard, prepared (1 Tbsp)
mustard powder
*pickles, dill/sour
pimiento (1 Tbsp)
pepper
lettuce, parsley, radishes, watercress, celery

* high in sodium — you can buy low-sodium brands

OPTION IV
TWO WEEKS OF SAMPLE MENUS
for 1000, 1200, and 1500 Calories

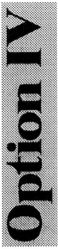

MENU TIPS

The following pages contain 14 days of menus to give you meal ideas at 3 different calorie levels. Please note the use of the Food Group System, which enables you to eat well-balanced, healthy, low-fat meals with the P-C-F mix per meal...and you don't need to count fat or calories...just food groups!

1. It helps to have a particular pattern of eating at meals, i.e. a fruit at breakfast, lunch, and snack; or 2-3 vegetables at supper. Patterns build consistency.

2. You may substitute favorite vegetables or fruit for those in menus.

3. You may add garlic, seasonings, or butter flavorings (i.e. Molly McButter) to any menu items. You may use non-stick vegetable oil cooking sprays whenever desired.

4. Drink 8-12 oz. water at every meal, and 32 oz. additional water throughout the day.

5. You may add "free" (calorie-free) foods as often as desired. See page 70 for "Freebies" listed.

6. You may add 3 "extra" foods a week (up to 100-150 calories each) and still lose weight — such as:

    - 1/2 cup (4 oz.) frozen fat-free, sugar-free yogurt or ice milk (80-110 calories)
    - 1/2 cup (4 oz.) fat-free chocolate pudding snack (Jello, Hunt's, etc.) (100 calories).
    - 1 frozen "ice cream" bar treat (80-100 calories)
    - 5 vanilla wafers (80 calories)
    - 2 Tbsp "lite" reduced calorie syrup (60 calories)
    - See page 69 for "Extra's" listed

7.
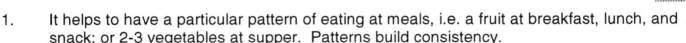

Mk = Milk	Vg = Vegetables
Mt = Meat	St = Starch/Bread
Fr = Fruit	Ft = Fat

8. With a little prior thought, you can plan delicious, healthy meals! Bon apetit!

14 - DAY SAMPLE MENUS
1000 CALORIES, 20-25 GRAMS FAT

2 Milk	4 Meat	4 Starches	2 Fruits	3 Vegetables	2 Fat
Tbsp = tablespoon			tsp = teaspoon	oz = ounce	

_____ DAY 1 _____

BREAKFAST
1/2 cup calcium-fortified orange juice (*1 Fr*)
1 wholewheat toast (*1 St*)
    with 1 tsp sugar-free jam/jelly (*free*)
1 cup skim milk (*1 Mk*)

LUNCH
Tuna Sandwich:
    2 slices reduced-calorie wholewheat bread (*1 St*)
    with 1/4 cup water-packed tuna (*1 Mt*)
    1 Tbsp fat-free mayonnaise (*free*) and
    1/4 cup chopped apple, celery, pickle (*free*)
    Lettuce and tomato slices (*free*)
1 small apple (*1 Fr*)
1 cup skim milk (*1 Mk*)

SUPPER
3 oz. skinless chicken breast, grilled (*3 Mt*)
1 small baked potato (*1 St*)
    with 1 Tbsp reduced-calorie margarine (*1 Ft*)
    (or Molly McButter sprinkles) (*free*)
1/2 cup carrots, steamed (*1 Vg*)
1/2 cup green beans, steamed (*1 Vg*)
1 cup green salad (*free*) with
    1 sliced tomato (*1 Vg*)
    2 Tbsp fat-free dressing (*free*)

SNACK
3 cups air-popped popcorn (*1 St*)
    with 1 Tbsp reduced-calorie margarine (*1 Ft*)

_____ DAY 2 _____

BREAKFAST
1 cup cubed or 1/3 of a cantaloupe (*1 Fr*)
1/2 wholewheat English muffin (*1 St*)
    with 1 tsp apple butter (*free*)
1 cup skim milk (*1 Mk*)

LUNCH
1/2 wholewheat bagel (*1 St*)
    w/1 oz. low-fat cheese (i.e., Weight Watchers) (*1 Mt*)
1 cup raw carrots, in sticks (*1 Vg*)
1 small pear (*1 Fr*)
1 cup nonfat yogurt (*1 Mk*)

SUPPER
3 oz. broiled fish w/lemon (*3 Mt*) and
    1 tsp melted margarine (*1 Ft*)
1/2 cup corn, steamed (*1 St*)
1/2 cup brussels sprouts, steamed (*1 Vg*)
1 cup Romaine salad (*free*) with
    1 tomato (*1 Vg*)
    1 Tbsp French dressing (*1 Ft*)

SNACK
38 pretzel sticks or 4 large pretzels (3/4 oz.) (*1 St*)

_____ DAY 3 _____

BREAKFAST
1/2 banana (*1 Fr*)
1/2 cup bran flakes (*1 St*)
1 cup skim milk (*1 Mk*)

LUNCH
Sandwich:
    2 sliced reduced-calorie wholewheat bread (*1 St*)
    1 oz. turkey (*1 Mt*)
    1 Tbsp fat-free mayonnaise (*free*)
    Lettuce, tomato slices (*free*)
1 small apple (*1 Fr*)
1 cup skim milk (*1 Mk*)
1/2 cup sugar-free jello (*free*)

SUPPER
3 oz. lean beef tenderloin (*3 Mt*)
1/3 cup rice (*1 St*)
    cooked in broth (*free*)
1/2 cup zucchini, steamed (*1 Vg*)
1/2 cup yellow squash, steamed (*1 Vg*)
1 spinach salad (*free*)
    with 1 small tomato (*1 Vg*)

SNACK
3 graham cracker squares (*1 St*)

_____ DAY 4 _____

BREAKFAST
1/2 grapefruit (*1 Fr*)
1/2 wholewheat bagel (*1 St*)
    with 1 1/2 Tbsp light cream cheese (*1 Ft*)
1 cup skim milk (*1 Mk*)

LUNCH
1 small baked potato (*1 St*) with
    1/4 cup low-fat cottage cheese (*1 Mt*)
1 large Romaine salad (*free*)
    with 2 Tbsp fat-free dressing (*free*)
1/2 cup asparagus, steamed (*1 Vg*)
1 1/4 cup strawberries (*1 Fr*)

SUPPER
Spaghetti:
    3 oz. extra lean (90% lean) ground beef, cooked
    and drained (*3 Mt*)
    1/2 cup spaghetti (*1 St*) over
    1/2 cup meatless spaghetti sauce (*1 St*)
1/2 cup spinach (*1 Vg*) and
1/2 cup mushrooms and onions, diced (*1 Vg*)
    sauteed in 1 tsp oil (*1 Ft*)
1/2 cup sugar-free jello (*free*)

SNACK
8 oz. carton lemon nonfat, sugar-free yogurt (*1 Mk*)

——————————— DAY 5 ———————————

BREAKFAST
1 orange (*1 Fr*)
1/2 cup oatmeal (*1 St*)
1 cup skim milk (*1 Mk*)

LUNCH
Pita Sandwich:
    1/2 pita pocket (*1 St*)
    1 oz. turkey (*1 Mt*)
    lettuce, tomato slices (*free*)
    1 Tbsp fat-free mayonnaise (*free*)
1 cup grapes (*1 Fr*)
1/2 cup V-8 or tomato juice (*1 Vg*)

SUPPER
3 oz. baked seafood (*3 Mt*)
1/2 cup mashed potatoes (*1 St*) with
    1 Tbsp reduced-calorie margarine (*1 Ft*)
1 cup broccoli-carrot-mushroom mix (*2 Vg*)
    stir-fried with 1 tsp olive oil (*1 Ft*)
Mixed green salad (*free*) with
    1 Tbsp fat-free dressing (*free*)
1 cup skim milk (*1 Mk*)

SNACK
2 large flavored rice cakes or
    1/2 cup dry Chex cereal mix (*1 St*)

——————————— DAY 6 ———————————

BREAKFAST
1 cup nonfat plain yogurt (*1 Mk*)
    mixed with 1/2 banana (*1 Fr*)
    and 3 Tbsp Grape Nuts or low-fat granola (*1 St*)

LUNCH
Chef's Salad:
    2 cups mixed salad greens (*free*)
    1/2 cup raw broccoli & 1/2 cup raw cauliflower (*1 Vg*)
    and 1 tomato, sliced (*1 Vg*)
    1 oz. turkey ham (*1 Mt*)
    1 oz. low-fat cheese (*1 Mt*)
    3-4 Tbsp fat-free dressing (5 cal/Tbsp) (*free*)
1 cup vegetable soup or 4 Rye Krisps (*1 St*)

SUPPER
2 slices of a medium cheese pizza (*2 Mt, 2 St, 2 Ft*)
1 cup cucumber, onion and tomato slices (*1 Vg*)
1 1/4 cup watermelon (*1 Fr*)

SNACK
8 oz. sugar-free, fat-free hot cocoa (*1 Mk*)

——————————— DAY 7 ———————————

BREAKFAST
1/2 cup calcium-fortified orange juice (*1 Fr*)
1 wholewheat pancake (*1 St*)
    topped with 1 Tbsp "lite" reduced-calorie syrup (*free*)
    and 1 Tbsp reduced-calorie margarine (*1 Ft*)
1 cup skim milk (*1 Mk*)

LUNCH
3 oz. roasted skinless chicken breast (*3 Mt*)
1/3 cup rice (*1 St*)
1/2 cup green beans (*1 Vg*)
1/2 cup carrots, steamed (*1 Vg*)
1/2 cup cabbage, shredded (slaw) (*free*) with
    2 Tbsp reduced-calorie dressing (*1 Ft*)

SUPPER
Taco Salad:
    1/3 cup pinto or kidney beans (*1 St*)
    1 oz. (3 Tbsp) grated low-fat cheese (*1 Mt*)
    1 cup raw vegetables (green pepper, carrots,
    red onion, mushrooms) (*1 Vg*)
    2 cups lettuce (*free*)
    1 corn tortilla, toasted and broken into chips (*1 St*)
    Picante sauce (*free*)
3/4 cup fresh pineapple chunks (*1 Fr*)

SNACK
1 cup nonfat, sugar-free raspberry yogurt (*1 Mk*)

DAY 8

BREAKFAST
1 fresh orange (*1 Fr*)
1/2 wholewheat English muffin (*1 St*)
    topped with 1 oz. (3 Tbsp) (1/4 cup) grated part-
    skim mozzarella cheese (*1 Mt*)
1 cup skim milk (*1 Mk*)

LUNCH
Fast food grilled chicken breast sandwich
    (no mayonnaise) (*2 St, 3 Mt*)
1 small apple (*1 Fr*)
1 cup skim milk (*1 Mk*)
(or occasional 4 oz. fat-free, sugar-free frozen yogurt)

SUPPER
Vegetarian Stir-fry:
    Heat in skillet in 2 tsp oil: (*2 Ft*)
        1 cup mixed frozen Japanese vegetables (*2 Vg*)
        1/2 cup diced onions and mushrooms (*1 Vg*)
1/3 cup steamed rice (*1 St*)
1 fortune cookie (*free*)

DAY 9

BREAKFAST
1/3 cantaloupe (*1 Fr*)
1/2 cinnamon-raisin bagel (*1 St*)
    with 1 Tbsp fat-free cream cheese (*free*)
8 oz. carton nonfat, sugar-free vanilla yogurt (*1 Mk*)

LUNCH
1 cup lentil or bean soup (*1 St, 1 Vg, 1 Mt*)
1 cup tossed salad (*free*)
    with 1 Tbsp Ranch dressing (*1 Ft*)
1 wholewheat roll (*1 St*)

SUPPER
3 oz. turkey or skinless chicken breast, roasted (*3 Mt*)
1/2 cup corn, steamed (*1 St*)
1/2 cup spinach (*1 Vg*), sautéed in 1 tsp olive oil (*1 Ft*)
1/2 cup carrots, steamed (*1 Vg*)
15-calorie frozen sugar-free popsicle (*free*)

SNACK
1 cup skim milk (*1 Mk*)
1 cup grapes (*1 Fr*)

DAY 10

BREAKFAST
1/2 banana (*1 Fr*)
1/2 cup shredded wheat (*1 St*)
1 cup skim milk (*1 Mk*)

LUNCH
Soft Tacos:
    2 corn tortillas (*2 St*)
    2 oz. skinless chicken, cooked (*2 Mt*)
    1/4 tomato, diced (*free*)
    lettuce, shredded (*free*)
    3 Tbsp picante sauce, optional (*free*)
1 fresh peach (*1 Fr*)

SUPPER
2 oz. red snapper (*2 Mt*)
    sautéed in 2 tsp oil (*2 Ft*)
1/2 cup red new potatoes, steamed (*1 St*)
1/2 cup yellow squash, steamed (*1 Vg*)
1/2 cup zucchini, steamed (*1 Vg*)
1 tomato, in wedges (*1 Vg*)

SNACK
1 cup fat-free, sugar-free hot cocoa
    or 8 oz. nonfat, sugar-free lemon yogurt (*1 Mk*)

DAY 11

BREAKFAST
1 1/4 cups fresh strawberries (*1 Fr*)
3 Tbsp Grapenuts on top of (*1 St*)
8 oz. plain, nonfat yogurt (*1 Mk*)

LUNCH
Tuna Sandwich:
    2 slices reduced-calorie wholewheat bread (*1 St*)
    1/4 cup water-packed tuna (*1 Mt*)
    1 Tbsp reduced-calorie mayonnaise (*1 Ft*)
    3 Tbsp chopped celery, apple, pickle (*free*)
    lettuce and tomato slices (*free*)
1 fresh small pear or apple (*1 Fr*)

SUPPER
Low-calorie frozen dinner
    (up to 300 cal., 10 gm fat) (*3 Mt, 1 St, 1 Vg*)
1/2 cup broccoli, steamed (*1 Vg*)
1 raw carrot, sliced (*1 Vg*)
1 wholewheat roll or bread slice (*1 St*)
    with 1 tsp margarine (*1 Ft*)

SNACK
1 cup skim milk (*1 Mk*)

DAY 12

BREAKFAST

1/2 grapefruit (*1 Fr*)
1 fat-free Eggo or Special K waffle (*1 St*)
    with 1 Tbsp "lite" reduced-calorie syrup (*free*)
8 oz. nonfat, sugar-free strawberry yogurt
    or 1 cup skim milk (*1 Mk*)

LUNCH

Hamburger:
    1 reduced-calorie bun (80 cal.) (*1 St*)
    3 oz. extra lean (90% lean) ground beef (*3 Mt*)
    lettuce, tomato, mustard (*free*)
1 1/4 cup watermelon slices (*1 Fr*)
1 cup skim milk (or occasional 4 oz fat-free,
    sugar-free chocolate pudding snack) (*1 Mk*)

SUPPER

Shrimp Creole:
    2 oz. (10 large) boiled shrimp (*1 Mt*)
    heated in 1/2 cup spaghetti sauce (*1 St*)
    served over 1/3 cup rice (*1 St*)
1 1/2 cups vegetable mix (broccoli, cauliflower,
    carrots, onions, mushrooms, etc.), (*3 Vg*)
    stir-fried in 2 tsp oil (*2 Ft*)

DAY 13

BREAKFAST

1/2 cup calcium-fortified orange juice (*1 Fr*)
1 wholewheat toast (*1 St*)
    with 1 tsp sugar-free jam (*free*)
1 poached egg (*1 Mt*)
1 cup skim milk (*1 Mk*)

LUNCH

Pasta Salad:
    1 cup pasta, cooked (*2 St*)
    1/2 cup cooked vegetables, sliced
    (broccoli, carrots, onions, red bell pepper) (*1 Vg*)
    3-4 Tbsp oil-free Italian dressing (5 cal/Tbsp) (*free*)
    1 oz. (3 Tbsp) Parmesan, grated (*1 Mt*)
Spinach salad (*free*)
    with 2 Tbsp reduced-calorie Catalina dressing (*1 Ft*)
1 cup skim milk (*1 Mk*)

SUPPER

Fajitas:
    1 soft wholewheat tortillas (*1 St*)
    2 oz. grilled flank steak, sliced (*2 Mt*)
        marinated in 2 tbsp lime juice (*free*)
        and 1/2 tsp fajita seasoning (*free*)
    1/2 cup onion slices, (*1 Vg*)
        grilled in 1 tsp oil (*1 Ft*)
    1/2 cup tomato, diced (*1 Vg*)
    1/2 cup lettuce, shredded (*free*)
3/4 cups fresh pineapple chunks (*1 Fr*)

DAY 14

BREAKFAST

1 1/4 cup strawberries (*1 Fr*)
2 wholewheat pancakes (4") (*2 St*)
    with 2 Tbsp "lite" reduced-calorie syrup (*free*)
1 cup skim milk (*1 Mk*)

LUNCH

3 oz. skinless chicken breast (*3 Mt*),
    marinated in 2 Tbsp oil-free Italian dressing (*free*)
    and baked, grilled, or broiled
1/2 cup cabbage, shredded (*free*)
    with 1 Tbsp coleslaw dressing (*1 Ft*)
1/2 cup green beans, steamed (*1 Vg*)
1/2 cup yellow squash, steamed (*1 Vg*)
1 1/4 cup watermelon slices (*1 Fr*)
1 cup skim milk (*1 Mk*)

SUPPER

Mini-pizzas:
    1 English muffin (2 halves) (*2 St*)
    2 Tbsp grated part-skim mozzarella cheese (*1 Mt*)
    1 oz. (3 Tbsp) mushrooms, sliced (*free*)
    2 Tbsp onion, diced (*free*)
    2 Tbsp green pepper, diced (*free*)
    1/4 cup pizza or spaghetti sauce (*free*)
1 cup raw vegetables (carrot sticks, celery, broccoli,
    tomato, cucumber, etc.) (*1 Vg*)
    with 2 Tbsp reduced-calorie Ranch dressing
    as dip (*1 Ft*)
15-calorie popsicle (*free*)

14-DAY SAMPLE MENUS
1200 CALORIES, 25 GRAMS FAT

2 Milk	5 Meat	5 Starches	3 Fruits	3 Vegetables	2 Fat
Tbsp = tablespoon		tsp = teaspoon		oz. = ounce	

_____ DAY 1 _____

BREAKFAST
1/2 cup calcium-fortified orange juice (1 Fr)
1 wholewheat toast (1 St)
    with 1 tsp sugar-free jam/jelly (free)
1 cup skim milk (1 Mk)

LUNCH
Tuna Sandwich:
    2 slices wholewheat bread (2 St) with
    1/2 cup water-packed tuna (2 Mt)
    1 Tbsp reduced-calorie mayonnaise (1 Ft) and
    1/4 cup chopped apple, celery, pickle (free)
    Lettuce and tomato slices (free)
1 small apple (1 Fr)
1 cup skim milk (1 Mk)

SUPPER
3 oz.skinless chicken breast, grilled (3 Mt)
1 small baked potato (1 St)
    with 1 Tbsp reduced-calorie margarine (1 Ft)
    (or butter-flavored sprinkles) (free)
1/2 cup carrots, steamed (1 Vg)
1/2 cup green beans, steamed (1 Vg)
1 cup green salad (free), with
    1 sliced tomato (1 Vg) and
    1 Tbsp fat-free dressing (free)
3/4 cup fresh pineapple chunks (1 Fr)

SNACK
3 cups air-popped popcorn (1 St) with
    1 Tbsp reduced-calorie margarine (1 Ft)

_____ DAY 2 _____

BREAKFAST
1 cup cubed or 1/3 of a cantaloupe (1 Fr)
1/2 wholewheat English muffin (1 St)
    with 1 tsp apple butter (free)
1 cup skim milk (1 Mk)

LUNCH
1 wholewheat bagel (2 St)
  with 2 oz. low-fat cheese (i.e., Weight Watchers) (2 Mt)
1 cup raw carrots, in sticks (1 Vg)
1 small pear (1 Fr)
1 cup nonfat yogurt (1 Mk)

SUPPER
3 oz. broiled fish w/lemon (3 Mt) and
    1 tsp melted margarine (1 Ft)
1/2 cup corn, steamed (1 St)
1/2 cup Brussels sprouts, steamed (1 Vg)
1 cup lettuce salad (free) with
    1 tomato, sliced (1 Vg) and
    1 Tbsp French dressing (1 Ft)
1/2 cup fresh fruit salad (1 Fr)

SNACK
38 pretzel sticks or 4 large pretzels (3/4 oz.) (1 St)

_____ DAY 3 _____

BREAKFAST
1/2 banana (1 Fr)
1/2 cup bran flakes (1 St)
1 cup skim milk (1 Mk)

LUNCH
Sandwich:
    2 slices wholewheat bread (2 St)
    2 oz. turkey (2 Mt)
    1 Tbsp fat-free mayonnaise (free)
    Lettuce, tomato slices (free)
1 small apple (1 Fr)
1 cup skim milk (1 Mk)
1/2 cup sugar-free jello (free)

SUPPER
3 oz. lean beef tenderloin (3 Mt)
1/3 cup rice (1 St)
    cooked in broth (free)
1/2 cup zucchini, steamed (1 Vg)
1/2 cup yellow squash, steamed (1 Vg)
1 spinach salad (free) with
    1 small tomato (1 Vg) and
    2 Tbsp dressing (2 Ft)
1 orange, in sections (1 Fr)

SNACK
3 graham cracker squares (1 St)

_____ DAY 4 _____

BREAKFAST
1/2 grapefruit (1 Fr)
1 wholewheat bagel (2 St)
    with 1 1/2 Tbsp light cream cheese (1 Ft)
1 cup skim milk (1 Mk)

LUNCH
1 small baked potato *(1 St)* topped with
    1/2 cup low-fat cottage cheese *(2 Mt)*
1 large Romaine salad *(free)*
    2 Tbsp fat-free dressing *(free)*
1/2 cup asparagus, steamed *(1 Vg)*
1 1/4 cup strawberries *(1 Fr)*

SUPPER
Spaghetti:
    3 oz. 90% lean ground beef, cooked & drained *(3 Mt)*
    1/2 cup meatless spaghetti sauce *(1 St)* over
    1/2 cup spaghetti *(1 St)*
1/2 cup spinach *(1 Vg)* and
    1/2 cup mushrooms & onions, diced *(1 Vg)*
    sauteed in 1 tsp oil *(1 Ft)*
1 cup melon, cubed *(1 Fr)*

SNACK
8 oz. carton lemon nonfat, sugar-free yogurt *(1 Mk)*

_____ DAY 5 _____

BREAKFAST
1 orange *(1 Fr)*
1/2 cup oatmeal *(1 St)*
1 cup skim milk *(1 Mk)*

LUNCH
Pita Sandwich:
    1 pita pocket *(2 St)*
    2 oz. turkey *(2 Mt)*
    lettuce, tomato slices *(free)*
    1 Tbsp fat-free mayonnaise *(free)*
1 cup grapes *(1 Fr)*
1/2 cup V-8 or tomato juice *(1 Vg)*

SUPPER
3 oz. baked seafood *(3 Mt)*
1/2 cup mashed potatoes *(1 St)*
    with 1 Tbsp reduced-calorie margarine *(1 Ft)*
1 cup broccoli-carrot-mushroom mix *(2 Vg)*
    stir-fried with 1 tsp olive oil *(1 Ft)*
Mixed green salad *(free)*
    with 1 Tbsp fat-free dressing *(free)*
1/2 cup fruit salad *(1 Fr)*
1 cup skim milk *(1 Mk)*

SNACK
2 large flavored rice cakes or
1/2 cup dry Chex cereal mix *(1 St)*

_____ DAY 6 _____

BREAKFAST
1 cup nonfat plain yogurt *(1 Mk)*
    mixed with 1/2 banana *(1 Fr)*
    and 3 Tbsp Grape Nuts or low-fat granola *(1 St)*

LUNCH
Chef Salad:
    2 cups mixed salad greens *(free)* with
    1/2 cup raw broccoli & 1/2 cup raw cauliflower *(1 Vg)*
    1 tomato, sliced *(1 Vg)*
    2 oz. turkey ham *(2 Mt)*
    1 oz. low-fat cheese *(1 Mt)*
    2 Tbsp fat-free dressing *(free)*
1 fresh peach *(1 Fr)*
1 cup vegetable soup or 4 Rye Krisps *(1 St)*

SUPPER
2 slices of a medium cheese pizza *(2 Mt, 2 St, 2 Ft)*
1 cup cucumber, onion and tomato slices *(1 Vg)*
2 4-inch bread sticks *(1 St)*
1 1/4 cup watermelon *(1 Fr)*

SNACK
8 oz. sugar-free, fat-free hot cocoa *(1 Mk)*

_____ DAY 7 _____

BREAKFAST
1/2 cup calcium-fortified orange juice *(1 Fr)*
1 wholewheat pancake *(1 St)*
    topped with 1 Tbsp "lite" reduced-calorie syrup *(free)*
    and 1 Tbsp reduced-calorie margarine *(1 Ft)*
1 cup skim milk *(1 Mk)*

LUNCH
3 oz. roasted skinless chicken breast *(3 Mt)*
1/3 cup rice *(1 St)*
1/2 cup green peas *(1 St)*
1/2 cup carrots, steamed *(1 Vg)*
1/2 cup cabbage, shredded (slaw) *(free)*
    with 2 Tbsp reduced-calorie dressing *(1 Ft)*
1 cup cubed or 1/3 of a cantaloupe *(1 Fr)*

SUPPER
Taco Salad:
    2/3 cup pinto or kidney beans *(1 St, 1 Mt)*
    1 oz. (1/4 cup) grated low-fat cheese *(1 Mt)*
    1 tomato, sliced *(1 Vg)*
    1 cup raw vegetables (green pepper, carrots, red
    onions, mushrooms) *(1 Vg)*
    1 cup lettuce *(free)*
    1 corn tortilla, toasted and broken into chips *(1 St)*
    Picante sauce *(free)*
3/4 cup fresh pineapple chunks *(1 Fr)*

SNACK
1 cup nonfat, sugar-free raspberry yogurt *(1 Mk)*

DAY 8

BREAKFAST
1 fresh orange *(1 Fr)*
1 wholewheat English muffin, in halves, *(2 St)*
    topped with 1 oz. (1/4 cup) grated part-skim
    mozzarella cheese *(1 Mt)*
1 cup skim milk *(1 Mk)*

LUNCH
Fast food grilled chicken breast sandwich
    (no mayonnaise) *(2 St, 3 Mt)*
1 small apple *(1 Fr)*
1 cup skim milk *(1 Mk)*
 (or occasional 4 oz. fat-free, sugar-free frozen yogurt)

SUPPER
Vegetarian Stir-fry:
    Heat in skillet in 2 tsp oil: *(2 Ft)*
        1 cup mixed frozen Japanese vegetables *(2 Vg)*
        1/2 cup diced onions and mushrooms *(1 Vg)*
1/3 cup steamed rice *(1 St)*
3/4 cup fresh pineapple chunks *(1 Fr)*
    topped with 1/4 cup low-fat cottage cheese *(1 Mt)*
1 fortune cookie *(free)*

DAY 9

BREAKFAST
1/3 cantaloupe *(1 Fr)*
1 cinnamon-raisin bagel *(2 St)*
    with 1 Tbsp fat-free cream cheese *(free)*
8 oz. carton nonfat, sugar-free peach yogurt *(1 Mk)*

LUNCH
1 cup lentil or bean soup *(1 St, 1 Vg, 1 Mt)*
1 cup tossed salad *(free)*
    with 1 Tbsp Ranch dressing *(1 Ft)*
    & 3 Tbsp Parmesan cheese *(1 Mt)*
1 wholewheat roll *(1 St)*
1/2 cup fresh fruit salad *(1 Fr)*

SUPPER
3 oz. turkey or skinless chicken breast, roasted *(3 Mt)*
1/2 cup corn *(1 St)*
1/2 cup spinach *(1 Vg)*, sauteed in 1 tsp olive oil *(1 Ft)*
1/2 cup carrots, steamed *(1 Vg)*
15 calorie frozen sugar-free popsicle *(free)*

SNACK
1 cup skim milk *(1 Mk)*
1 cup grapes *(1 Fr)*

DAY 10

BREAKFAST
1 banana *(2 Fr)*
1 cup shredded wheat *(2 St)*
1 cup skim milk *(1 Mk)*

LUNCH
Soft Tacos:
        2 corn tortillas *(2 St)*
        2 oz. skinless, cooked chicken *(2 Mt)*
        1/4 tomato, diced *(free)*
        lettuce, shredded *(free)*
        3 Tbsp picante sauce, optional *(free)*
1 fresh peach *(1 Fr)*

SUPPER
3 oz. red snapper *(3 Mt)*
    sauteed in 2 tsp oil *(2 Ft)*
1/2 cup red new potatoes, steamed *(1 St)*
1/2 cup yellow squash, steamed *(1 Vg)*
1/2 cup zucchini, steamed *(1 Vg)*
1 tomato, in wedges *(1 Vg)*

SNACK
1 cup fat-free, sugar-free hot cocoa
    or 8 oz. nonfat, sugar-free lemon yogurt *(1 Mk)*

DAY 11

BREAKFAST
1 1/4 cups fresh strawberries *(1 Fr)*
3 Tbsp Grapenuts on top of *(1 St)*
8 oz. plain, nonfat yogurt *(1 Mk)*

LUNCH
Tuna Sandwich:
        2 slices reduced-calorie wholewheat bread *(1 St)*
        1/2 cup water-packed tuna *(2 Mt)*
        1 Tbsp reduced-calorie mayonnaise *(1 Ft)*
        3 Tbsp chopped celery, apple, pickle *(free)*
        lettuce and tomato slices *(free)*
1 fresh small pear or apple *(1 Fr)*

SUPPER
Low-calorie frozen dinner (up to 300 cal.,
    10 gm fat) *(3 Mt, 1 St, 1 Vg)*
1/2 cup broccoli, steamed *(1 Vg)*
1 raw carrot, sliced *(1 Vg)*
1 wholewheat roll or bread slice *(1 St)*
    with 1 tsp margarine *(1 Ft)*

SNACK
1 cup skim milk *(1 Mk)*
1 cup grapes *(1 Fr)*
3 graham cracker squares *(1 St)*

_____DAY 12 _____

BREAKFAST
1/2 grapefruit *(1 Fr)*
1 fat-free Eggo or Special K waffle *(1 St)*
    with 1 Tbsp reduced-calorie syrup *(free)*
8 oz. nonfat, sugar-free strawberry yogurt
    or 1 cup skim milk *(1 Mk)*

LUNCH
Hamburger:
    1 bun *(2 St)*
    3 oz. lean (90% lean) ground beef *(3 Mt)*
    1 slice low-fat cheddar cheese (40 cal/oz.) *(1 Mt)*
    lettuce, tomato, mustard *(free)*
1 1/4 cup watermelon slices *(1 Fr)*
1 cup skim milk *(1 Mk)*
    (or occasional 4 oz. fat-free, sugar-free chocolate
    pudding snack)

SUPPER
Shrimp Creole:
    2 oz. (10 large) boiled shrimp *(1 Mt)*
    heated in 1/2 cup spaghetti sauce *(1 St)*
    served over 1/3 cup rice *(1 St)*
1 1/2 cups vegetable mix (broccoli, cauliflower,
    carrots, onions, mushrooms, etc.), *(3 Vg)*
    stir-fried in 2 tsp oil *(2 Ft)*
1 cup cantaloupe slices (1/3 melon) *(1 Fr)*

_____DAY 13 _____

BREAKFAST
1/2 cup calcium-fortified orange juice *(1 Fr)*
1 wholewheat toast *(1 St)*
    with 1 tsp sugar-free jam *(free)*
1 poached egg *(1 Mt)*
1 cup skim milk *(1 Mk)*

LUNCH
Pasta Salad:
    1 cup pasta, cooked *(2 St)*
    1/2 cup cooked vegetables, sliced
        (broccoli, carrots, onions, red bell pepper) *(1 Vg)*
    3 Tbsp fat-free Italian dressing *(free)*
    2 Tbsp Parmesan, grated *(1 Mt)*
Spinach Salad *(free)*
    with 2 Tbsp reduced-calorie Catalina dressing *(1 Ft)*
1/2 cup fresh fruit salad *(1 Fr)*
1 cup skim milk *(1 Mk)*

SUPPER
Fajitas:
    2 soft wholewheat tortillas *(2 St)*
    3 oz. grilled flank steak, sliced *(3 Mt)*
        marinated in 2 Tbsp lime juice *(free)*
        and 1/2 tsp fajita seasoning *(free)*
    1/2 cup onion slices, *(1 Vg)*
        sauteed in 1 tsp oil *(1 Ft)*
    1/2 cup tomato, diced *(1 Vg)*
    1/2 cup lettuce, shredded *(free)*
3/4 cups fresh pineapple chunks *(1 Fr)*

_____DAY 14 _____

BREAKFAST
1 1/4 cup strawberries *(1 Fr)*
2 wholewheat pancakes (4") *(2 St)*
    with 2 Tbsp "lite" reduced-calorie syrup *(free)*
1 cup skim milk *(1 Mk)*

LUNCH
3 oz. skinless chicken breast, *(3 Mt)*
    marinated in 2 Tbsp fat-free Italian dressing *(free)*
    and baked, grilled, or broiled
1/2 cup mashed potatoes *(1 St)* with
    1 tsp (or 1 Tbsp reduced-calorie) margarine *(1 Ft)*
1/2 cup cabbage, shredded *(free)*
    with 1 Tbsp coleslaw dressing *(1 Ft)*
1/2 cup yellow squash, steamed *(1 Vg)*
1/2 cup green beans, steamed *(1 Vg)*
1 1/4 cup watermelon slices *(1 Fr)*
1 cup skim milk *(1 Mk)*

SUPPER
Mini-pizzas:
    1 English muffin (2 halves) *(2 St)*
    1 oz. (1/4 cup) grated part-skim mozzarella cheese *(1 Mt)*
    1 oz. Canadian bacon or smoked turkey *(1 Mt)*
    2 Tbsp mushrooms, sliced *(free)*
    2 Tbsp onion, diced *(free)*
    2 Tbsp green pepper, diced *(free)*
    1/4 cup pizza sauce *(free)*
1 cup raw vegetables *(1 Vg)*
    (carrot sticks, celery, broccoli, tomato, cucumber, etc.)
1 fresh orange, in slices *(1 Fr)*

14-DAY SAMPLE MENUS
1500 CALORIES, 25-40 GRAMS FAT

2 Milk	6 Meat	7 Starches	3 Fruits	3 Vegetables	4 Fat
Tbsp = tablespoon			tsp = teaspoon	oz. = ounce	

_____ DAY 1 _____

BREAKFAST
1/2 cup calcium-fortified orange juice *(1 Fr)*
2 wholewheat toast or 1 bagel *(2 St)*
    with 2 tsp sugar-free jam/jelly *(free)*
1 cup skim milk *(1 Mk)*

LUNCH
Tuna Sandwich:
    2 slices wholewheat bread *(2 St)* with
    1/2 cup water-packed tuna *(2 Mt)*
    1 Tbsp reduced-calorie mayonnaise *(1 Ft)* and
    1/4 cup chopped apple, celery, pickle *(free)*
    Lettuce and tomato slices *(free)*
1 small apple *(1 Fr)*
1 cup skim milk *(1 Mk)*

SUPPER
4 oz. skinless chicken breast, grilled *(4 Mt)*
1 small baked potato *(1 St)* with
    1 Tbsp reduced-calorie margarine *(1 Ft)*
    (or butter-flavored sprinkles) *(free)*
1/2 cup carrots, steamed *(1 Vg)*
1/2 cup green beans, steamed *(1 Vg)*
1 cup green salad *(free)* with
    1 sliced tomato *(1 Vg)* and
    2 Tbsp fat-free dressing *(free)*
1 roll *(1 St)* with
    1 tsp margarine *(1 Ft)*
3/4 cup fresh pineapple chunks *(1 Fr)*

SNACK
3 cups air-popped popcorn *(1 St)* with
    1 Tbsp reduced-calorie margarine *(1 Ft)*

_____ DAY 2 _____

BREAKFAST
1 cup cubed or 1/3 of a cantaloupe *(1 Fr)*
1 wholewheat English muffin *(2 St)* with
    2 tsp apple butter *(free)*
1 cup skim milk *(1 Mk)*

LUNCH
1 cup vegetable soup *(1 St)*
1 wholewheat bagel *(2 St)* with
    2 oz. low-fat cheese (i.e., Weight Watchers) *(2 Mt)*
1 raw carrot, in sticks *(1 Vg)*
1 small pear *(1 Fr)*
1 cup nonfat yogurt *(1 Mk)*

SUPPER
4 oz. broiled fish w/ lemon *(4 Mt)* and
    2 tsp melted margarine *(2 Ft)*
1/2 cup corn, steamed *(1 St)*
1/2 cup brussels sprouts, steamed *(1 Vg)*
1 cup Romaine salad *(free)* with
    1 tomato, sliced *(1 Vg)* and
    2 Tbsp French dressing *(2 Ft)*
1/2 cup fresh fruit salad *(1 Fr)*

SNACK
38 pretzel sticks or 4 large pretzels (3/4 oz.) *(1 St)*

_____ DAY 3 _____

BREAKFAST
1/2 banana *(1 Fr)*
1/2 cup bran flakes *(1 St)*
1 cup skim milk *(1 Mk)*

LUNCH
Sandwich:
    2 slices wholewheat bread *(2 St)*
    2 oz. turkey *(2 Mt)*
    2 tsp mayonnaise *(2 Ft)*
    Lettuce, tomato slices *(free)*
1 small apple *(1 Fr)*
1 cup skim milk *(1 Mk)*
1/2 cup sugar-free jello *(free)*

SUPPER
4 oz. lean beef tenderloin *(4 Mt)*
2/3 cup rice *(2 St)*
    cooked in broth *(free)*
1/2 cup zucchini, steamed *(1 Vg)*
1/2 cup yellow squash, steamed *(1 Vg)*
1 spinach salad *(free)* with
    1 small tomato *(1 Vg)* and
    2 Tbsp dressing *(2 Ft)*
1 orange, in sections *(1 Fr)*

SNACK
6 graham cracker squares *(2 St)*

_____ DAY 4 _____

BREAKFAST
1/2 grapefruit *(1 Fr)*
1 wholewheat bagel *(2 St)*
1 cup skim milk *(1 Mk)*

LUNCH
1 small baked potato *(1 St)* topped with
    1/2 cup low-fat cottage cheese *(2 Mt)*
1 large Romaine salad *(free)* with
    2 Tbsp French dressing *(2 Ft)*
1/2 cup asparagus, steamed *(1 Vg)*
1 1/4 cup strawberries *(1 Fr)*

SUPPER
Spaghetti:
    3 oz. 90% lean ground beef, cooked & drained *(3 Mt)*
    1/2 cup meatless spaghetti sauce *(1 St)* over
    1 cup spaghetti *(2 St)*
    3 Tbsp grated Parmesan cheese *(1 Mt)*
1/2 cup spinach, steamed *(1 Vg)* and
    1/2 cup mushrooms & onions, diced *(1 Vg)*
    sautéed in 1 tsp oil *(1 Ft)*
1 wholewheat bread *(1 St)* with
    1 tsp melted margarine and garlic *(1 Ft)*
1 cup melon, cubed *(1 Fr)*

SNACK
8 oz. carton lemon nonfat, sugar-free yogurt *(1 Mk)*

_____ DAY 5 _____

BREAKFAST
1 orange *(1 Fr)*
1 cup oatmeal *(2 St)*
1 cup skim milk *(1 Mk)*

LUNCH
Pita Sandwich:
    1 pita pocket *(2 St)*
    3 oz. turkey *(3 Mt)*
    lettuce, tomato slices *(free)*
    1 Tbsp reduced-calorie mayonnaise *(1 Ft)*
1 cup grapes *(1 Fr)*
1/2 cup V-8 or tomato juice *(1 Vg)*

SUPPER
3 oz. baked seafood *(3 Mt)*
1 cup mashed potatoes *(2 St)*
    with 1 Tbsp reduced-calorie margarine *(1 Ft)*
1 cup broccoli-carrot-mushroom mix *(2 Vg)*
    stir-fried with 1 tsp olive oil *(1 Ft)*
Mixed green salad *(free)*
    with 1 Tbsp Italian dressing *(1 Ft)*
1/2 cup fruit salad *(1 Fr)*
1 cup skim milk *(1 Mk)*

SNACK
2 large flavored rice cakes or
1/2 cup dry Chex cereal mix *(1 St)*

_____ DAY 6 _____

BREAKFAST
1 cup nonfat plain yogurt *(1 Mk)*
    mixed with 1/2 banana *(1 Fr)*
    and 6 Tbsp Grape-Nuts or low-fat granola *(2 St)*

LUNCH
Chef Salad:
    2 cups mixed salad greens *(free)* with
    1/2 cup raw broccoli & 1/2 cup raw cauliflower *(1 Vg)*
    1 tomato, sliced *(1 Vg)*
    3 oz. turkey ham *(3 Mt)*
    1 oz. low-fat cheese *(1 Mt)*
    3-4 Tbsp fat-free dressing (5 cal a Tbsp)*(free)*
1 roll *(1 St)* with
    1 tsp margarine *(1 Ft)*
1 fresh peach *(1 Fr)*
1 cup vegetable soup *(1 St)*

SUPPER
2 slices of a medium cheese pizza *(2 Mt, 2 St, 2 Ft)*
1 cup cucumber, onion and tomato slices *(1 Vg)* with
    1 Tbsp French dressing *(1 Ft)*
2 4-inch bread sticks *(1 St)*
1 1/4 cup watermelon *(1 Fr)*

SNACK
8 oz. sugar-free, fat-free hot cocoa *(1 Mk)*

_____ DAY 7 _____

BREAKFAST
1/2 cup calcium fortified orange juice *(1 Fr)*
2 wholewheat pancakes *(2 St)*
    topped with 2 Tbsp "lite" reduced-calorie syrup *(free)*
    and 2 Tbsp reduced-calorie margarine *(2 Ft)*
1 cup skim milk *(1 Mk)*

LUNCH
4 oz. roasted skinless chicken breast *(4 Mt)*
1/3 cup rice *(1 St)*
1/2 cup green peas, steamed *(1 St)*
1/2 cup carrots, steamed *(1 Vg)* with
    1 tsp margarine *(1 Ft)*
1/2 cup cabbage, shredded (slaw) *(free)*
    with 2 Tbsp reduced-calorie dressing *(1 Ft)*
1 cup cubed or 1/3 of a cantaloupe *(1 Fr)*

SUPPER
Taco Salad:
    2/3 cup pinto or kidney beans *(1 St, 1 Mt)*
    1 oz. (3 Tbsp) grated low-fat cheese *(1 Mt)*
    1 tomato, sliced *(1 Vg)*
    1 cup raw vegetables (green pepper, carrots,
    red onions, mushrooms) *(1 Vg)*
    1 cup lettuce *(free)*
    1 corn tortilla, toasted and broken into chips *(1 St)*
    Picante sauce *(free)*
3/4 cup fresh pineapple chunks *(1 Fr)*

SNACK
1 cup nonfat, sugar-free raspberry yogurt *(1 Mk)*
3 Gingersnaps or 2 Bordeaux cookies *(1 St)*

_____ DAY 8 _____

BREAKFAST
1 fresh orange *(1 Fr)*
1 English muffin, in halves, *(2 St)*
    topped with 1 oz. (1/4 cup) grated part-skim
    mozzarella cheese *(1 Mt)*
1 cup skim milk *(1 Mk)*

LUNCH
Fast food grilled chicken breast
    sandwich (no mayonnaise) *(2 St, 3 Mt)*
1 small apple *(1 Fr)*
1 cup skim milk *(1 Mk)*
    (or occasional 4 oz. fat-free, sugar-free frozen yogurt)

SUPPER
Vegetarian Stir-fry:
    Heat in skillet in 3 tsp oil: *(3 Ft)*
        1 cup mixed frozen Japanese vegetables *(2 Vg)*
        1/2 cup diced onions and mushrooms *(1 Vg)*
1 cup steamed rice *(3 St)*
3/4 cup fresh pineapple chunks *(1 Fr)*
    topped with 1/2 cup low-fat cottage cheese *(2 Mt)*
1 fortune cookie *(free)*

_____ DAY 9 _____

BREAKFAST
1/3 cantaloupe *(1 Fr)*
1 cinnamon-raisin bagel *(2 St)*
    with 1 Tbsp cream cheese *(1 Ft)*
8 oz. carton nonfat, sugar-free vanilla yogurt *(1 Mk)*

LUNCH
1 cup lentil or bean soup *(1 St, 1 Vg, 1 Mt)*
1 cup tossed salad *(free)*
    with 1 Tbsp Ranch dressing *(1 Ft)*
    & 3 Tbsp Parmesan cheese *(1 Mt)*
1 wholewheat roll *(1 St)*
    with 1 tsp margarine *(1 Ft)*
1/2 cup fresh fruit salad *(1 Fr)*

SUPPER
3 oz. turkey or skinless chicken breast, roasted *(3 Mt)*
1 cup corn, steamed *(2 St)*
1/2 cup spinach *(1 Vg)*, sautéed in 1 tsp olive oil *(1 Ft)*
1/2 cup carrots, steamed *(1 Vg)*
15 calorie frozen sugar-free popsicle *(free)*

SNACK
Half Sandwich:
    1 slice wholewheat bread *(1 St)*
    1 oz. turkey ham *(1 Mt)*
    mustard, lettuce, tomato *(free)*
1 cup grapes *(1 Fr)*
1 cup skim milk *(1 Mk)*

_____ DAY 10 _____

BREAKFAST
1 banana *(2 Fr)*
1 cup shredded wheat *(2 St)*
1 cup skim milk *(1 Mk)*

LUNCH
Soft Tacos:
    3 corn tortillas *(3 St)*
    3 oz. skinless, cooked chicken, *(3 Mt)*
        browned in 1 tsp oil *(1 Ft)*
    1/4 tomato, diced *(free)*
    lettuce, shredded *(free)*
    3 Tbsp picante sauce, optional *(free)*
1 fresh peach *(1 Fr)*

SUPPER
3 oz. red snapper *(3 Mt)*
    sautéed in 2 tsp oil *(2 Ft)*
1/2 cup red new potatoes, steamed *(1 St)*
1 small raw tomato, in wedges *(1 Vg)*
1/2 cup yellow squash, steamed *(1 Vg)*
1/2 cup zucchini, steamed *(1 Vg)*
1 Tbsp reduced-calorie margarine
 on vegetables *(1 Ft)*

SNACK
1 cup fat-free, sugar-free hot cocoa
    or 8 oz. nonfat, sugar-free lemon yogurt *(1 Mk)*
3 graham cracker squares *(1 St)*

_____ DAY 11 _____

BREAKFAST
1 1/4 cups fresh strawberries *(1 Fr)*
1 slice wholewheat toast *(1 St)*
    with 1 tsp margarine *(1 Ft)*
3 Tbsp Grape Nuts *(1 St)* on top of
    8 oz. plain, nonfat yogurt *(1 Mk)*

LUNCH
Tuna Sandwich:
    2 slices wholewheat bread *(2 St)*
    1/2 cup water-packed tuna *(2 Mt)*
    1 Tbsp reduced-calorie mayonnaise *(1 Ft)*
    3 Tbsp chopped celery, apple, pickle *(free)*
    lettuce and tomato slices *(free)*
1 fresh small pear or apple *(1 Fr)*

SUPPER
Low-calorie frozen dinner (up to 300 cal.,
    10 gm fat) *(3 Mt, 1 St, 1 Vg)*
1/2 cup broccoli, steamed *(1 Vg)*
  with 1 tsp margarine *(1 Ft)*
1 raw carrot, sliced *(1 Vg)*
1 wholewheat roll or bread slice *(1 St)*
    with 1 tsp margarine *(1 Ft)*
1 cup grapes *(1 Fr)*

SNACK
1 cup skim milk *(1 Mk)*
1/2 bagel *(1 St)*
1 oz. low-calorie cheese (i.e. Laughing Cow) *(1 Mt)*

—————————————**DAY 12**—————————————

BREAKFAST
1/2 grapefruit *(1 Fr)*
2 fat-free Eggo or Special K waffle *(2 St)*
    with 2 Tbsp "lite" reduced-calorie syrup *(free)*
    and 1 Tbsp reduced-calorie margarine *(1 Ft)*
8 oz. nonfat, sugar-free strawberry yogurt
    or 1 cup skim milk *(1 Mk)*

LUNCH
Hamburger:
    1 bun *(2 St)*
    3 oz. extra lean (90% lean) ground beef *(3 Mt)*
    1 slice low-fat cheddar cheese (40 cal./oz.) *(1 Mt)*
    lettuce, tomato, mustard *(free)*
1 1/4 cup watermelon slices *(1 Fr)*
1 cup skim milk *(1 Mk)*
    (or occasional 4 oz. fat-free, sugar-free chocolate
    pudding snack)

SUPPER
Shrimp Creole:
    2 oz. (10 large) boiled shrimp *(1 Mt)*
    heated in 1/2 cup spaghetti sauce, *(1 St)*
    served over 2/3 cup rice *(2 St)*
1 1/2 cups vegetable mix (broccoli, cauliflower,
    carrots, onions, mushrooms, etc.), *(3 Vg)*
    stir-fried in 3 tsp oil *(3 Ft)*

SNACK
1 cup cantaloupe slices (1/3 melon) *(1 Fr)*
    with 1/4 cup low-fat cottage cheese *(1 Mt)*

—————————————**DAY 13**—————————————

BREAKFAST
1/2 cup calcium-fortified orange juice *(1 Fr)*
1 wholewheat toast *(1 St)*
    with 1 Tbsp reduced-calorie margarine *(1 Ft)*
1 poached egg *(1 Mt)*
1 cup skim milk *(1 Mk)*

LUNCH
Pasta Salad:
    1 cup pasta, cooked *(2 St)*
    1/2 cup cooked vegetables, sliced
      (broccoli, carrots, onions, red bell pepper) *(1 Vg)*
    4 Tbsp fat-free Italian dressing (5 cal a Tbsp)*(free)*
    3 Tbsp Parmesan, grated *(1 Mt)*

Spinach Salad *(free)*
    with 2 Tbsp reduced-calorie Catalina dressing *(1 Ft)*
1/2 cup fresh fruit salad *(1 Fr)*
1 cup skim milk *(1 Mk)*

SUPPER
Fajitas:
    3 soft wholewheat tortillas *(3 St)*
    4 oz. grilled flank steak, sliced *(4 Mt)*
      marinated in 2 Tbsp lime juice *(free)*
      and 1/2 tsp fajita seasoning *(free)*
    1/2 cup onion slices, *(1 Vg)*
      sauteed in 1 tsp oil *(1 Ft)*
    1/2 cup tomato, diced *(1 Vg)*
    1/2 cup lettuce, shredded *(free)*
3/4 cups fresh pineapple chunks *(1 Fr)*

SNACK
3 cups air-popped popcorn, *(1 St)*
    with 1 Tbsp reduced-calorie margarine *(1 Ft)*
    (or 3 cups microwave "light" popcorn)

—————————————**DAY 14**—————————————

BREAKFAST
1 1/4 cup strawberries *(1 Fr)*
3 wholewheat pancakes (4") *(3 St)*
    with 2 Tbsp "lite" reduced-calorie syrup *(free)*
    and 1 tsp margarine *(1 Ft)*
1 cup skim milk *(1 Mk)*

LUNCH
3 oz. skinless chicken breast, *(3 Mt)*
    marinated in 2 Tbsp oil-free Italian dressing *(free)*
    and baked, grilled, or broiled
1/2 cup mashed potatoes *(1 St)*
    with 1 tsp (or 1 Tbsp reduced-calorie) margarine *(1 Ft)*
1/2 cup cabbage, shredded *(free)*
    with 1 Tbsp coleslaw dressing *(1 Ft)*
1/2 cup yellow squash, steamed *(1 Vg)*
    with 1 tsp margarine *(1 Ft)*
1/2 cup green beans, steamed *(1 Vg)*
1 1/4 cup watermelon slices *(1 Fr)*
1 cup skim milk *(1 Mk)*

SUPPER
Mini-pizzas:
    1 English muffin (2 halves) *(2 St)*
    1 oz. (1/4 cup) grated part-skim mozzarella cheese *(1 Mt)*
    2 oz. Canadian bacon or smoked turkey *(2 Mt)*
    2 Tbsp mushrooms, sliced *(free)*
    2 Tbsp onion, diced *(free)*
    2 Tbsp green pepper, diced *(free)*
    1/4 cup pizza or spaghetti sauce *(free)*
1 cup raw vegetables (carrot sticks, celery,
    broccoli, tomato, cucumber, etc.) *(1 Vg)*
    w/ 2 Tbsp reduced-calorie Ranch dressing as dip *(1 Ft)*
1 fresh orange, in slices *(1 Fr)*

SNACK
38 pretzel sticks or 12 3-ring twists (3/4 oz.) *(1 St)*
    (or 1 cup Cheerios)

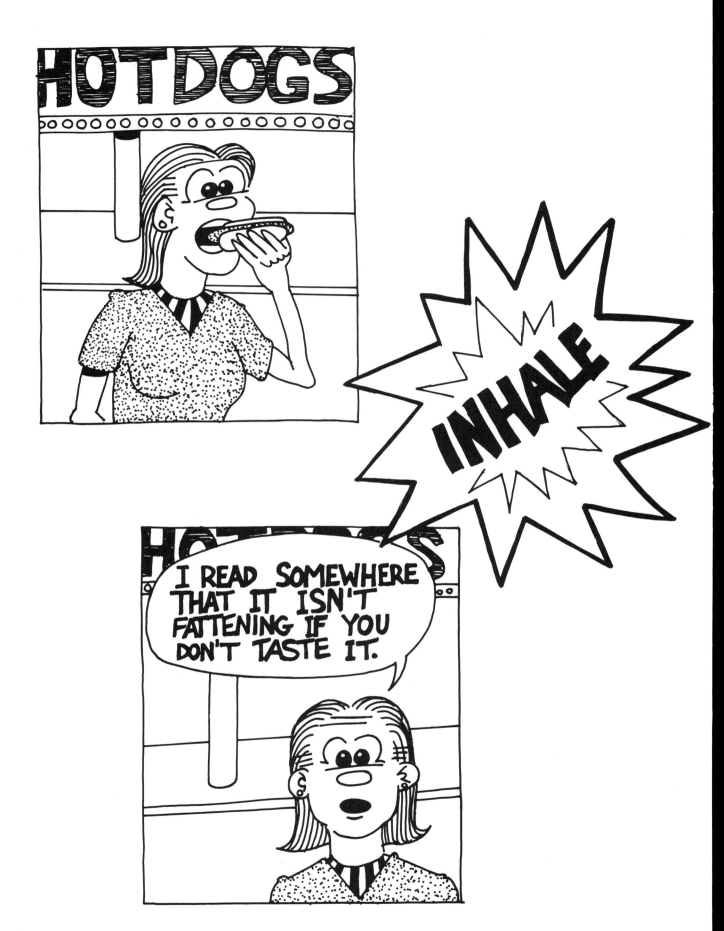

© 1993, *The Balancing Act Nutrition and Weight Guide*, G. Kostas, M.P.H., R.D., Dallas, Texas

OPTION V

MIX-AND-MATCH P-C-F MEALS

This system allows you to choose well-balanced, low-fat, high-fiber P-C-F meals very easily. Combine any of the following breakfast, lunch, or supper meals and you'll consume your desired 1000-1500 calories/day, and 20-30 grams fat per 1000 calories. Most meals are conveniently "assembled" with little or no cooking.

Our recommendations for weight loss:

WOMEN: Eat 1000-1200 calories a day and 20-30 grams fat as:

                  Breakfast: 250-300 calories, 0-5 gms fat
                  Lunch: 300-400 calories, 5-10 gms fat
                  Supper: 450-500 calories, 10-15 gms fat

MEN: Eat 1500-1800 calories a day and 30-60 grams fat as:

                  Breakfast: 300-400 calories, 0-10 gms fat
                  Lunch: 600-700 calories, 10-25 gms fat
                  Supper: 600-700 calories, 10-25 gms fat

For weight maintenance, we recommend:

WOMEN: Eat 1500-1800 calories, 30-60 grams fat

                  Breakfast: 300 calories, 0-5 grams fat
                  Lunch: 600-700 calories, 10-25 grams fat
                  Supper: 600-700 calories, 10-25 grams fat

                  Snack: 100 calories, 0-5 grams fat

MEN: Eat 2000-2500 calories, 50-75 grams fat

                  Breakfast: 500 calories, 0-10 grams fat
                  Lunch: 700-900 calories, 15-30 grams fat
                  Supper: 700-900 calories, 15-30 grams fat
                  Snack: 200 calories, 0-10 grams fat

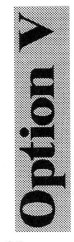

MIX-AND-MATCH P-C-F MEALS
Quick and Easy Breakfast Ideas
(200 - 300 Calories) (≤ 10 grams Fat)

Healthy breakfast meals include fruit, wholegrains, and protein (milk or meat) for the P-C-F balance. Note: meals with the same food groups tend to have the same number of calories and fat.

C = Complex Carbohydrate		P = Protein		F = Fat (in grams)		Cal = Calories	
tsp = teaspoon	Tbsp = tablespoon		c = cup	tr = trace amount		red = reduced	

FOOD GROUP

		Cal.	Fat		Cal.	Fat		Cal.	Fat
Fruit (C)	2 Tbsp raisins	60		1/2 banana	60		3/4 c blueberries	60	
Starch (C)	2/3 c bran flakes	80	tr	3/4 c oat flakes	80	1	1/2 c shredded wheat	80	tr
Milk (P,C,F)	1 c skim milk	90	tr	3/4 c 2% milk	90	4	1/2 c whole milk	75	4
		___	___		___	___		___	___
TOTALS		230	tr		230	5		215	4
Fruit (C)	1/2 cup applesauce	60		1/3 cantaloupe	60		1 1/4 c strawberries	60	
Starch (C)	1/2 wholewheat tortilla topped with	80	1	1/2 whole-wheat pita pocket	80	tr	3 Tbsp grapenuts	80	tr
Milk (P,C) or **Meat** (P,F)	1/4 c part-skim ricotta cheese	90	5	1/2 c low-fat cottage cheese	80	2	1 c nonfat yogurt	90	tr
Fat (F)	(put fruit and cinnamon over cheese;broil)			3 tsp diet margarine	50	5	1 Tbsp chopped nuts	50	5
		___	___		___	___		___	___
TOTALS		230	6		270	7		280	5
2 Fruit (C)	1 cup fruit salad	120		1/2 banana + 1 1/4 c strawberries	60 60		1 banana	120	
Starch (C)	1 small baked potato	80	tr	4 rye crackers*	80	1	2 slices red.-cal. wholewheat bread	80	tr
Milk (P,C) or **Meat** (P,F)	1 ounce (3 Tbsp) mozzarella cheese, grated	80	5	1 c skim milk (Blend fruit and milk as shake)	90	tr	1 Tbsp peanut butter	100	8
		___	___		___	___		___	___
TOTALS		280	5		290	1		300	8
Fruit (C)	1/2 c orange juice	60		1 apple	60		1 orange	60	
Starch (C)	1 wholewheat toast	80	1	4 wholewheat crackers	80	1	1/2 c oatmeal	80	tr
Milk (P,C) or **Meat** (P,F)	1 egg, poached/boiled	80	5	1 ounce mozzarella cheese	80	5	1 cup skim milk	90	tr
Fat (F)	1 tsp margarine or 1 Tbsp jam	45	5				1 tsp margarine or 2 tsp sugar	45	5
		___	___		___	___		___	___
TOTALS		265	11		220	6		275	5

FOOD GROUP		Cal.	Fat		Cal.	Fat		Cal.	Fat
Fruit (C)	1/2 grapefruit	60		6 oz. tomato juice	35		1 pear	60	
Starch (C)	1/2 bagel	80		1/2 English muffin	80	tr	1 corn tortilla	80	1
Meat (P,F)	1 ounce turkey	50	1	1 ounce lean ham	50	2	1 ounce red.-fat cheese,* grated, melted	80	5
Fat (F)	1 Tbsp Neufchatel cheese	40	3	1 tsp margarine (or 1 oz. low-fat cheese)	45	5			
TOTALS		230	4		210	7		220	6
Fruit (C)	1 small pear	60		1 medium peach	60		1 small apple	60	
2 Starch (C)	1 c dry Chex cereal mix (rice, wheat, corn, bran chex, shredded wheat, pretzels)	160	1	1 c canned vegetable soup	80	2	1 wholewheat English muffin or 1 bagel	160	1
				5 melba toast	80	2	1 wedge Laughing Cow cheese	50	3
Milk (P,C) or Meat (P,F)	1 oz. wedge red.-cal. Laughing Cow cheese	50	2	1 c skim milk	90	tr			
TOTALS		270	3		310	4		270	4
Fruit (C)	1/8 honeydew	60		1 orange	60		1/3 cup pineapple	60	
Starch (C)	1/2 English muffin	80	tr	1 wholewheat toast	80	1	1 wholewheat toast	80	1
Meat (P,F)	1 egg, poached	80	5	1 egg (or egg substitute) blended with	80	5	1 oz. red.-fat Kraft cheddar cheese	80	5
	1 oz. low-fat cheese*	40	3	1/4 c low-fat cottage cheese	40	1	1 oz. Canadian Bacon	40	2
	(Open-faced sandwich)			(Omelet, cooked with nonstick spray)					
TOTALS		260	8		260	7		260	8
Fruit (C)	1 c grapes	60		1/2 grapefruit	60		1/2 c orange juice	60	
Starch (C)	2 slices red.-cal. wholewheat bread	80	tr	1/2 wholewheat English muffin	80	tr	2 red.-cal. wholewheat bread	80	tr
2 Meat (P,F) 1/2 Fat (F)	1 oz. low-fat cheese*	35	2	2 oz. Canadian Bacon	80	4	2 oz. hamburger patty, broiled	160	10
	1 oz. lean ham (grill or broil)	50	1	1/2 Tbsp red.-cal. margarine	25	2	tomato, lettuce, mustard	0	
TOTALS		225	4		245	6		300	10

*NOTE: **Nonfat** cheeses (fat-free) refer to Kraft Free slices, etc.

Low-fat cheeses (fat-free) ($\leq$ 3 gm. fat per oz.) refer to Weight Watcher's slices, Laughing Cow red.-cal. wedges, etc.

Reduced-fat cheeses ($\leq$ 5 gm. fat per 1 oz.) refer to part-skim mozzarella, Parmesan, Kraft reduced-fat Cheddar or Swiss, etc., Weight Watcher's Natural cheeses, etc.

Reduced-calorie refers to 35-40 calories per slice bread and 50 calories per tablespoon margarine or mayonnaise.

Quick and Easy Brown-Bag Lunches
(300-500 Calories) (≤ 13 grams Fat)

C = Complex Carbohydrate	P = Protein	F = Fat (in grams)	Cal = Calories
tsp = teaspoon Tbsp = tablespoon	c = cup	tr = trace amount	red = reduced

SANDWICHES

	Cal.	Fat		Cal.	Fat
2 slices wholewheat bread (C)	160	tr	2 slices red.-cal. wholewheat bread (C)	80	tr
1/2 c tuna in water (P,F)	70	2	2 oz. chicken, turkey or lean beef (P,F)	100	2
3 tsp diet mayonnaise (F)	45	5	1 tsp mayonnaise (F)	45	5
lettuce, pickle	0		lettuce, tomato slices	0	
1 large apple or			1 small orange (C)	60	
8 ounces apple juice (C)	120		25 stick pretzels (C)	80	tr
TOTALS	**395**	**7**	**TOTALS**	**365**	**7**

	Cal.	Fat		Cal.	Fat
2 slices red.-cal. wholewheat bread (C)	80	tr	1 wholewheat pita pocket (C)	160	1
1 Tbsp peanut butter (P,F)	100	8	1 c vegetables, cooked (C)	50	
1 banana (C)	120		1 oz grated mozzarella cheese (P,F)	80	5
1 c skim milk (P,C)	90		1 peach (C)	60	
TOTALS	**390**	**8**	**TOTALS**	**350**	**6**

	Cal.	Fat		Cal.	Fat
2 slices wholewheat bread (C)	160	2	fast food hamburger (P,C,F)	350	10
2 oz. lean ham (P,F)	100	4	(1/4 pound meat, no mayonnaise)		
1 Tbsp fat-free mayonnaise (F)	15		1 small apple (from home) (C)	60	0
lettuce	0		water		0
carrot sticks (C)	25				
1 small pear (C)	60				
TOTALS	**360**	**6**	**TOTALS**	**410**	**10**

COLD SALADS

Pasta Salad:	Cal.	Fat	Fruit Salad:	Cal.	Fat
1/2 c spaghetti (C)	80		1/2 c low-fat cottage cheese (P,F)	100	2
1 c raw vegetables (C)	25		1/3 c pineapple chunks (C)	60	
1 ounce grated mozzarella cheese (P,F)	80	5	3/4 c strawberries (C)	30	
3 Tbsp nonfat Italian dressing* (F)	25		1/2 banana, sliced (C)	60	
1 fresh fruit (C)	60		topping: 3 Tbsp grapenuts (C)	80	
TOTALS	**270**	**5**	**TOTALS**	**330**	**2**

Rice-Vegetables Salad:	Cal.	Fat	Chef Salad:	Cal.	Fat
2/3 c cooked rice (C)	160		2 c mixed salad greens (C)	20	
1 c raw vegetables (C)	25		1 tomato	25	
1 ounce cooked chicken (P,F)	50	1	2 oz. turkey ham (P,F)	100	2
3 tsp red.-cal. mayonnaise	45	5	1/2 c low-fat cottage cheese (P,F)	80	2
1 fresh fruit (C)	60		2 Tbsp red.-cal. dressing (F)	45	5
			4 rye crisps (C)	80	tr
TOTALS	340	6	TOTALS	350	9

OTHERS

	Cal.	Fat		Cal.	Fat
1 c plain skim milk yogurt (P,C)	90		Salad (C)	25	
1 1/4 c fresh strawberries (C)	60		1 Tbsp salad dressing (F)	80	6
4 graham crackers or			1 medium baked potato (C)	160	
8 wholewheat crackers (C)	160	1	1oz. (3 Tbsp) mozzarella cheese (P,F)	80	5
TOTALS	310	1	TOTALS	345	11

	Cal.	Fat		Cal.	Fat
1 c minestrone soup (C,F)	80	2	Low-calorie frozen meal ($\leq$ 300 cal,	300	9
6 wholewheat crackers* (C,F)	120	1	$\leq$ 10 gm fat) (such as Lean Cuisine,		
1 ounce low-fat cheese (P,F)	50	3	Weight Watchers, etc.) (P,C,F)		
12 grapes (C)	60		1 fruit (C)	60	
TOTALS	310	6	TOTALS	360	9

	Cal.	Fat
1/2 ounce box raisins (4 tablespoons) (C)	120	
5 graham crackers or 1 c dry cereal mix (shredded wheat, bran, rice, corn chex, pretzels) (C)	160	4
1 c skim milk (P,C)	90	
TOTALS	370	4

OTHER IDEAS

1. Pick up sandwich at local deli at lunch or before work (some deli's are in grocery stores). Add fresh fruit from home.
2. Pack leftovers.
3. Keep supply of soup, frozen meals, cheese and crackers, peanut butter, fruit and juice at work.
4. See breakfast and supper ideas.
5. Choose salad, potato, soup bars at local grocery store deli's.

*NOTE: **Nonfat** cheeses (fat-free) refer to Kraft Free slices, etc.

Low-fat cheeses ($\leq$ 3 gm. fat per oz.) refer to Weight Watcher's slices, Laughing Cow red.-cal. wedges, etc.

Reduced-fat cheeses ($\leq$ 5 gm. fat per 1 oz.) refer to part-skim mozzarella, Parmesan, Kraft red.-fat Cheddar, Swiss, etc., Weight Watcher's Natural cheeses, etc.

Reduced-calorie refers to 35-40 calories per slice bread and 50 calories per tablespoon margarine or mayonnaise.

Nonfat salad dressings ("fat-free" or "no oil") contain 5-20 calories per tablespoon.

Quick and Easy Supper Ideas
(250-500 Calories, ≤ 15 grams Fat)

C = Complex Carbohydrate	P = Protein		F = Fat (in grams)	Cal = Calories
tsp = teaspoon Tbsp = tablespoon	c = cup		tr = trace amount	red = reduced

MINI PIZZA and FRUIT

	Cal.	Fat
2 oz. Canadian Bacon (P,F)	80	4
1 oz. (3 Tbsp) mozzarella (P,F)	80	5
1/2 c raw mushrooms (C)	15	
1/2 c tomato sauce* (C) on	35	
2 pita pocket halves, or 2 tortillas or		
2 English muffin halves (C)	160	
1 large fruit (C)	120	
TOTALS	**490**	**9**

STUFFED VEGETABLES, FRUIT, BREAD

	Cal.	Fat
Fill and bake tomato, green pepper,		
squash, or eggplant (C)	25	
with 2 oz. lean ground turkey,	100	2
cooked and added to		
1/3 c cooked rice (C) and	80	
1/2 c chopped onions and green	25	
peppers in 1/2 c tomato sauce (C)	35	0
1 fruit (C)	60	
1 wholewheat dinner roll (C)	80	1
TOTALS	**405**	**3**

CHALUPA OR TACO

	Cal.	Fat
1 corn tortilla (C)	80	1
2 ounces lean ground beef, drained (P,F)	160	10
1 ounce (3 Tbsp) low-fat cheddar* (P,F)	40	3
1/2 c diced tomato, 2 Tbsp chopped onion (C)	25	
lettuce, pepper, picante sauce	0	
1 c skim milk (P,C)	90	
1 1/4 c strawberries (C)	60	0
TOTALS	**455**	**14**

BAKED POTATO, SALAD AND FRUIT

	Cal.	Fat
1 medium potato (C) with	160	tr
1 oz. (3 Tbsp) red.-fat cheddar		
cheese (P,F)	80	5
Tossed salad with raw vegetables (C)	25	
with 1 Tbsp French dressing (F)	60	6
1 1/4 c watermelon	60	
TOTALS	**385**	**11**

SOUP, SALAD AND FRUIT

	Cal.	Fat
1 c vegetable soup (C)	80	2
Tossed salad with raw vegetables (C) with	25	
2 Tbsp red.-cal. Italian dressing* (F) and	45	5
1 ounce grated Parmesan cheese (P,F)	80	5
1 slice French bread (C)	80	5
1/2 c fruit salad (C)	60	
TOTALS	**370**	**12**

SOUP, SANDWICH AND FRUIT

	Cal.	Fat
1 c chicken noodle soup (C)	80	2
2 slices wholewheat bread(C)	160	2
3 ounces lean meat (P,F)	160	10
mustard, lettuce, tomato	0	
1 small pear or apple	60	
TOTALS	**460**	**4**

CHEESE TOAST, FRUIT SALAD

	Cal.	Fat
1 slice wholewheat toast (C)	80	1
1 oz. red.-cal. Laughing Cow cheese	50	3
1 c fruit salad (C)	120	
1 c V-8 juice (C)	50	
TOTALS	**300**	**4**

COLD PLATE

	Cal.	Fat
1 c raw vegetables (C)	25	
with 1/2 c nonfat plain yogurt (P,C)	45	
dip mixed with herbs and spices	0	
2 oz. red.-fat Swiss cheese* (P,F)	160	10
8 wholewheat crackers (C)	160	2
1 c grapes (C)	60	
TOTALS	**450**	**12**

CHICKEN & RICE DINNER

	Cal.	Fat
3 oz. chicken breast (no skin) or fish (P,F),	150	3
seasoned with 2 Tbsp red.-calorie Italian		
dressing* (F) and grilled or baked	45	5
1/2 c steamed spinach, etc. (C)	25	
1/2 c steamed carrots, etc. (C)	25	
2/3 c brown or wild rice (C)	160	
1/3 cantaloupe (C)	60	
TOTALS	**465**	**8**

TACO SALAD AND FRUIT

	Cal.	Fat
Lettuce	0	
1/2 tomato or 1 small, sliced	25	
2 oz. lean ground turkey or chicken	100	3
(P,F) cooked in 1/2 c picante sauce (C)	0	
2/3 c pinto or kidney beans (P,C)	160	
with optional chili powder added		
1 oz. grated low-fat cheese* (P,C)	40	3
1 1/4 c strawberries (C)	60	
TOTALS	**465**	**6**

STEAMED VEGETABLES W/RICE

	Cal.	Fat
2 c mixed steamed vegetables (C)	100	
1 c rice (C)	240	tr
1 c plain nonfat yogurt (P,C)	90	tr
and 1/2 c mixed fruit (C)	60	
(Optional sugar substitute)		
TOTALS	**490**	**tr**

TUNA-NOODLE CASSEROLE

Mix and heat until cheese melts:

	Cal.	Fat
3 oz. water-packed tuna (P,F)	105	3
1 c cooked noodles (C)	160	tr
1 c steamed carrots (C)	50	
1 oz. grated red.-fat cheese* (P,F)	80	5
1/4 c skim milk (P,C)	25	tr
1 small apple (C)	60	
TOTALS	**455**	**8**

BEEF DINNER

	Cal.	Fat
3 oz. beef tenderloin (P,F)	170	8
Corn on cob (6" long) (C)	80	tr
Tossed lettuce with raw vegetables (C)	25	
with 1 Tbsp fat-free dressing (C)	15	
1/2 c steamed green beans with mushrooms (C)	25	
2 tsp red.-cal. margarine (F)	30	3
TOTALS	**345**	**11**

SPAGHETTI

	Cal.	Fat
1 c spaghetti (C), topped with	160	tr
1/2 c meatless spaghetti sauce (C,F) and	80	2
2 Tbsp grated parmesan cheese	50	4
Fresh spinach salad (C)	20	
with 2 Tbsp fat-free Italian dressing (C)	30	
1 slice Italian bread (C)	80	
1 c skim milk (P,C)	90	tr
TOTALS	**510**	**6**

STIR-FRY

	Cal.	Fat
2 c frozen vegetables (C)	100	
(Japanese style) cooked in		
1 tsp canola oil (F) with	45	5
3 oz. skinless chicken breast, sliced (P,F)	150	3
1/2 c linguini (C)	80	tr
1/2 c fresh fruit salad (C)	60	
TOTALS	**435**	**8**

HAM DINNER

	Cal.	Fat
3 oz. lean ham (P,F)	150	7
Small baked sweet potato (C)	90	tr
1 c broccoli/cauliflower, steamed (C)	50	
2 tsp red.-cal. margarine (F)	30	3
1 c pineapple/orange fruit mix (C)	120	
TOTALS	**440**	**10**

FROZEN DINNER

	Cal.	Fat
Low-cal. frozen meal (P,C,F)	300	10
(≤ 300 calories, ≤ 10 gm fat)		
(Lean Cuisine, Healthy Choice, etc.)		
1 c steamed vegetables (fresh or frozen) (C)	50	
1 c fresh fruit salad (C)	120	
TOTALS	**470**	**10**

TUNA MELT SANDWICH

	Cal.	Fat
1 wholewheat English muffin (C,F)	160	1
3 oz. water-packed tuna (P,F) mixed	105	3
with 1 Tbsp red.-cal. mayonnaise (F)	45	5
2 Tbsp part-skim grated mozzarella cheese (P,F)	50	4
1 c raw vegetables (C) (carrots, celery, tomato slices)	25	
1/2 banana (C)	60	
TOTALS	**445**	**13**

SHRIMP CREOLE

	Cal.	Fat
Mix & heat: 2/3 c white rice (C)	160	
1 c tomato sauce (C)	70	
steamed celery, onion, seasonings	0	
Add: 2 oz. (10) frozen cooked shrimp (P,F)	90	2
Romaine salad with mushrooms & tomatoes, with	25	
2 Tbsp red.-cal. dressing* (F)	45	5
1 sliced fresh peach	60	
TOTALS	**450**	**7**

VEGETARIAN DINNER

	Cal.	Fat
2/3 c beans (P,C)	160	tr
2/3 c rice (C)	160	
Tossed salad with raw vegetables (C)	25	
with 2 Tbsp red.-cal. dressing* (F)	45	5
1 c cantaloupe (1/4 melon) (C)	60	
TOTALS	**450**	**5**

*NOTE: **Nonfat** cheeses (fat-free) refer to Kraft Free slices, etc.
Low-fat cheeses (≤ 3 gm. fat per oz.) refer to Weight Watcher's slices, Laughing Cow red.-cal. wedges, etc.
Reduced-fat cheeses (≤ 5 gm. fat per 1 oz.) refer to part-skim mozzarella, Parmesan, Kraft red.-fat Cheddar, Swiss, etc., Weight Watcher's Natural cheeses, etc.
Reduced-cal. refers to 35-40 calories per slice bread and 50 calories per tablespoon margarine or mayonnaise.
Nonfat salad dressings ("fat-free" or "no oil") contain 5-20 calories per tablespoon.

III
BE CALORIE-WISE
AND FAT-SMART

NUTRITION FOCUS

1. Compare calories and fat (94-95)
2. Select "Low-Calorie Snacks" (96-97) and "Recipes" (98)
3. Watch out for "Anonymous Calories" and choose "Alternatives." You can have your chocolate and eat it too! (99)
4. When you "Trim Fat - Save Calories!" (100-102)
5. Shop for "Lower-Calorie Foods" (103-109), which generally have less fat
6. Use this condensed Fat Gram Counter as a quick reference guide (108-110)
7. Learn "Shopping Criteria At-A-Glance" to select foods wisely and quickly (p. 111)

HABIT FOCUS

Practice two new habits.

EXERCISE FOCUS

Keep exercising! The more you do, the better you feel.

RECORDS

Keep those records going - they help you progress!

GOALS

HABIT: keep low-calorie snacks and foods available
FOOD: try new low-calorie products, snacks, and recipes
EXERCISE: burn at least 200 calories per day, average
RECORDS: food, exercise, weight - count new low-calorie foods tried

---

CALORIE & FAT COMPARISONS

MEAT AND SUBSTITUTES

	Cal.	Fat (gm)
Chicken (3 oz)		
baked, broiled (w/o bone, skin)	120	3
+ 2 Tbsp barbecue sauce	145	3
fried	220	11
Beef Steak (3 oz)		
Sirloin, flank	180	8
T-bone, porterhouse	180	8
Hamburger, medium fat	250	18
Prime rib	250	17
Brisket	350	27
Fish (3 oz) - cod, trout, snapper, etc.		
baked or broiled	100	2
+ 1 Tbsp butter	200	12
or 1 Tbsp tartar sauce	200	12
fried	200	12

VEGETABLES

	Cal.	Fat (gm)
Potato (1 small, 1/2 medium, or 1/2 c)		
baked or broiled	80	0
+ 1 Tbsp butter (100 cal.)	180	10
+ 1 Tbsp sour cream (30 cal.)	210	13
+ 1 Tbsp grated cheese (30 cal.)	240	16
hash browns (1/2 c)	170	9
French fried (20), small order	220	13
potato chips (25)	250	17
Okra (1/2 c)		
boiled	20	0
fried	200	12
Onions (1)		
boiled	50	0
fried rings (10)	400	26

MISCELLANEOUS

	Cal.	Fat (gm)
Taco (1 medium)	200-300	13
Pizza (1/8 of 12-in. pizza)	150-250	5-10
Chili (1 c)	300-400	22
Soups (1 c)		
broth, bouillon	40	1
broth-based (i.e., chicken noodle)	70	2
creamed	180	7
Coleslaw with mayonnaise (1/2 c)	120	7
Pasta salad	130	6
Tuna salad (1/2 c)	150	12
Potato or macaroni salad (1/2 c)	175	10
Beef stew (1 c)	220	10
Macaroni & cheese (3/4 c)	325	17
Lasagna (1 c)	700	36
Chicken a la King (1 c)	300	20

SANDWICHES

	Meat Only Cal.	Fat	*Sandwich Cal.	Fat
Chicken or turkey (3 oz baked or smoked	150	3	490	25
Bacon (1 oz or 3 strips)	150	12	490	34
Hot dog (1)	150	13	490	35
Chopped ham (3 oz.)	150	8	540	30
Hamburger patty (3 oz)	250	18	565	40
Bologna (3 oz.)	270	24	610	46
Cheese (2 oz. or 2 slices)	200	20	565	44
Tuna (1/2 c)				
in water	100	2	440	24
in oil	225	9	565	31

Made with 2 slices bread + 2 Tbsp mayonnaise which add 340 calories and 22 gms fat. Omit mayo and save 200 calories and 22 gms fat.

SNACKS

	Cal.	Fat (gm)
Peanut butter (1 Tbsp)	90	10
Candy, chocolate (1 oz.)	150	10
Nuts, seeds (1 oz.)	180	10
Chips (1 oz. or 1 small bag)	150	10
Yogurt (8 oz.)		
plain, nonfat	90	0
plain, low-fat	160	5
fruit flavored	250-300	0
fruit flavored, nonfat, sugar-free	100	0

SWEETS, DESSERTS

	Cal.	Fat (gm)
Cookies		
ginger snaps, vanilla wafers (3)	50	1
chocolate chip (2 small)	100	6
creme-filled (2), oreos (2)	100	6
homemade (choc. chip, oatmeal) (1)	100	3
fat-free (oatmeal, fruit, etc.) (3)	75	0
Pound cake (no icing, 3x3x1 1/2 in.)	115	6
Glazed donut (1)	180	11
Sweet roll, tart, pastry (1)	270	15
Cheese cake (3x2x1 1/2 in.)	365	24
Cake with icing (2-layer, 2 3/8 in. arc)	350-500	15-20
Pie (1/8 pie, all types)	300-400	15-20

cal. = calories	oz. = ounce	Tbsp = tablespoon	gm = grams	g = grams	c = cup

FROZEN DESSERTS

	Cal.	Fat (gm)
Ice cream (1/2 c)		
regular	130	7
rich (i.e. Baskin Robbins)	165	9
soft-serve	165	10
very rich (i.e. Hagen Daaz)	300	20
Ice milk, fruit ice, sorbet	100	0
Frozen yogurt	110	2
Sherbet	130	2
Ice cream bar or sandwich (avg.)	160	11
Milkshake (8 oz)	350	10
Hot fudge sundae	650	30

LOWER CALORIE SNACKS and DESSERTS

	Cal.	Fat (gm)
Sugar-free jello (1/2 c)	10	0
Vegetable (1)	25	0
Chocolate low-cal shake or hot cocoa (8 oz; i.e. Alba '77)	70	0
Popsicle, twin pop	70	0
Frozen fruit bar	70	0
Jello (1/2 c) or low-fat pudding (1/2 c)	70	0
Popcorn (3 c) popped without fat or microwave "light"	80	1
Pretzels (38) (or 3/4 oz)	80	1
Fruit (1 medium)	80	0
Shredded wheat (1/2 c)	90	0
Angel food cake, sponge cake (1/12 of cake or 1 1/2-in. arc)	110	0
Milkshake (8 oz skim milk + 1/2 c unsweetened fruit)	120	0

CEREALS (1/2 CUP)

	Cal.	Fat (gm)
Puffed wheat	25	0
Corn flakes	50	0
Shredded wheat, bran flakes	90	0
Grapenuts	210	0
Granola	250-300	12
low-fat	175-210	3
Granola Bar	235	8
low-fat	80-110	2

SAUCES (1 TABLESPOON)

	Cal.	Fat (gm)
Au Jus, Tabasco, hot sauce, steak sauce, picante, salsa	0	0
Barbecue, catsup, mustard, teriyaki, soy, Worcestershire, sweet and sour	10-15	0
Tartar	95	9
Fat-free tartar	16	0

SAUCES (1/4 CUP)

	Cal.	Fat (gm)
Tomato	25	0
Light tomato spaghetti sauce	25-45	0-2
Spaghetti (meat-free)	35-50	1
Barbecue, catsup	50	1
Brown gravy (mix)	30	2
Brown gravy mix (nonfat)	25	0
Brown gravy (homemade)	165	14
Cheese	125	10
Hollandaise	260	28

DIPS (1/4 CUP)

	Cal.	Fat (gm)
Fat-free commercial dips	60	0
Bean Dip	80	4
Onion Dip	100	8
Guacamole	115	10
Cheese Dip	125	10

SALAD DRESSINGS (1 TABLESPOON)

	Cal.	Fat (gm)
Vinegar, lemon, hot sauce, picante	0	0
Fat-free dressings	6	0
Reduced-cal dressings, all types	15-40	2-4
Ranch, French	55	6
Bleu Cheese, roquefort, Italian, Russian, Caesar, oil & vinegar, etc.	70-80	8-9
Nonfat mayonnaise	12	0
Reduced-fat mayonnaise	50	5
Mayonnaise	100	10

CONDIMENTS (1 TABLESPOON)

	Cal.	Fat (gm)
Low-calorie jelly, etc.	8-25	0
Lite syrup	30	0
Sugar, honey, syrup	50	0
Jelly, jam, marmalade, spreadable fruit	55	0
Reduced-fat margarine	50	5
Whipped butter or margarine	85	8
Butter or margarine	100	10
Skim milk	5	0
Non-dairy creamer, powder	30	2
Non-dairy creamer, liquid	20	1
Half and half	20	2
Fat-free, plain yogurt	6	0
Sour cream	30	3
Nonfat sour cream	15	0

BEVERAGES (8 OUNCES)

	Cal.	Fat (gm)
Water, mineral water, tea, coffee, club soda, diet drinks, Kool-aid without sugar	0	0
Ginger ale	50	0
Soft drinks, punch	100	0
Tomato, V-8 juice	50	0
Orange, grapefruit juice	100	0
Grape, prune juice	200	0
Skim milk (1/2% fat)	80	1
Low-fat milk (2% fat)	120	5
Whole milk (4% fat)	150	10
Carnation Instant Breakfast (w/ skim milk)	220	1
Sugar-free Carnation Instant Breakfast	160	1

ALCOHOL

	Cal.	Fat (gm)
Beer (12 oz)		
lite	100	0
regular	150	0
Wine, champagne (4 oz)	100	0
Gin, rum, vodka, etc. (1 1/2 oz)	100	0
Martini, daiquiri (4 oz)	200	0
Margarita	450	0
Non-alcoholic beer (12 oz)	70	0
Non-alcoholic wine (8 oz)	70	0

LOW-CALORIE SNACKS

If you are truly hungry, eat a snack now to prevent binging later. Eat calorie-free snacks in limitless quantities. If the snacks you choose do contain calories, eat a smaller entre at your next meal. Or, plan a daily snack as part of your daily eating. A planned snack prevents you from feeling "deprived", hungry, or unnecessarily "guilty".

WHEN CHOOSING A SNACK, REMEMBER THESE POINTERS:

1. Keep low-calorie snacks on hand. Clean and prepare raw vegetables and fruits immediately after purchase. Have them handy in the regrigerator for those quick food "snack attacks".

2. Liquids can fill an "empty feeling" quickly ... especially warm beverages sipped slowly. Try water, diet drinks, clear soup, tea, coffee.

3. Foods high in water and/or fiber content are lowest in calories, (i.e., popcorn, fruit, raw vegetables, shredded wheat, baked potato).

4. The more crunchy and chewable the snack, the more satisfying it is.

5. Make a snack attractive - something colorful or served in an attractive manner: a salad with lettuce, red cabbage, tomato, carrots, yellow squash, etc.; or a drink in a beautiful glass; or fruit or vegetable in a pretty sherbet dish.

6. Choose snacks that require preparation (i.e. popcorn) or are slow to eat (i.e., raw fruits and vegetables, sliced).

7. Pause 10 minutes before snacking. Chances are, a delay can ward off a binge. Drink a tall glass of water before a snack. You'll eat less!

See "Snack Ideas" on pages 97-98.

FREEBIES (No Calories)

refreshing water!
unsweetened tea, coffee
sugar-free soft drinks
lemonade with sugar substitute
sugar-free gelatin made with sugar-free
  soda for "tangy" taste
unflavored gelatin
bouillon, broth
club soda
Perrier water
herb teas
fresh cranberries

sour or dill pickles
cucumbers, radishes
lettuce, watercress
celery, rhubarb
Tabasco
hot sauce
Worcestershire sauce
soy sauce
steak sauce
herbs, spices
lemon, lime
vinegar

60 OR LESS CALORIES (No Fat)

1 small fruit-apple, orange, etc	40	1/2 c orange juice	60
1 c cooked non-starchy vegetables	50	1/2 c tomato, V-8 juice	35
2 c raw non-starchy vegetables,		1 carrot	25
i.e. broccoli stalks, cauliflowerettes	50	1 small tomato	25
1/2 banana (may freeze)	60	1 small green salad with 1 Tbsp	
1/4 cantaloupe, 1/2 grapefruit	60	fat-free dressing	20
1 1/4 c strawberries, 10 cherries	60	1 rice cake	35
1/2 c sugar-free canned or frozen fruit	50	1 slice low-calorie bread	35
1 small baked apple, with cinnamon	60	1 bread stick	40
1/2 c applesauce, without sugar	50	4 pieces melba toast	40
1 package low-cal dried fruit snack,		3 wheat crackers	45
apple, cinnamon, strawberry	40	1 c puffed wheat	40
1 slice, 3/4 oz, fat-free cheese	40	6 mini fat-free cookies	60
1/2 oz (2 Tbsp) regular cheese* or	50	1 c onion soup	35
1 oz (1 wedge), skim gruyere cheese*	50	1 c egg drop soup	30
1 oz part-skim ricotta cheese*	40	4 oz ginger ale	40

*All snacks are fat-free, except cheeses marked, which contain 2-5 gms. fat.

100 OR LESS CALORIES (No Fat)

1 c skim milk	90	1 1/2 oz box raisins	100
1/2 c nonfat cottage cheese	80	1/2 c gelatin or low-cal pudding	70
(add seasonings and use as spread)		1 small slice angel food cake	
1/2 c nonfat plain yogurt		(1 1/2 inch arc)	110
(add seasonings and use as dip)	100	1 c homemade or canned soup	70-90
1 oz mozzarella cheese*	80	1 packet low-cal hot cocoa mix	50-70
3 c unbuttered popcorn	75	1 packet low-cal milkshake mix -	
1 shredded wheat biscuit (or 2/3 c)	90	(vanilla, strawberry, chocolate)	70
2 c puffed wheat or rice	80	1 popsicle, twin pop, frozen fruit bar	70
3 graham crackers (2 in. square each)	80	1/2 c fat-free ice milk or fruit ice	100
38 pretzel sticks (3 1/8 in. long)	80	1/2 c fat-free frozen yogurt	100

*All snacks are virtually fat-free, except mozzarella, with 5 gms. fat.

LOW-CALORIE SNACK RECIPES

1. Hot cocoa: mix: 1 cup skim milk, sugar substitute and 1 tablespoon cocoa powder = 1 milk serving = 110 calories, 0 fat

2. Chocolate milkshake: blend together in blender: 1 cup skim milk, 1 tablespoon cocoa powder, sugar substitute, crushed ice, = 1 milk serving = 110 calories, 0 fat

3. Fruit flavored milkshake: blend in blender: 1/2 cup unsweetened fruit, sugar substitute (as desired), 1 cup skim milk, (crushed ice), flavor extract (such as rum, almond, vanilla, walnut, etc.) = 1 milk + 1 fruit = 150 calories, 0 fat

4. Fruit yogurt: 1/2 cup commercial nonfat plain yogurt + 1 serving fruit = 1 milk + 1 fruit = 150 calories, 0 fat

5. Homemade custard: mix together: 1 egg (beaten), 1 cup skim milk, pinch of salt, 1 package of sugar substitute, 1/4 teasoon vanilla extract. Pour into 2 custard cups and sprinkle with nutmeg. Set cups in pan of water and bake at 350 degrees for 45 minutes. Other flavors such as almond, lemon or orange may be used in place of vanilla. One serving (1 custard cup) = 1 milk serving = 90 calories, 0 fat

6. Marinated vegetables with wine vinegar.

7. Fat-free plain yogurt with cinnamon, vanilla extract and sugar substitute (can freeze).

8. Homemade vegetable soup made with V-8 juice.

9. Sugar-free carbonated drink or herb tea served in chilled crystal goblet.

10. Milkshake: skim milk, cinnamon, almond extract, crushed ice.

11. Add herbed vinegar (i.e. tarragon vinegar) or wine vinegar to vegetables or salads.

12. Fat-free, sugar-free yogurt, 100 calories for 8 ounces.

13. Apple pie spice added to oatmeal.

14. Colorful fresh fruit salad.

15. Baking tip: If a recipe calls for 12 muffins (or cookies, etc.), use smaller tins and make 24, for half the calories! Also, decrease the sugar by 1/4 cup - no one will notice the difference in taste ... only in calories.

16. Hot Spiced Tea: 4 cups water, 1 cinnamon stick, 1 whole clove, 1 strip lemon peel (4 inches long), 1 strip orange peel (6 inches long), dash nutmeg, 3 or 4 tea bags.

       Method: In saucepan, combine all ingredients except tea. Simmer 5-10 minutes. Add tea bags and steep to taste. Serve hot or chill for iced tea.

ANONYMOUS CALORIES

THESE ADD UP FAST!!!

CHOCOLATE	Cal.	Fat (gm)	FROZEN DESSERTS	Cal.	Fat (gm)
Chocolate chips, 1 oz	150	8	Frozen yogurt, 1/2 c	120	3
Chocolate kisses, 6 pieces	150	10	Weight Watcher's English Toffee Bar	120	8
Chocolate fudge, 1 oz	150	10	Sherbet, 1/2 c	130	3
Brownie, 1 small	150	6	Soft serve ice cream, 1/2 c	180	6
Cream filled chocolate cookies, 3	150	6	Ice cream sandwich	170	8
Chocolate pudding, 1/2 c	150	6	Sugar-free ice cream sandwich	180	6
Chocolate icing, 2 Tbsp	170	7	Chocolate coated ice cream bar	175	10
Chocolate coated ice cream bar	175	6	Sugar-free chocolated-coated ice cream bar	150	11
Chocolate cupcake with icing	175	6			
Chocolate cookies, 2	180	7	Cholesterol-free chocolate-coated ice cream bar	130	7
Chocolate milk, 1 c	230	10			
M & M's, plain, 1.7 oz package	240	10	Tofutti, 1/2 c	220	1-12
Chocolate bar, 2 oz	300	15	Ice cream, 1/2 c	165-300	7-14
Chocolate ice cream 1/2 c	165-300	10-20	Very rich specialty ice cream, 1/2 c	300	8
Chocolate cake with icing, 1 slice	425	21			

ALTERNATIVES

THESE ADD UP MORE SLOWLY!!

CHOCOLATE	Cal.	Fat (gm)	FROZEN DESSERTS	Cal.	Fat (gm)
Ande's chocolate mint, 1	25	1	Popsicle, sugar-free (2-bar)	15-35	0
Tootsie roll (2 1/2" x 3/8")	30	1	Popsicle, 2-bar	70	0
Estee's milk chocolate candy bar (2 squares)	60	5	Creamsickle, sugar-free	25	1
Chocolate teddy graham cracker, 11	60	2	Weight Watcher's Double Fudge bar	35	0
Snackwell's Devil's Food cake cookie	50	0	Sugar-free Fudgesicle	35	1
Snackwell's Double Fudge cookie	50	1	Fudgsicle	70	1
Snackwell's Chocolate sandwich cookie	50	1	Weight Watcher's Chocolate Mousse bar	70	1
Low-calorie hot cocoa, 1 c	50	0	Dole frozen fruit bar	70	0
Alba chocolate milkshake	70	0	Weight Watcher's chocolate fat-free frozen dessert, 1/2 c	80	0
Pepperidge Farm Bordeaux cookies, 2	70	4			
Chocolate "snap" cookies, 4	100	3	Jello chocolate pudding pop, 1	80	2
Lovin' Lite Chocolate brownie	100	2	Blue Bell Chocolate fat-free fudge bar	80	0
Weight Watcher's brownie	100	3	Blue Bell Chocolate fat-free frozen dessert, 1/2 c	80	0
Entenmann's Fudge Brownie, fat-free	110	0			
Weight Watcher's Chocolate eclair	120	4	Weight Watcher's Chocolate Treat Bar	100	1
Hostess Lite Cupcake (1.5 oz)	130	2	Fat-free frozen yogurt, 1/2 c	100	0
Entenmann's Chocolate Loaf cake, 1 oz	70	0	Fruit ice, 1/2 c	100	0
Nabisco's Devil's Food cake, 1	70	1	Fruit sorbet, 1/2 c	100	0
Chocolate fat-free pudding snack pack, (Jello, Hunt's, Hershey's), 1/2 c	100	0	Ice milk, 1/2 c	100	3
			Diet Ice Cream, 1/2 c	100	0
Chocolate syrup, 1 Tbsp.	50	2	Haagen Daas Frozen Yogurt bar	100	1
Fudge topping, 1 Tbsp	60	2	Klondike Lite Ice Cream Sandwich	100	2
Smucker's Light Fudge Topping, 1 Tbsp	35	0	McDonald's fat-free frozen yogurt	100	0
Braum's Light Fudge Topping, 1 Tbsp	35	0			

TRIM FAT - SAVE CALORIES!

INSTEAD OF THIS ...			SUBSTITUTE ...			SAVE	
	Cal.	Fat (g)		Cal.	Fat (g)	Cal.	Fat (g)
whole milk, 8 oz	160	8	skim milk, 8 oz	90	0	70	8
sour cream, 4 oz	240	24	nonfat yogurt, 4 oz	60	0	180	24
rich ice cream, 1 c	300	20	nonfat ice milk, 1 c	200	0	100	20
ham, 2 oz	100	5	turkey breast, 2 oz	70	2	30	3
croissant, 1 large	300	15	English muffin	140	1	160	14
party crackers, 4	80	4	rye wafers, 2 triple	40	0	40	4
butter or margarine, 1 Tbsp	100	12	Parmesan cheese, 1 Tbsp	25	2	75	10
chocolate bar, 1 1/2 oz	240	15	granola bar, 1	130	4	110	11
chocolate chip cookie, 1	50	2	gingersnap, 1	15	0	25	2
yellow cake with icing, 1/12 cake	450	18	angel food cake, 1/12 cake	120	0	330	18
danish pastry	275	15	bran muffin, medium	160	5	115	10
apple pie, 1/6 of 9" pie	400	18	baked apple with 1 Tbsp nuts, raisins	155	4	245	14
peanuts, 1 c	840	72	popcorn, 1 c dry	30	0	810	72
potato chips, 1 oz (15 chips)	150	10	pretzels, 8 triple-ring (medium)	100	1	50	9
peanut butter, 2 Tbsp	190	16	low-fat ricotta cheese, 2 Tbsp	40	3	150	13

INSTEAD OF THIS ...	Cal.	Fat (gm)
Breakfast		
orange juice, 6 oz	90	0
1 egg, fried	110	10
toast, 1 slice	80	0
butter, 1 pat	35	4
jam, 1 Tbsp	55	0
coffee	0	0
half 'n half, 1 Tbsp	20	2
	380	16
Lunch		
chef salad -		
lettuce, 1 c	10	0
avocado, 1/6	70	7
tomato, 1/2 medium	20	0
roast beef, 2 oz	130	6
cheddar cheese, 2 oz	230	20
black olives, 3	30	3
dressing, 2 Tbsp	160	18
crackers, 6 rounds	110	6
chocolate chip cookies, 2	100	4
iced tea with lemon	0	0
TOTALS	860	64
Dinner		
Prime Rib, 4 oz	400	36
green beans		
with cheese sauce, 2 Tbsp	60	5
cornbread, 2 1/2" x 2 1/2" square	190	5
butter, 1 pat	35	4
cake with icing, 1/12th cake	350	15
beer, 12 oz	150	0
	1,185	65
TOTALS	2,525	145

TRY THIS ...	Cal.	Fat (gm)
Breakfast		
orange juice, 6 oz	90	0
1 egg, poached	80	6
toast, 1 slice	70	0
ricotta cheese, 2 Tbsp	40	3
jam, 1 Tbsp	55	0
coffee	0	0
milk, skim, 1 Tbsp	5	0
	340	9
Lunch		
chef salad -		
lettuce, 1 c	10	0
asparagus, 2 1/2" spears	10	0
tomato, 1/2 medium	20	0
chicken, 2 oz	100	5
cottage cheese, 2 oz (1/2 c)	120	5
dressing, 1 Tbsp	80	9
rye wafers, 2 triple	40	0
vanilla wafers, 3	50	2
iced tea with lemon	0	0
TOTALS	430	21
Dinner		
flank steak, 4 oz	220	8
green beans, 1/2 c	25	0
baked potato	200	0
margarine, 1 pat	35	4
(or 1 Tbsp sour cream)		
pound cake, 1/2" slice	110	9
wine spritzer, 4 oz	100	0
	690	21
TOTALS	1,460	51

CALORIES SAVED = 1,065   **GRAMS FAT SAVED = 94**

INSTEAD OF THIS ...			TRY THIS ...		
	Cal.	Fat (gm)		Cal.	Fat (gm)
Breakfast			**Breakfast**		
orange juice, 6 oz	90	0	cantaloupe, 1/4 medium	60	0
cereal, dry, 1 c	150	0	cereal, cooked, 1 c	140	0
sugar, 1 Tbsp	50	0	raisins, 1 Tbsp	20	0
banana, 1/2 medium	50	0	maple extract, 1/4 tsp	0	0
milk, whole, 4 oz	75	5	milk, skim, 4 oz	45	0
coffee	0	0	coffee	0	0
half 'n half, 1 Tbsp	20	2	milk, skim, 1 Tbsp	5	0
	435	**7**		**260**	**0**
Lunch			**Lunch**		
sandwich -			sandwich -		
bologna, 2 oz	200	17	chicken, 2 oz	100	6
Swiss cheese, 1 oz	100	10	low-calorie cheese, 1 oz.	50	3
bread, 2 slices	140	1	bread, 2 slices	140	0
mayonnaise, 2 tsp	65	8	mayonnaise, 2 tsp	65	8
mustard, 2 tsp	0	0	mustard, 2 tsp	0	0
lettuce, 1 leaf	0	0	lettuce, 1 leaf	0	0
coleslaw, 1/2 c	120	10	tomato, 1/2 medium	25	0
			w/wine vinegar, basil	0	0
cola-type drink, 12 oz	150	0	apple juice, 4 oz	80	0
			with soda water, 6 oz	0	0
	775	**46**		**460**	**17**
Dinner			**Dinner**		
Polish pork sausage, 1 link (3 oz.)	275	24	pork tenderloin (lean),	140	4
			applesauce, 2 Tbsp	15	0
acorn squash, 1 c	140	0	boiled, roasted potato (small)	100	0
brown sugar, 1 Tbsp	50	0	with wine-herb baste	0	0
creamed peas and onions, 2/3 c	100	5	braised peas, onions, mushrooms, 1/2 c	70	0
			margarine, 1 pat	35	4
apple pie, 1/6 of 9" pie	400	18	baked apple with cinnamon	80	0
	965	**47**		**440**	**8**
TOTALS	**2,175**	**100**	**TOTALS**	**1,160**	**25**

```
┌──────────────────────────────────────────────────────────────────┐
│   CALORIES SAVED = 1,015      GRAMS FAT SAVED =75                   │
└──────────────────────────────────────────────────────────────────┘
```

LOWER CALORIE FOODS*

LUNCHEON MEAT (1 oz) †	Cal.	Fat (gm)
Boar's Head		
Turkey, Ham, Beef	30	0
Corned Beef/Brisket	40	2
Louis Rich		
Chicken or Turkey Breast (Smoked or Oven Roasted)(96-98% fat-free)	30	<1
Turkey Ham, Pastrami or Turkey Bacon	60	2
Pure ground turkey (4 oz.)	200	12
Hormel Light 'n Lean		
Lemon Peppered Smoked Breast of Turkey	30	1
Ham, Cooked or Smoked	25	1
Rotisserie Smoked Chicken	10	1
Healthy Choice		
Turkey Breast; Ham	60	2
Chicken Breast (6 slices = 1 oz)	50	0
Frank (97% fat-free)	50	1
Extra lean low-fat grnd. beef (3 oz)	90	2
Plantation		
Turkey Breast, Smoked or Oven-Cooked	30	0
Turkey Pastrami	40	2
Hillshire Farm Deli Select		
Smoked Chicken & Roasted Ham	50	0
Smoked Ham (97% Fat-Free)	60	2
Food Club		
Corned Beef, Smoked Beef	40	2
Ham, Turkey, Chicken	45	2
Carl Buddig (4 slices - sliced extra thin)		
Pastrami	40	2
Smoked Beef	45	2
Smoked Chicken, Smoked Turkey	50	4
Oscar Meyer (97% Fat-free)		
Chicken	25	<1
Smoked Cooked Ham (1 slice)	25	1
Corned Beef, Smoked Beef	30	1
Bacon (2 slices)	60	5
Sara Lee Light		
Chicken, Turkey, Beef, Pork, Ham	30-35	0-1
Ham, 3 varieties	40-45	0-2
Corned Beef/Brisket	35-40	2
Beef Pastrami	50	3

MISCELLANEOUS MEATLESS OPTIONS	Cal.	Fat (gm)
Green Giant Harvest Burgers (1)	140	4
Morning Star Farms		
Meatless Chicken Patties (4)	170	10
Better 'n Burgers (1)	70	0

	Cal.	Fat (gm)
Breakfast Links (2)	60	3
Breakfast Pattie (1)	70	3
Breakfast Strips (2)	60	5
TUNA AND FISH FILETS		
Chicken of the Sea Tuna (6 1/2 oz)		
Chunk Light in Spring Water	185	3
Star Kist Tuna (6 1/8 oz)		
Solid White in Spring Water	200	3
Healthy Choice Breaded Fish Filet (1)	180	4
Mrs. Paul's Healthy Treasures Fish Filet (1)	170	3
Gorton's Grilled Filets (1)	130	6
CANNED CHICKEN		
Swanson White Chicken in Water (2 oz.)	70	1
EGG SUBSTITUTES		
Egg Beaters (1/4 c = 1 egg)	25	0
Scramblers (1/4 c = 1 egg)	35	0
CHEESE (1 oz)		
Alpine Lace Free 'n Lean		
American (1 oz = 1 1/3 slices)	40	0
Cheddar (1 oz = 1 1/3 slices)	40	0
Borden Fat-Free American, Swiss	40	0
Borden Liteline Slices		
Swiss, Sharp, Cheddar, Colby, American (1 slice = 3/4 oz = 35 cal.)	50	2
American-Sodium Lite (1 slice = 3/4 oz = 35 cal.)	50	2
Kraft Light 'n Lively Slices		
Swiss, American, Sharp Cheddar (3/4 oz = 1 slice = 50 cal.)	70	4
Kraft		
Fat-free Cream Cheese (1 oz = 2 Tbsp)	25	0
Light Cream Cheese (1 oz = 2 Tbsp)	60	5
Light Neuchaftel (1 oz)	70	6
Light Mozzarella, shredded or block (1 oz = 1/4 c)	80	4
Parmesan (1 oz = 3 Tbsp)	80	5
Velveeta Light (1 oz)	70	4
Kraft Free (1 oz)	45	0
Laughing Cow (Reduced Calories)		
Mini-Bonbel Rounds (1 oz)	50	3
Gruyere Cheese Wedges (1 oz wedge)	50	3
Healthy Choice (1 oz)		
Fat-Free Cream Cheese (2 Tbsp)	25	0
American Slices (1 slice)	25	0
Shredded nonfat Cheddar (1/4 c)	45	0
Nonfat Mozzarella String Cheese (1 oz)	45	0

† **Note:** *Food labels describe **2 oz** servings; the above numbers describe **1 oz** servings.*

© 1993, *The Balancing Act Nutrition and Weight Guide*, G. Kostas, M.P.H., R.D., Dallas, Texas

	Cal.	Fat (gm)
Frigo		
Fat-free ricotta (1/2 c)	40	0
Food Club		
Mozzarella, part-skim (1 oz)	80	5
Precious		
Ricotta, low-fat (1/2 c)	140	6
Ricotta, fat-free (1/2 c)`	80	0

COTTAGE CHEESE (1/2 C)

	Cal.	Fat (gm)
Borden Nonfat	70	0
Weight Watcher's (1% fat)	90	1
Breakstone Free	80	0
Schepps (1% fat)	80	1

BREAD (1 SLICE)

Very thin sliced bread ("diet", low-calorie, or "light"):

Pepperidge Farm, Orowheat, Lightstyle, Earth Grains, Less (white or wholewheat),

	Cal.	Fat (gm)
Country Hearth diet sliced, **Mrs. Baird's**	35	0
Stella D'Oro Zweibeck toast (3 sticks)	60	0

BAGELS

	Cal.	Fat (gm)
Small (2 oz)	160	1
Large (3-5.5 oz)	250-400	2

PIZZA

	Cal.	Fat (gm)
Tombstone Light		
Supreme (8")	250	9
Vegetable (12") 1/2 pizza	220	6
Healthy Choice Supreme French Bread Pizza (1/2 pizza)	340	6

MARGARINE (1 TABLESPOON)

"Liquid oil" listed as first ingredient:

	Cal.	Fat (gm)
Chiffon (whipped), **Shedd's Spread**	90	10
I Can't Believe It's Not Butter	90	10
Fleischman's Reduced-calorie	70	8
Fleischmann's Lower fat	40	5
Promise Light	50	6
Weight Watcher's Light	45	4

BUTTER SUBSTITUTES

	Cal.	Fat (gm)
Butter Buds, Molly McButter sprinkles	12	0
I Can't Believe It's Not Butter pump spray	0	0
Fleischman's Low-cal spread (1 Tbsp)	5	0

COOKING OILS (1 TABLESPOON)

	Cal.	Fat (gm)
All Brands	120	14
Corn, Sunflower, Safflower, Olive, Canola		

COOKING SPRAY OILS (per spray)

	Cal.	Fat (gm)
Pam, Baker Joy, Weight Watcher's, Mazola, Wesson's Butter-flavor sprays	0	0

SOUR CREAM (2 TABLESPOONS)

	Cal.	Fat (gm)
Land O Lakes No-fat sour cream	30	0
Daisy Light low-fat sour cream	60	5

MAYONNAISE (1 TABLESPOON)

	Cal.	Fat (gm)
Weight Watcher's		
Light mayonnaise	25	2
Fat-free mayonnaise	12	0
Kraft		
Miracle Whip "Light"	35	3
Miracle Whip "Free"	15	0
Light mayonnaise	50	5
"Free" Mayonnaise	10	0

SALAD DRESSINGS (1 TABLESPOON)

	Cal.	Fat (gm)
Kraft Low-Cal and Kraft Free		
Italian, 1/3 less fat	35	3
Italian, fat-free	10	0
Blue Cheese, fat-free	16	0
Catalina, 1/3 less fat	35	2
Catalina, fat-free	18	0
Ranch, 1/3 less fat	60	6
Ranch, fat-free	18	0
French, fat-free	20	0
Creamy Italian, fat-free	20	0
Thousand Island, fat-free	16	0
Good Seasons (No oil)		
Zesty Herb	6	0
Creamy Italian, fat-free	8	0
Honey Mustard	10	0
Hidden Valley Fat Free		
Blue Cheese	12	0
Italian Parmesan	16	0
Caesar	20	0
Honey Dijon	30	0
Ranch	35	0
Wish Bone Lite		
Thousand Island	20	0
Creamy Roasted Garlic	20	0
Italian	15	0
Ranch, Blue Cheese	45	4
Seven Seas		
Italian	30	3
Creamy Italian, 1/3 less fat	45	4
Italian, fat-free	4	0
Lite Ranch	50	5
Weight Watchers		
Italian, Fat-free	6	0
Caesar, Fat-free	10	0
Creamy Cucumber, Fat-free	18	0
Creamy Italian, Fat-free	30	0
Ranch	35	0
French	40	0
Honey Dijon	45	0

	Cal.	Fat (gm)
Creamy Italian, fat-free	12	0
Italian, fat-free	6	0

BEVERAGES

	Cal.	Fat (gm)
Herb Teas (8 oz)	0	0
Sugar-Free Soft Drinks (12 oz)	0	0
Lipton Tea		
Lemon-flavored, Sugar-free, instant (8 oz)	2	0
Instant Tea (8 oz)	2	
Low-Calorie, Sugar-free (8 oz)	4	0
Crystal Light all flavors (8 oz)	4	0
Country Time Lemonade,		
Unsweetened (8 oz)	4	0
Kool-Aid all flavors with Nutrasweet (8 oz)	4	0
Lite-Line - all flavors with Nutrasweet (8 oz)	6	0
Tang, Sugar-free (8 oz)	7	0
Ocean Spray		
Cranapple Juice, low-calorie (6 oz)	30	0

HOT COCOA OR SHAKES

	Cal.	Fat (gm)
Carnation Diet Hot Cocoa (1 packet)	50	0
Swiss Miss Lite (1 packet)	50	0
Alba 66		
Hot cocoa mix (1 packet)	60	0
Alba 77		
Thick-N-Frosty Shake - strawberry, vanilla, chocolate (1 packet)	70	0

CHIPS, POPCORN, SNACKS

	Cal.	Fat (gm)
Burnes & Ricker Bagel Crisps (1 oz = 5 crisps)		
Regular	130	4
Fat-free	100	0
Guiltless Gourmet		
Baked Tortilla Chips (1 oz = 20 chips)	110	1
Black Bean or Pinto Bean Dips (1 oz)	25	0
Fat-free queso (1 oz)	25	0
Frito Lay		
Baked Tostitos Tortilla Chips (1 oz = 13 chips)	110	1
Baked Potato Chips (1 oz = 12 chips)	110	1
Health Valley Fat-Free Puffs		
50 Cheese Puffs (1 oz)	100	0
50 Caramel Corn Puffs (1 oz)	100	0
Hain's		
Mini rice cakes, 6 flavors (6-8 cakes)	60	0
Blueberry apple (1 bar)	140	0
Louise's Fat-free Potato Chips, no salt (1 oz. = 30 chips)	110	0
Orville Redenbacker Smart Pop (Light Popcorn) (3 cups)	50	1
Rold Gold Pretzels (1 oz = 10 pretzels)	110	0

	Cal.	Fat (gm)
Skinny Munchies (1 package)		
Crispy Onion, Wheat, Toasted Coconut, Nacho Cheese, Smokey Barbecue	59	2
Weight Watcher's		
Caramel popcorn (1 oz)	100	1
Microwave popcorn (1 oz)	90	1
Vic's Corn Popper, low-fat		
White Cheddar (1 oz = 2 1/2 cups)	110	3
Caramel (1 oz = 1 cup)	110	0
Cracker Jack Butter Toffee Glazed Popcorn, fat-free (1 cup)	110	0

CEREAL/GRANOLA BARS (1)

	Cal.	Fat (gm)
Carnation Breakfast Bar	150	6
Health Valley Fat-free Granola Bar	140	0
Kellogg's Low-fat Crunchy Granola Bar	80	1
Nature Valley Granola Bar		
Chewy low-fat bar	110	2
Wholegrain low-fat fruit bar	80	1
Nutrigrain Cereal Bar	140	3
Quaker Low-fat Granola Bar	110	2
Healthy Choice Fat-free Granola Bar	100	0
Snackwell Cereal Bar	120	0
Nestle's Sweet Success Bar	120	4
Kellogg's Rice Krispie Treat	90	2

DIPS (2 TABLESPOON)

	Cal.	Fat (gm)
Land O Lakes Fat-free dips		
Ranch, French onion, salsa	30	0
Kraft		
Green onion, avacado, French onion, ranch	60	4

SOUPS

	Cal.	Fat (gm)
Campbell's (one 10 1/2 oz can)		
Broth, Beef (bouillon)	40	0
Beef, Consomme	60	0
Broth, Chicken	90	5
Won Ton	100	3
Beef Mushroom, Chicken Gumbo, Chicken with Stars, Chicken with Rice, Old Fashion Vegetable, Vegetarian Vegetable	150	5
Clam Chowder (Manhattan Style), Chicken Vegetable, Chicken Noodle, Cream of Potato, French Onion, Vegetable Beef	175	6
Alphabet Vegetable, Clam Chowder (New England Style)	200	8
Borden - MBT (1 packet)		
Beef Broth	12	0
Chicken Broth	12	0
Onion Soup	16	0
Lipton dehydrated soups (8 oz)		
Beefy Onion	30	0
Onion Mushroom	45	0

	Cal.	Fat (gm)
Herb Ox (1 cube)		
Bouillon	50	0
Lipton Cup-A-Soup (1 packet)		
Chicken Noodle	50	1
Lipton Cup-A-Soup Lite (1 packet), all flavors	45	1
Healthy Choice Soups		
Chunky Beef Vegetable (15 oz)	220	2
Chunky Chicken Noodle/Veg. (15 oz)	320	8
Chili w/Beans/Ground Turkey (15 oz)	400	10
Spicy Chili w/Beans/Ground Turkey (15 oz)	440	10
Health Valley Soups/Beans		
5-Bean Soup (15 oz)	200	0
3-Bean Chili (10 oz)	180	0
Organic Black Beans/Tofu Weiners (15 oz)	320	6
Organic Lentils/Tofu Weiners (15 oz)	340	6
Western Black Beans/Veg. (15 oz)	210	2
Hearty Lentils/Veg. (15 oz)	240	2

FRUIT

	Cal.	Fat (gm)
Food Club "Light" (1/2 c)		
Fruit Cocktail, Cling Peaches and Peaches	50	0
Pear Halves	60	0
Pineapple	70	0
Libby's "Light" (1/2 c)		
Fruit Cocktail, Peaches and Pear Halves	50	0
Featherweight (1/2 c)		
Apricots (water packed); Mandarin Oranges	35	0
Grapefruit Segments	40	0
Applesauce, Peaches, Fruit Cocktail, Fruits		
for Salads (all water packed)	50	0
Sliced Pineapple	70	0
Weight Watcher's Dried Fruit Snack (1 packet)		
Dried Apple, Dried Peaches,		
Dried Pineapple and Dried Strawberries	25-50	0
Mott's or Lucky Leaf (1/2 c)		
Applesauce, sugar-free	50	0

SWEETS, EXTRAS

	Cal.	Fat (gm)
SUGAR-FREE JELLY (1 TEASPOON)		
Knott's Light Fruit Spread	8	0
Smucker's Simply Fruit	16	0
Smucker's Light Fruit Spread	7	0
SYRUP (1 TABLESPOON)		
Aunt Jemima Light	25	0
Butterworth's Light	30	0
PANCAKE MIX		
Aunt Jemima Light Buttermilk	130	2
Hungry Jack Extra Light	120	2
WAFFLES		
Kellogg's Special K	80	0
NON-DAIRY CREAM TOPPINGS (1 TABLESPOON)		
Dream Whip	8	0

	Cal.	Fat (gm)
Cool Whip, La Creme	16	1
Fat-Free Cool Whip	6	0
SUGAR TWIN Diet Brown Sugar (1 Tbsp)	2	0

FROZEN DESSERTS

	Cal.	Fat (gm)
Weight Watcher's		
Ice Milk, all flavors (4 oz) (1/2 c)	120	4
Ice Cream Treats, all flavors (1 bar)	100	7
Fat-free Frozen Dessert Bars (1 bar)	30-90	0
Ice Cream Sandwich (1 bar)	130	8
Hot Fudge Sundae (1)	160	4
Blue Bell		
Diet Ice Cream, all	100	0
Fat-free frozen yogurt (1/2 c)	120	4
Fat-free fudge bar (1)	120	4
Cream Pops (1)	60	1
Mini light sandwich (1)	80	2
Frozen Bars		
All Flavors (1 bar)	70	0
Sugar-free (1 bar)	15-35	0
Dreyer's		
Frozen yogurt (1/2 c)	110	4
Fat-free dessert (1/2 c)	100	0
Dannon		
Frozen yogurt	110	0
Crystal Light		
Double Chocolate Fudge Bar (1 bar)	50	2
Dole		
Fruit and Juice Bars (1)	70	0
Fruit and Yogurt Bars (1)	60	0
Sorbet (1/2 c)	70	0
Welch's		
Fruit Juice Bar	25	0
Creamsicle, sugar-free (1 bar)	25	1
Fudgesicle		
1 bar	70	1
Sugar-free bar (1)	35	0
Jell-O		
Pudding Pops (1 bar)	80	2
Borden		
Eskimo Bar, sugar-free (1 bar)	150	11
non-fat (1 bar)	130	7
All Natural Ice Milk (4 oz) (1/2 c)	100	2
Orange Sherbet (1/2 c)	100	1
Klondike Light		
Ice Cream Sandwich	100	2
Chocolate Bar	110	6
Haagen-Daas		
Frozen Yogurt Bar	100	1

	Cal.	Fat (gm)
Healthy Choice (1/2 c)		
Frozen Desserts, all flavors	130	2
Ultra Slim-Fast		
Frozen Dessert (1/2 c)	100	0
Fudge Bar (1 bar)	70	10
Breyer's		
Light Ice Milk (1/2 c)	125	4
Blue Bunny (1/2 c)		
Frozen yogurt, low-fat	115	3
TCBY Yogurt (1/2 c)		
Sugar-free, non-fat	72	0
Nonfat	100	0
Regular	120	1

CAKES/PIES/PASTRIES

	Cal.	Fat (gm)
Entenmann's Fat-Free (1 slice)		
Chocolate Loaf Cake	70	0
Louisiana Crunch Cake	80	0
Hostess		
Light Cupcakes, all flavors (1)	130	2
Light Twinkies (1)	110	2
Pepperidge Farm Desserts Light		
Apple 'N Spice Bake (1 slice)	170	2
Fudge Brown, fat-free	120	0
Sara Lee Free & Light (1 slice)		
Apple Danish	130	0
Pound Cake	70	0
Apple Crisp	150	2
Apple Pie	190	4
Pillsbury Lovin'Lites		
Fudge Brownie Mix (1/24)	100	2
Blueberry Muffin Mix (1/12)	100	1
Weight Watcher's		
Strawberry Cheesecake (4 oz)	180	4
Apple Pie (3.5 oz)	165	4
Brownie (1)	100	3
LIGHT CAKE MIXES (1/12TH CAKE)		
Betty Crocker Supermoist Light	185	4
Pillsbury Lovin'Lites	170	3
Duncan Hines Delights	180	4
LIGHT FROSTINGS (2 TBSP)		
Betty Crocker low-fat, all	120	1
Pillsbury Light, all	120	2

GELATINS, PUDDINGS

	Cal.	Fat (gm)
D-Zerta Gelatin, all flavors (1/2 c)	8	0
Jell-O with Nutrasweet, all flavors (1/2 c)	8	0
D-Zerta Pudding, all flavors (1/2 c)	60	0
Hunt's, Hershey's, Jello Fat-free Puddings, all flavors (1/2 c)	100	0

COOKIES

	Cal.	Fat (gm)
Entenmann's		
Fat-free cookies (1)	80	0
Health Valley		
Fat-free Apricot Cookies, etc. (3)	75	0
Nabisco		
Devil's Food Cakes (1)	70	1
Fig newtons (2)	120	2
Nilla Wafers (7)	120	4
Snackwell's		
Mini Chocolate Chip Cookies (6)	60	1
Oatmeal Raisin or Choc. Sandwich cookies (1)	60	1
Devil's Food or Double Fudge (1)	50	0
Cinnamon Grahams (9)	50	0
Sunshine		
Animal Crackers (13)	120	3
Teddy Grahams (1/2 oz)	60	2

CRACKERS

	Cal.	Fat (gm)
Hain Ryecrackers (6)	60	1
Health Valley		
Rice Bran crackers (3)	50	2
Wholewheat Crackers (1 oz)	80	1
Nabisco		
Harvest Crisps (oat, rice, 5-grain) (6)	60	2
Fat-free saltines (5)	50	0
Saltines, reg. or wholewheat (5)	60	2
Triskets, reg. or unsalted (3)	60	2
OLD LONDON Onion Rounds (5)	50	0
PEPPERIDGE FARM tiny goldfish (22)	60	2
SUNSHINE Oyster & Soup Crackers (16)	60	1
SNACKWELL'S		
Cheese Crackers (18)	60	1
Wheat Crackers (5)	50	0
RALSTON-PURINA Rykrisps (2)	40	0
WASA Crispbreads, all types (1)	45	0

*NOTE:
1. Check "Gourmet Foods" section, "Diet Foods" section, and "Health Foods" section at your grocery store, along with regular food sections for these special low-calorie, low-fat, low-sugar, low-sodium products.
2. Check for your local brand names. Take a grocery store tour with a dietitian in your city.
3. New specialty foods arrive every week. Keep checking labels & finding new products.

FAT GRAM COUNTER

Mark the foods you eat often and seek lower-fat alternatives, if needed.

MEAT, FISH, POULTRY (3 oz.)	Grams of Fat	Total Calories
Beef, cooked (visible fat removed)		
corned beef	16	215
eye of round, roasted (select)	5	185
London broil, braised (choice)	12	210
porterhouse steak, broiled (choice)	9	185
rib, broiled (prime)	16	240
rib eye (Delmonico) steak, broiled (choice)	10	190
T-bone steak, broiled (choice)	9	180
top loin (filet) steak, broiled (select)	6	160
wedge-bone sirloin steak, broiled (choice	8	180
Luncheon meats (1 slice)		
Louis Rich 96% Fat Free Turkey Pastrami	0	25
Louis Rich Oven Roasted Turkey Breast	0	30
Oscar Meyer Bologna	4	50
Oscar Meyer Hard Salami	3	35
Oscar Meyer 95% Fat Free Smoked Cooked Ham	1	25
Seafood, cooked		
anchovies, canned in oil, drained, 5	2	40
Atlantic cod	1	90
haddock	1	95
lobster	1	85
salmon, pink, canned with bone and liquid	5	120
smoked salmon (lox)	4	100
swordfish	4	130
tuna, canned in oil, drained	7	160
tuna, canned in water, drained	0	110
shrimp	1	85
shrimp, breaded, fried	10	200
Poultry, cooked		
chicken breast, w/skin	7	165
chicken breast, no skin	3	145
chicken drumstick w/skin, batter fried	11	190
chicken drumstick, no skin	2	75

	Grams of Fat	Total Calories
chicken wing, no skin	2	45
turkey, light meat with skin	7	170
turkey, light meat, no skin	3	135
turkey, dark meat with skin	10	190
turkey, dark meat, no skin	6	160
Eggs		
1 large	5	75
Fleishmann's Egg Beaters, 1/4 c	0	25
Healthy Choice Egg Substitute	3	60
MILK & DAIRY PRODUCTS		
Milk (1 c)		
whole	8	150
2 % fat	5	120
1% fat	3	100
skim	0	90
buttermilk	2	100
Cream (1 tbsp)		
half and half	2	20
heavy whipping cream	6	50
sour cream	3	25
Cheese		
American, 1 oz.	9	110
cheddar, 1 oz.	9	110
cottage cheese, creamed, 1 cup	9	200
cottage cheese, 1% fat, 1 cup	2	160
cottage cheese, fat-free, 1 cup	0	140
cream cheese, 1 oz.	10	100
mozzarella, part-skim, 1 oz.	5	70
Parmesan, grated, 1 tbsp	2	25
ricotta, 1/2 cup	16	200
ricotta, part-skim, 1/2 cup	10	170
ricotta, fat-free, 1/2 cup	0	80
Swiss, 1 oz.	8	110
Weight Watchers American Pasteurized Process Cheese Product, 1 slice	2	45
Yogurt		
plain, 8 oz.	7	150
plain nonfat, sugar-free, 8 oz.	0	110
flavored (coffee, lemon, vanilla), 8 oz.	3	200-250
flavored, nonfat, sugar-free, 8 oz.	0	100

	Grams of Fat	Total Calories

BREADS, GRAINS, ETC.

Breads

	Grams of Fat	Total Calories
bagel, 1	1	160
English muffin, 1	1	140
wholewheat bread, 1 slice	1	70

Cereals

Cheerios, 1 1/4 cups	2	110
Corn Flakes, 1 cup	0	100
Raisin Bran, 3/4 cup	1	120
Cream of Wheat, 1 cup	0	100
Shredded Wheat, 1 biscuit	0	80
Oatmeal, 2/3 cup cooked	2	100
Granola, 1/4 cup	5	130
Puffed Rice, 1 cup	0	50

Crackers

Cheez-It Snack Crackers, 12	4	70
Graham crackers, 2 squares	1	60
Ritz, 4	4	70
Oyster crackers, 10	1	33

Other

pasta, 1 cup cooked	1	200
white rice, 1 cup cooked	0	225
pancakes, 4" plain	2	60
waffles, 7" plain	8	200
French toast, 1 slice	7	150
Bran Muffin, large	11	350
Sara lee Golden Corn Muffin	13	250

Fruits & Vegetables

apple, 1 medium	1	80
banana, 1 medium	1	105
fruit cocktail, canned in heavy syrup, 1/2 cup	0	90
orange, 1 medium	0	65
raisins, 1/3 cup	0	150
avocado, 1/2 medium	15	155
broccoli, 1/2 cup cooked	0	25
carrot, raw, 1 medium	0	30
corn, canned, 1/2 cup	1	65
green beans, 1/2 cup cooked	0	20
peas, 1/2 cup cooked	0	70

Beans, Nuts, & Seeds

kidney beans, 1/2 cup boiled	0	115
lentils, 1/2 cup boiled	0	115
cashews, dry roasted, 1/4 cup	16	200
coconut, flaked, 1/4 cup	6	90
peanuts, 1/4 cup	18	210

	Grams of Fat	Total Calories
peanut butter, 1 tbsp	8	95
pistachios, dry roasted, 1/4 cup	17	195
sesame seeds, 1/4 cup	21	220
tahini (sesame butter), 1 tbsp	7	90
walnuts, 1/4 cup	18	190

Spreads, Oils

butter, 1 tsp	4	35
whipped butter, 1 tsp	3	30
margarine, stick & tub, 1 tsp	4	35
diet margarine, tub, 1 tsp	2	17
vegetable oils (corn, olive, etc.), 1 Tablespoon	14	120 (average)
vegetable oil spray	1	6

Salad Dressings

blue cheese, 1 tbsp	8	75
French, 1 tbsp	6	70
Italian, 1 tbsp	7	70
Russian, 1 tbsp	8	75
thousand island, 1 tbsp	6	60

Soups

canned Chicken Noodle, 1 cup	2	70
canned Cream of Mushroom, 1 cup	7	100
Lipton Noodle, 1 cup	2	70
Progresso Green Split Pea, 1 cup	3	150
Progresso Beef Minestrone, 1 cup	3	135
Ramen Pride Oriental Noodles & Pork Flavor, 10 oz.	8	200

Sweets

Cadbury's Milk Chocolate with Fruit & Nuts, 1 oz.	8	150
Hershey Chocolate Kisses, 5	8	125
Milky Way bar	11	280
Milky Way II bar	8	190
Snicker's Bar, 2.16 oz.	14	290
Three Musketeers Bar, 2.13 oz.	9	260
angel food cake, 1/12 cake	0	125
brownie with nuts (3x2x7/8")	12	200
cheesecake, 1/8 cake	13	280
Hostess Ding Dong, 1	9	170
Hostess Twinkie, 1	5	160
pound cake, 1/2" slice	6	150
Almost Home Chocolate Chip Cookie	25	130
Fig Newton, 1	1	50
Gingersnaps, 4	3	120
apple pie, 1/8	12	280
banana cream pie, 1/8	12	235
pumpkin pie, 1/8	13	240
chocolate pudding, 1 cup	12	385

	Grams of Fat	Total Calories
Chocolate cake with icing	22	450
Nature Valley Granola Bar	5	120
Sara Lee Cheese Danish	8	130

Frozen Desserts
Ice cream
Breyers, 1/2 cup	8	160
Haagen Daz, 1/2 cup	18	300
Sealtest, 1/2 cup	6	140

Other
Fruit 'N Yogurt Bar	0	70
Fruit sorbet, 1/2 cup	0	100
Eskimo Pie, 3 oz. bar	12	180
Chocolate Pudding Pop	2	80
Ice Milk, 1/2 cup	3	120
Sherbet, 1/2 cup	3	135
Popsicle	0	70
Tofutti, 1/2 cup	12	210
Fat-free Frozen yogurt, 3 fl. oz.	0	80

Toppings
chocolate syrup, 2 tbsp	1	90
fudge topping, 2 tbsp	5	125
whipped cream, 2 tbsp	1	16

Dry Snack Foods
Potato chips, 1 oz. (15 chips)	10	150
Orville Redenbacher's Natural Microwave Popping Corn, 4 cups popped	7	110
popcorn, air-popped, 1 cup	0	25
Light Potato Chips, 1 oz. (15 chips)	8	150
pretzels, 1 oz. (50)	1	111
Guiltless Gourmet Chips, 1 oz.	0	130

 © 1993, *The Balancing Act Nutrition and Weight Guide,* G. Kostas, M.P.H., R.D., Dallas, Texas

SHOPPING CRITERIA AT-A-GLANCE

Food Category		Serving Size	Per Serving Fat (gm)	Per Serving Sodium (mg)
Beverages		8 oz	≤3	
Dinners/Entrees		300 cal.	≤ 10	≤ 800
Frozen, Canned, Packaged		200 cal.	≤ 6	≤ 600
Soups		per serving	≤ 3	≤ 600
Packaged Side Dishes*		per serving	≤ 5	≤ 400
(as prepared)				
Sauces/Coatings		per serving	≤ 2	≤ 500
Breads, Crackers, Snacks		per serving	≤ 2	
Cereal		per serving	≤ 2	
Muffins		1 piece	≤ 5	
Cheese,	reduced-fat	1 oz	≤ 5	
	low-fat	1 oz	≤ 3	
Yogurt,	low-fat	8 oz	≤ 3	
	non-fat	8 oz	0	
Milk,	low-fat	8 oz	≤ 3	
	skim	8 oz	0	
Meat		1 oz	≤ 3	
Margarine,	reduced-calorie	1 Tbsp	≤ 7	
	low-calorie	1 Tbsp	≤ 5	
Salad Dressing,	reduced-calorie	1 Tbsp	≤ 3	
	fat-free	1 Tbsp	0	
Mayonnaise,	reduced-calorie	1 Tbsp	≤ 5	
	fat-free	1 Tbsp	0	
Sour Cream,	reduced-calorie	2 Tbsp	≤ 3	
	fat-free	2 Tbsp	0	
Cream Cheese,	reduced-calorie	2 Tbsp	≤ 6	
	fat-free	2 Tbsp	0	
Frozen Desserts,	low-fat	per serving	≤ 5	
	fat-free	per serving	0	

Abbreviations: ≤ means "less than or equal to" the number of grams of fat specified; gm = grams; mg = milligrams
* To prepare side dish (such as macaroni & cheese, specialty rice, etc.) without fat, omit the recommended butter, margarine or oil called for in the recipe. The fat content is listed on the label, "as packaged", before fat is added.

IV
EXERCISE AND COOKING

EXERCISE FOCUS

1. "Why Exercise" (115) What "Types"? (116).

2. Rate your Heart Rate (117) and perceived exercise exertion.

3. Discover new idease on "How to Begin to Exercise" (118).

4. Create your "Balanced Fitness Plan" (119-125).

5. How much exercise will burn off that pizza?! (126).

NUTRITION FOCUS

1. Continue your healthy Eating Plan.

2. Create delicious meals with these "Cooking Tips" (127) and ingredient substitutions (128).

3. Enjoy "Your Favorite Foods Made Healthy!" (129) and "Fun Foods" (130).

4. Find creative ways to eat more veggies! (131).

5. Try a new cookbook with low-calorie recipes (Appendix B).

RECORDS

Continue your food, exercise, weight records daily.

GOALS

HABIT: exercise— incorporate the aerobic fitness goals into your lifestyle

FOOD: prepare foods in a healthy way with less calories, fat, sugar, salt

EXERCISE: pick up your pace — keep progressing!

RECORD: food, exercise, weight— how many calories did you burn this week?

IV EXERCISE/COOKING

WHY EXERCISE?

Benefits of an Aerobic Exercise Program

WEIGHT CONTROL:

- accelerates weight loss by increasing **CALORIES** you burn (this helps especially when you reach a plateau).
- increases your **METABOLIC RATE** — even hours after you stop exercising
- decreases **APPETITE** — naturally
- decreases body **FAT** stores and promotes **FAT-BURNING**
- builds **LEAN BODY MASS** (muscle) which speeds up your metabolism
- reduces **STRESS AND BOREDOM** which can lead to excessive eating
- **MOTIVATES** adherence to your calorie-controlled eating program
- **CHANGES** your appetite, so you desire more light, low-fat foods

PHYSIOLOGICAL (Cardiovascular):

- improves **CARDIOVASCULAR HEALTH** (your heart, blood vessels and lungs work more efficiently)
- improves **CIRCULATION OF OXYGEN** and nutrients
- increases **HDL-cholesterol** blood levels — to reduce coronary risk
- decreases blood **CHOLESTEROL, TRIGLYCERIDES and GLUCOSE** and decreases **BLOOD PRESSURE** — to reduce coronary risk
- improves your **MUSCLE TONE, AGILITY, and STRENGTH**
- increases your **STAMINA and ENDURANCE**
- increases your **RESISTANCE** to stress and illness
- builds **STRONGER BONES** and joints to prevent osteoporosis

PSYCHOLOGICAL:

- builds **SELF-CONFIDENCE** and a **POSITIVE SELF**
- reduces **EMOTIONAL STRESS and DEPRESSION**
- increases **ALERTNESS**
- enables a **SENSE OF WELL-BEING and ENJOYMENT OF LIFE**
- helps you **FEEL and LOOK YOUR BEST**
- improves the **QUALITY OF YOUR LIFE**

SOCIAL:

- opens up a new world of **FRIENDS**
- creates a new **RECREATIONAL** interest

Aerobic Fitness Goals For Weight Loss

1. **F** — Frequency - 4-5 times per week
2. **I** — Intensity - moderate
3. **T** — Time - 30-45 minutes per workout

For best weight loss results, burn approximately 250 calories per day. (See Calorie Expenditure Tables - Appendix C.)

EXERCISE IS NOT A CHOICE — IT'S A MUST!

TYPES OF EXERCISE

WHAT TYPES OF EXERCISE SHOULD YOU DO FOR BEST RESULTS?

AEROBIC EXERCISES —

- Strengthen the heart, blood vessels, and lung capacity
- Build endurance through sustained vigorous activity (walking, jogging, dancing, swimming).
- Promote oxygen transport through the body, which leads to fitness and more fat-burning

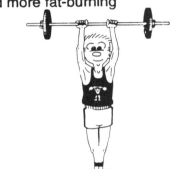

ANAEROBIC EXERCISES —

- Increase stamina by demanding maximum energy for brief periods (a sudden sprint or jump or movement)
- Increase muscle tone (through calisthenics)
- Increase muscular strength by tensing one set of muscles against a resistance (pushing against a door jam, push-ups, sit-ups, etc.) or by using free weights or weight machines
- Build lean body mass (muscle), helping you burn fat better

FLEXIBILITY STRETCHING EXERCISES —

- Increase muscle agility and prevent muscle injury
- Before and after exercise, always warm up and cool down gradually for 5 minutes to prevent rapid heart rate changes or muscle changes. Stretch **after** a warm-up and cooldown.

Studies show that a **combination** of **AEROBIC EXERCISES AND ANAEROBIC CONDITIONING EXERCISES** work together to promote fitness and provide the most effective means of short-term and long-term weight loss and maintenance. See a fitness specialist to help you design the best program for you. You may wish to start with an aerobic program, as described on page 122.

Two landmark studies at the Cooper Institute for Aerobics Research have shown that:

- Even the **smallest improvement** in cardiovascular fitness from exercise can significantly reduce your risk of heart disease, hypertension, stroke, and cancer. You don't have to run a marathon to be healthy! Brisk walking 30 minutes a day, 5 days a week will **improve** fitness.
- Walking at a **faster pace** (a 12-minute mile) speeds your fitness conditioning; but at a slower pace (a 20-minute mile), you reap the same cardiovascular benefits — a "good" or HDL-cholesterol and an 18% reduced risk of coronary heart disease!
- So it's worth it to pick up your pace! A 12-minute mile brisk pace burns 53% more calories than a 20-minute mile pace, and promotes greater overall fitness and aerobic conditioning.

ALWAYS CHECK WITH YOUR PHYSICIAN BEFORE BEGINNING AN EXERCISE PROGRAM!

TWO TIPS: 1) In your DAILY PLANNER, schedule an exercise appointment with yourself!
2) Rise and shine! Morning exercisers tend to be the most consistent.

EXERCISE HEART RATE

You exercise more comfortably and safely when you exercise at the appropriate intensity, called your **TARGET HEART RATE** range. How do you know what intensity is best for you, and if you are exercising at this level?

There are two methods you can use to find out:
1. Simplest way: if you perceive yourself to be "exerting", but not "over-doing", and can carry on a conversation while exercising, most likely you are exercising right on "target"! Use the Borg Scale below to rate your level of intensity. Strive to exercise at perceived levels 2-4.
2. Technical way: Use a heart pulse meter under medical supervision to measure your heart rate.

Exercise in your **TARGET HEART RATE** (safe heart rate); avoid your **MAXIMUM** (unsafe):

AGE	SAFE RANGE	MAXIMUM
20	140-170	200
30	130-162	190
40	126-158	180
50	119-145	170
60	112-136	160
70	105-128	150

Remain in your Target Heart Range for at least 20 minutes for the best aerobic and cardiovascular conditioning. **NEVER** exceed your maximum heart rate!

Borg Rating of Perceived Exertion (RPE) Scale

This scale rates the level of exertion you are experiencing from 0 (rest) to 10 (extreme effort).

10	VERY, VERY HARD
8	VERY HARD
6	HARD
4	SOMEWHAT HARD
3	MODERATE
2	LIGHT
1	VERY LIGHT
0	NO EXERTION

© 1992, Gunnar Borg. Reprinted by permission. Adapted from *Medicine and Science in Sports and Exercise*, 1982, Vol 14, No. 5, pg. 377-381

REMINDERS:

AEROBIC EXERCISE MUST BE:
- **STEADY:** non-stop, rhythmic
- **DURATION:** 20 + minutes, (30 minutes best for weight loss)
- **INTENSITY:** moderate (Borg scale 2-4)

FITNESS IS:
- **LOST** — if 2 days or less per week of exercise
- **MAINTAINED** — if 3 days per week of exercise
- **IMPROVED** — if 5-6 days per week of exercise

HOW TO BEGIN TO EXERCISE

WONDERING WHERE TO BEGIN? FIND WAYS TO HABITUALLY MOVE MORE DAILY:

1. **Incorporate more "natural" activity in your DAILY ROUTINE:**

    1.   Sit instead of lying down.
    2.   Stand instead of sitting
    3.   Walk instead of drive. (Many local errands can be fun when done on foot or bike.)
    4.   Take stairs instead of elevators.
    5.   Pick up your walking pace.
    6.   Stoop, bend, reach — use your muscles ("Use it or lose it").
    7.   Park your car farthest from your destination.
    8.   Choose the farthest phone, bathroom, or path between two points.
    9.   Visit with a friend or family member on a walk.
    10. Make an "after-dinner walk" part of your lifestyle.
    11. Clean that closet, vacuum or mop, do yard work or home repairs.
    12. Use "coffee breaks" at work to walk or climb staircases.
    13. Make your own list of ways to move more daily.

2. **Establish a REGULAR EXERCISE PROGRAM:**

    1.   Set up a personal **DAILY** program of walking, biking, swimming, jogging, etc.
    2.   Join an exercise class, dancing class, or team sport.
    3.   Find an exercise partner and set goals together.
    4.   Involve yourself in active hobbies — gardening, carpentry, dancing, etc.
    5.   Try your hand at a new recreational sport — tennis, volleyball, badminton, ping pong, bowling, racquetball, golf, etc. Take lessons!

3. **Work out your PERSONAL PROGRAM:**

    1.   Choose activities you like, and are convenient to you.
    2.   Start out slowly and avoid strain. Increase your goals weekly.
    3.   Have a plan of action. See pages 119-122.
    4.   Remember that you need sustained exercise of at least 20 minutes to reap cardiovascular benefits, and 30-45 minutes to burn body fat stores.
    5.   Set aside a regular time daily for exercise — and keep with it!
    6.   Set a goal to burn at least 250 calories a day (see page 126 + Appendix C).
    7.   Keep a daily activity log (see sample, page 121) and monitor your progress.

4. **BALANCE your program:**

    1.   Exercise **aerobically** 30-45 minutes daily. Follow the PROGRESSIVE AEROBIC FITNESS GOALS (p. 122) to build up to 30-45 minutes exercise daily.
    2.   Warm up and cool down for 5 minutes **before** and **after** exercise, then stretch for **flexibility**. (See Diagram A, page 123.)
    3.   Condition your muscles with **strength training** 2-3 times a week, 20-30 minutes per session. Seek a qualified trainer to help you or see Diagram B, page 124.
    4.   Add to your agility and easier exercise with **flexibility stretching** (Diagram C, page 125).
    5.   Follow the **BALANCED FITNESS PROGRAM** (page 119) for maximum results.

© 1993, *The Balancing Act Nutrition and Weight Guide*, G. Kostas, M.P.H., R.D., Dallas, Texas

A BALANCED FITNESS PLAN

BALANCED FITNESS means AEROBIC FITNESS and STRENGTH and FLEXIBILITY.

YOUR ACTION PLAN SUMMARY:

DAYS 1,3: DO PROGRESSIVE-PACED AEROBIC EXERCISE + STRENGTH CONDITIONING
DAYS 2,4: ENJOY YOUR-OWN-PACED AEROBIC EXERCISE + FLEXIBILITY STRETCHING
DAY 5:   SELECT LIGHTER, LONGER AEROBIC EXERCISE

---

1. **AEROBICALLY EXERCISE** FIVE DAYS A WEEK. ALTERNATE PROGRESSIVE-PACED AND YOUR-OWN-PACED DAYS OF EXERCISE TO BUILD FITNESS FASTER. CHOOSE AN AEROBIC ACTIVITY YOU ENJOY: walk, jog, bike, swim, aerobic dance, stair-climb (machine), jump rope, etc.

DAYS 1,3:   PROGRESSIVE-PACED AEROBIC EXERCISE

- Exercise 20-40 minutes at a brisk pace (BORG 4 = somewhat hard), 2 days a week.
- Select a standard route or distance. Increase your pace each week by 15-20 seconds (covering the same distance in a shorter time span).
- You may use the PROGRESSIVE AEROBIC FITNESS GOALS on page 122 as a guide. Select your current and desired level of fitness. Work toward your goal.
- Example: a walker may work toward walking 3 miles in 45 minutes (at a 15 minutes-a-mile pace).
- As you become more fit, you'll burn more calories (from 200-300 to 400-600 calories per session).

DAYS 2,4:   YOUR-OWN-PACED AEROBIC EXERCISE

- Exercise 30-45 minutes **at your own pace** (BORG 2 = light exertion), 2 days a week.
- There is no emphasis on speed or distance.

DAY 5:   LIGHTER, LONGER AEROBIC EXERCISE

- Perform an aerobic activity or **EVERYDAY ACTIVITY,** as long as you move continuously, non-stop, for 45 to 90 minutes (BORG 1-2 = very light to light exertion). Start with 45 minutes. Add 5 minutes weekly till you reach a maximum of 90 minutes.
- Examples: long walk, hike, bike ride, dancing, shopping, yard work, lawn-mowing, gardening, washing/waxing car, raking leaves, shoveling snow, sweeping/vacuuming/mopping, sight-seeing on foot, active hobbies, etc.

2. ### DAYS 1,3:   STRENGTH CONDITIONING EXERCISES

- Needed for muscle strength and endurance.
- Allow 20-30 minutes, 2 days a week; you'll burn 100-200 calories each time.
- Do home calisthenics (Diagram B), or free weights or weight machines (with guidance).

3. ### DAYS 2,4:   FLEXIBILITY STRETCHING EXERCISES

- Needed for muscle flexibility, agility, toning, injury prevention, and relaxation.
- Allow 5-7 minutes, 2 days a week.
- See Diagram C or attend a stretch class. Also stretch 3 to 5 minutes each time you exercise (before and after).

Exercise Plan developed by Philip Walker, MS, Fitness Management Consultant, Cooper Clinic. Printed with permission.

4. | EVERY TIME YOU EXERCISE: |

- **WARM-UP** (pre-exercise), 5 minutes
  - a. Walk or cycle slowly 3 minutes; then stretch 1 minute (see Diagram A).
  - b. This warms up your joints and muscles to prevent injury, increase endurance, and help you ease into exercise comfortably.
- **COOL-DOWN** (post-exercise), 5 minutes
  - a. Slow down your pace for 3 minutes after completing your desired exercise and stretch muscles used for 1-2 minutes (see Diagram A).
  - b. This slows your heart rate gradually (safely) and relaxes your muscles. You'll feel great!

5. | EXAMPLE OF 5-DAY EXERCISE PLAN |

EXAMPLE OF BASIC 5-DAY EXERCISE PLAN

DAY 1	DAY 2	DAY 3	DAY OFF	DAY 4	DAY 5	DAY OFF
PROGRESSIVE PACED AEROBICS + STRENGTH	YOUR-OWN-PACE AEROBICS + FLEXIBILITY	PROGRESSIVE PACED AEROBICS + STRENGTH	OFF	YOUR-OWN-PACE AEROBICS + FLEXIBILITY	PROGRESSIVE LIGHT, LONGER AEROBICS	OFF

SPECIFIC EXAMPLE: WEEK ONE - MARY JONES

DAY 1	DAY 2	DAY 3	DAY OFF	DAY 4	DAY 5	DAY OFF
PROGRESSIVE Walk 1 mile in 20 minutes + STRENGTH	YOUR-OWN-PACE Bike 30 minutes (5 miles) + FLEXIBILITY	PROGRESSIVE Walk 1 mile in 20 minutes + STRENGTH	OFF	YOUR-OWN-PACE Bike 30 minutes (5 miles) + FLEXIBILITY	PROGRESSIVE LIGHT, LONGER Walk 45 minutes in a park (visiting with a friend)	OFF

SPECIFIC EXAMPLE: WEEK TWO - MARY JONES

DAY 1	DAY 2	DAY 3	DAY OFF	DAY 4	DAY OFF	DAY 5
PROGRESSIVE Walk 1 mile in 19 minutes, 45 seconds + STRENGTH	YOUR-OWN-PACE Swim 30 minutes + FLEXIBILITY	PROGRESSIVE Walk 1 mile in 19 minutes, 45 seconds + STRENGTH	OFF	YOUR-OWN-PACE Aerobic dance class 60 minutes including FLEXIBILITY	OFF	PROGRESSIVE LIGHT, LONGER Wash/Wax/ Clean Car 50 minutes

 © 1993, *The Balancing Act Nutrition and Weight Guide*, G. Kostas, M.P.H., R.D., Dallas, Texas

6. CREATE YOUR OWN PLAN, BASED ON THE PRINCIPLES DESCRIBED. FILL IN THIS CHART.

DAY 1	DAY 2	DAY 3	DAY 4	DAY 5	DAY 6	DAY 7

7. **WHAT TO EXPECT:**

- Each week, your fitness will improve as you pick up your pace. A faster metabolism results. Allow 6-12 weeks to see vast improvements in your pace, strength, and endurance as well as your inches and weight.

- Allow approximately 3 hours a week to exercise.

- You'll lose 1/2 lb. fat each week when you burn approximately 1,500 calories a week (200-300 calories daily) from becoming active 3 hours a week.

YOU DON'T FEEL LIKE EXERCISING TODAY?

Tell Yourself:

"Every little bit helps."

"Something is better than nothing."

PROGRESSIVE AEROBIC FITNESS GOALS

These are gradually progressive exercise levels of fitness. Use these as a guide as you work toward improving your fitness level, using the PROGRESSIVE-PACED exercise system.

WALKING EXERCISE PROGRAM

LEVEL	DISTANCE (miles)	TIME (min.)
1	1.0	20:00
2	1.0	18:00
3	1.0	16:00
4	1.0	15:00
5	1.5	27:00
6	1.5	26:00
7	1.5	25:00
8	1.0	14:25
9	2.0	33:00
10	2.0	32:00
11	1.5	21:40
12	2.0	28:50
13	2.0	28:30
14	2.5	37:00
15	2.5	35:00
16	2.0	27:00
17	2.5	34:00
18	3.0	45:00

BEGINNER JOGGING PROGRAM

LEVEL	ACTIVITY	DISTANCE (miles)	TIME (min.)
1	Walk/Jog	1.0	12:00
2	Walk/Jog	1.0	11:00
3	Walk/Jog	1.0	10:00
4	Jog	1.0	9:00
5	Jog	1.5	16:00
6	Jog	1.5	15:00
7	Jog	1.5	14:00
8	Jog	1.5	13:00
9	Jog	2.0	21:00
10	Jog	2.0	20:00
11	Jog	2.0	19:00
12	Jog	2.0	18:00
13	Jog	2.5	27:00
14	Jog	2.5	26:00
15	Jog	2.5	25:00
16	Jog	3.0	32:00
17	Jog	3.0	31:00
18	Jog	3.0	30:00

SWIMMING EXERCISE PROGRAM

LEVEL	DISTANCE (yards)	TIME (min.)
1	300	15:00
2	300	12:00
3	400	15:00
4	400	13:00
5	500	16:00
6	500	14:00
7	600	17:00
8	600	15:00
9	700	20:00
10	700	18:00
11	800	22:00
12	800	20:00
13	900	24:00
14	900	22:00
15	1000	26:00
16	1000	25:00

STATIONARY CYCLING EXERCISE PROGRAM

LEVEL	LOAD	SPEED (mph/rpm)	TIME (min.)
1	1.5	15/55	4:00
2	1.5	15/55	6:00
3	1.5	15/55	8:00
4	1.5	15/55	10:00
5	2.0	15/55	10:00
6	2.0	15/55	12:00
7	2.0	15/55	14:00
8	2.0	15/55	16:00
9	2.0	15/55	18:00
10	2.0	15/55	20:00
11	2.5	17.5/65	18:00
12	2.5	17.5/65	20:00
13	2.5	20/75	20:00
14	2.5	20/75	20:00
15	2.5	20/75	25:00
16	3.0	20/75	30:00

You'll burn 200-300 calories (approximately) per session initially; 400-600 as you become more fit.

DIAGRAM A — EASY PRE-EXERCISE WARM-UP (5 MINUTES)

Guidelines: Before you exercise vigorously, prepare your body as follows:

- *Walk or cycle at slow rate for 3-5 minutes to warm up your muscles to prevent injury.*
- *Then spend 5-10 seconds per stretch below stretching slowly, relaxed, and with a controlled, fluid motion.*
- *Your warmed up muscles will help you move more easily, safely, longer, and faster.*

1. TO-THE-SIDE HEAD TURNS (4)

Standing erect, look slowly to the left; hold for 2 seconds. Look to the right; hold for 2 seconds.

4 LEFT/RIGHT HEAD TURNS

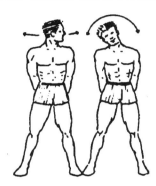

2. SHOULDER ROTATIONS (10)

Stand with arms hanging to your side. Rotate shoulders forward to rear.

10 ROTATIONS FORWARD/REAR

3. ELBOW ROTATIONS (15)

Place fingertips on shoulders, elbows pointing out to side. Draw large circles with both elbows forward to rear.

15 ROTATIONS REAR

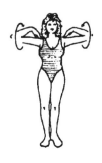

7. KNEE TO CHEST PULLS (2)

Lie down. Support knee with hands under the knee. Raise leg to bring knee to chest. Lower back to the ground. Hold for 10 seconds. Relax and repeat with second leg.

2 KNEE TO CHEST - 10-SECOND HOLD

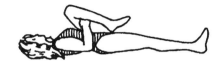

6. CALF RAISES (10)

Stand erect with feet shoulder-width apart. Raise heels as high as possible, then relax.

10 RAISES - 2-SECOND HOLD

5. THIGH STRETCHES (2)

Stand facing a wall. Brace yourself with left arm. Hold the top of your right foot behind you with your right hand. Gently pull your heel toward your buttocks. Hold 5 seconds. Repeat for the other side.

4 STRETCHES - 5-SECOND HOLD

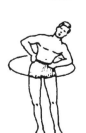

4. SMALL TRUNK CIRCLES (10)

Place hands on hips, keeping trunk still. Form small circle with upper body. Keeping shoulders still, draw circle with hips to left and right. Avoid giant circles.

10 CIRCLES LEFT AND RIGHT

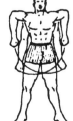

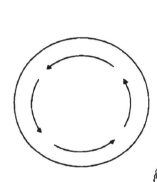

Program developed & sketches reprinted with permission from Philip Walker, M.S., Cooper Clinic Fitness Management Consultant.

© 1993, *The Balancing Act Nutrition and Weight Guide*, G. Kostas, M.P.H., R.D., Dallas, Texas   123

DIAGRAM B — STRENGTH CONDITIONING EXERCISES (30 MINUTES)
for muscle strength and endurance

Guidelines:

1. *Start with a comfortable number of repititions per exercise.*
   Beginners: *1-5 repititions.* ***Intermediates:*** *10-12 repetitions.* ***Conditioned:*** *18-20 repetitions.*
2. *As the exercise becomes easier, increase the number of repetitions.*

To Maximize Conditioning:

1. *Attempt the maximum repetitions (reps) you can do in 30 seconds for each exercise.*
2. *To strengthen your muscles, do 60-70% of your maximum reps. For example, if you can do 10 leg raises in 30 seconds, take (10 x .6) or 10 x .7) and do 6-7 repetitions.*
3. *As the exercise becomes easier, do steps 1 and 2 again.*

1. REAR LEG RAISES

Position yourself as below. Push leg to rear of body (to protect back, lift no higher than shoulder level) and return. After a set number of repetitions, change legs and repeat.

2. LATERAL LEG LIFTS

Lie on your side, lower leg slightly bent and hand supporting your head. Raise upper leg, keeping it straight. After a set number of repetitions, change legs.

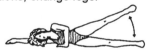

3. LATERAL LEG BEND

Lie on your back, arms out to sides with legs bent 90° and together. Keep shoulders flat, then lower legs to floor left and return; then lower to floor right. Repeat. After a set number of repetitions, change legs.

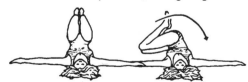

4. CALF RAISES

Stand erect, feet shoulder width apart and balls of feet on block or step. Raise heels to full extension. Then, lower heels. Repeat.

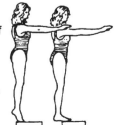

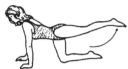

9. MODIFIED PUSH-UPS

Lie in prone position, hands under shoulders. Lift legs vertically, keeping your back straight. Push to full extention of arms. Relax to floor.

8. COORDINATED JUMPING (PARTIAL JUMPING JACKS)

Stand erect with hands by sides and feet together. With a jump, raise hands to horizontal position with feet opened. Jump to return. Repeat.

7. ABDOMINAL CRUNCHES

Lie on your back. Bend both legs 70-90° so the soles are flat on the floor and place your hands crossed over your chest. Slowly lift your upper body half way to vertical and slowly relax. Repeat.

6. LEG SWINGING

Stand, resting your left hand on a chair for support, feet shoulder width apart. Avoid high backkicks. Tighten your lower back and hip muscles to support lower back. Slowly swing your right leg forward and slightly backwards, keeping your toes pointed at all times. After a set number of repetitions, change legs.

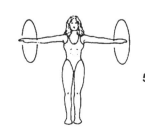

5. ARM CIRCLES

Stand erect with feet together and arms horizontal to side. Make a rapid small circle action to the rear, keeping arms and wrists locked.

Program developed & sketches reprinted with permission from Philip Walker, M.S., Cooper Clinic Fitness Management Consultant.

© 1993, *The Balancing Act Nutrition and Weight Guide*, G. Kostas, M.P.H., R.D., Dallas, Texas

DIAGRAM C — FLEXIBILITY STRETCHING EXERCISES (5-7 minutes)
for muscle flexibility, agility and relaxation

Guidelines:

1. *Select 6-10 exercises.*
2. *Do 1 of each exercise you selected.*

1. SEATED SHOULDER PRESS (1)

From a sitting position, raise your legs 90° and place both hands behind, resting on the floor, palms down. Keeping your feet firmly on the floor and your hands in the same position, raise your buttocks a few inches and move slowly towards your heels. Hold for 5 seconds and return to the relaxed position.

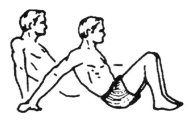

2. TRUNK TWISTING (1)

Lie on your back, resting on your elbows. Bend both legs fully. Keeping legs together and shoulders square, lower to the left. Use slow and controlled motions. Return and repeat to right. Hold position for 10 seconds. **DO NOT DO THIS IS YOU HAVE BACK PROBLEMS.**

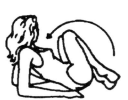

3. KNEE TO CHEST PULL (1)

Lie on your back. Support knee with hands under the knees. Raise bent left leg to chest. Lower your back to the ground. Hold for 10 seconds. Relax and repeat with right side.

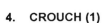

4. CROUCH (1)

Kneel, sitting forward on your heels. Do not sit on knees. Lean forward with hands as far forward as possible. Push downwards with your chest. Hold for 10 seconds. Relax and repeat.

8. HEAD ROTATIONS (3)

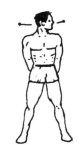

Kneeling or standing, slowly place chin to chest and roll head from left to right towards each shoulder.

7. SIDE BENDING (1)

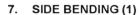

Stand erect with feet shoulder width apart, knees bent. Raise right arm over your head with left hand supported on leg. Bend body slowly to left, keeping your back straight. Hold for 5 seconds and repeat to right.

6. CALF STRETCH

Stand 2 full paces from a wall/tree. Lean forward placing hands above head. Place right leg (bent) forward and left leg outstretched to rear. Push downwards on left heel. Hold for 10 seconds. Relax and repeat with left leg.

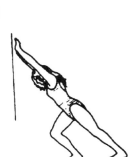

5. THIGH STRETCH (1)

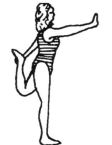

Stand facing a wall. Brace yourself with left arm. Hold the top of your right foot behind you with your right hand. Gently pull your heel toward your buttocks. Hold 5 seconds. Repeat for the other side.

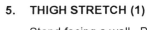

Program developed & sketches reprinted with permission from Philip Walker, M.S., Cooper Clinic Fitness Management Consultant.

EXERCISE EQUIVALENTS OF FOOD CALORIES

	Food	Calories	MINUTES OF ACTIVITY		
			Walking 3 mph 5 cal./min.	Bike Riding 8 cal./min.	Jogging/ Swimming 10 cal./min.
FRUIT	Apple, Banana, etc.				
	Large	100	20	12	10
	Medium	80	14	9	7
	Small	40	8	5	4
DAIRY	Cheese, American, 1 oz.	110	22	13	11
	Ice cream, rich, 1/2 cup	300	60	38	30
	Ice milk, 1/2 cup	100	20	12	10
	Malted milkshake, 12 oz.	400	80	50	40
	Milk, whole, 1 cup	150	30	19	15
	Milk, skim, 1 cup	90	16	10	8
VEGETABLE	Green beans, 1/2 cup cooked	15	3	2	1.5
	Carrot, raw	25	5	3	3
	Green peas, 1/2 cup cooked	70	14	9	7
STARCH	Bread, 1 slice	70	14	9	7
	Cereal, 3/4 cup, dry	100	20	12	10
	Pancake with 1 tablespoon syrup	150	30	19	15
	Potato, medium	160	28	18	14
MEAT	Bacon, 2 strips	100	20	12	10
	Chicken, fried, 1/2 breast	300	60	38	30
	Egg, fried	100	20	12	10
	Ribs (2 oz.)	200	40	24	20
	Pork chop, loin (3 oz.)	200	40	24	20
	Steak, T-bone (8 oz.)	640	130	80	64
	Fish, baked (3 oz.)	150	30	19	15
COMBI-NATIONS	Pizza (13"), cheese, 1/8	150	30	19	15
	Club sandwich	600	120	75	60
	Hamburger with bun	650	130	81	65
	Spaghetti with meat sauce, 1 cup	500	100	63	50
SWEETS and DESSERTS	Angel food cake, 1/12	140	28	18	14
	Cake with icing, 1/12	500	100	63	50
	Chocolate candy bar, 2 oz.	300	60	38	30
	Cookie, vanilla wafer, 6	100	20	12	10
	Doughnut, jelly	250	50	31	25
	Pie, Apple, 1/6	450	90	64	45
	Pie, Pecan, 1/6	750	150	94	75
MISC.	Soft drink, 12 ounces	150	30	19	15
	Mayonnaise, 1 tablespoon	100	20	12	10
	Salad dressing, 1 tablespoon	80	16	10	8

COOKING TIPS

HERE'S HOW TO INCREASE FLAVOR AND NUTRITION WHILE REDUCING CALORIES, FATS, SUGAR, AND SALT:

1. Choose fish, poultry and lean cuts of meat (see Meat group on page 59).

2. Eat more fish, poultry, veal (30-50 calories and 1-2 grams fat per ounce) and lean meat cuts like tenderloin, round (60 calories and 2-3 grams fat per ounce). Avoid cuts of high-fat red meat with visible fat (100 calories and 10 grams fat per ounce).

3. Trim excess fats from meats before cooking.

4. Remove skin from poultry before cooking.

5. Use water-packed tuna and salmon.

6. Bake, broil or boil rather than fry. (Frying can add 200 calories).

7. Use non-stick sprays and non-stick pans to replace oil for sautéing or stir-frying.

8. Chill soups and stews and lift off congealed fat or use a strainer to pour off fat.

9. Make gravies with fat-free broth, skim milk and cornstarch.

10. Prepare vegetables without added fat or sauces.

11. Cook onions, green pepper and other vegetables in a little broth instead of sautéing them in fat. Add garlic powder and onion powder to enhance flavor.

12. Season vegetables with herbs and spices and unsalted chicken or beef broth rather than bacon, butter, ham hocks or salt pork.

13. In cheese sauces, use skim milk and non-fat or low-fat cheese rather than whole milk, regular cheese and butter. Also, use evaporated skim milk for thicker sauces.

14. Serve foods simply, without added sauces.

15. Use evaporated **skim** milk instead of evaporated milk or light cream in a recipe.

16. Eliminate dabs of butter in casseroles. Use reduced-fat margarines or fat-free butter-flavored granules to season foods.

17. Instead of sour cream or vegetable dips, use plain non-fat yogurt blended with non-fat cottage cheese and seasonings, or mix plain non-fat yogurt and a ranch dressing packet. Also, use on baked potatoes and salads.

18. Use non-fat cottage cheese (blended) in place of cream cheese or sour cream in recipes. Or, use new fat-free sour cream and cream cheese products.

19. Replace oil in cake, brownie, and muffin recipes or packaged mixes with an equal portion of applesauce or strained fruit (baby food), or non-fat yogurt or low-fat buttermilk.

20. Reduce sugar in recipes 1/4 to 1/3 without affecting the final product; reduce fat by 1/2.

21. Use naturally sweet flavors instead of excess sugar such as vanilla, cinnamon, almond and cherry extracts, raisins, banana or concentrated apple juice.

22. Select fresh fruits as sweet desserts.

ADDITIONAL TIPS TO REDUCE SODIUM:

1. Omit salt in recipes. Other seasonings are much more flavorful.

2. Use pure herbs and spices or an herb-and-spice blend to enhance the flavor of foods.

3. Buy **unsalted** broth, bouillon, tomato juice, crackers, pretzels, catsup, mustard, salad dressings, etc. READ THE LABELS!!

4. Make your own chicken broth. Freeze in cubes for later use.

5. Use onion and garlic powder rather than onion and garlic salt.

6. Buy fresh, frozen or low-sodium canned vegetables.

7. Replace 1 cup of buttermilk with 1 cup of non-fat milk + 1 tablespoon lemon juice in recipes.

LOW-FAT COOKING SUBSTITUTES

Recipe calls for:	Substitute:
1 whole egg	1/4 c egg substitute or 2 egg whites
1 c shortening or butter (baking)	3/4 c liquid oil or 1 c margarine (2 sticks)
1 Tbsp oil/butter (sautéing)	2 Tbsp broth or wine, or 1 tsp oil with non-stick cooking spray and non-stick pan, or diet margarine
1 Tbsp shortening or butter	2 tsp liquid oil or 1 Tbsp margarine or 1 Tbsp diet margarine
1 Tbsp butter (seasoning)	1 Tbsp reduced-fat margarine or fat-free butter-flavored granules (i.e. Molly McButter)
1 square chocolate (1 oz.)	3 Tbsp dry cocoa powder + 1/2 Tbsp liquid oil
1 c whole milk or cream	1 c skim milk or 1 c skim evaporated milk
1 c sour cream	1 c nonfat yogurt or fat-free or low-fat cottage cheese (blenderized) or 1 c nonfat sour cream
1 oz. cream cheese	1 oz. low-fat cottage cheese (blenderized) or 1 oz. fat-free or low-fat cream cheese
1/4 c oil (in baking) (cake mixes, brownies, muffins, pancakes)	2 Tbsp oil + 2 Tbsp nonfat yogurt or 1/4 c applesauce or 1/4 c mashed banana or 1/4 c strained fruit (baby food) or 1/4 c pureed or strained prunes or 1/4 c nonfat yogurt
1 egg + 3 Tbsp oil (in cake or brownie mix)	1/2 c nonfat plain yogurt
1 Tbsp mayonnaise	1 Tbsp fat-free or reduced-fat mayonnaise, or 2 Tbsp nonfat yogurt (in tuna or potato salad, etc.)
1 c cream soup	1 c reduced-fat cream soup (i.e. Campbell's Healthy Request Cream Soup)
1 oz. cheese (American, cheddar, etc.)	1 oz. of reduced-fat or fat-free cheese, or 3/4 oz. regular cheese (or grate cheese to use less)
1/2 c nuts	1/2 cup Grapenuts or omit completely

YOUR FAVORITE FOODS MADE HEALTHY!!

1. Baked potato — add low-fat or nonfat yogurt + low-fat mozzarella cheese; or diet margarine; or soy sauce, or spaghetti or picante sauce; or fat-free Ranch dressing; or "butter" granules.

2. Pizza — use pita bread or flour tortilla for crust + lean ground meat (drained) or chicken; or a vegetarian pizza with low-fat cheese.

3. Lasagna — use chicken or make a vegetarian lasagna.

4. Taco shell — hang flour tortilla over 2 rods in the oven and bake at 400 degrees until crisp.

5. Tortilla chips — cut flour tortillas into quarters and bake at 400 degrees until crisp; or toast tortilla in toaster; then break into chips.

6. French fries — spray pan with non-stick spray and slice a red potato very thin; place slices on a pan (do not overlap); sprinkle with parmesan cheese and seasonings of choice. Broil until tender or bake 1 hour, turning once.

7. Stir-fry vegetables in fat-free broth, water or wine instead of oil until just crisp-tender.

8. A milkshake can be made by blending 1 cup of skim milk (2 percent), fresh or frozen fruit, flavor extract, cinnamon and ice. This is a refreshing dessert without the excess sugar or fat calories. Also make a juice shake with fruit and fruit juice.

9. Granola can be homemade without the excess sugar, honey or fats.

10. Snack on air-popped or microwave "light" popcorn or unsalted pretzels rather than deep fried chips. Save about 200 calories.

11. Blend air-popped and microwave "light" popcorn to cut fat and increase flavor.

12. Blend 1 commercial box of chex mix with other cereals, i.e. bran chex, corn chex, wheat chex, rice chex. You'll dilute fat and salt per cup.

13. Blend unsalted and salted pretzels to cut salt.

FUN FOODS

1. Veggies and Dip — 1 cup raw vegetables + 1/2 cup yogurt-based dip.
2. Nachos — 1 corn tortilla (quartered and toasted) + 1 ounce nonfat or low-fat cheese + jalepeno pepper slices.
3. Tortilla chips — cut flour tortillas into quarters and bake at 400 degrees until crisp.
4. Taco shell — place flour tortilla over 2 rods in oven and bake at 400 degrees until crisp.
5. Wholewheat crackers — toasted Shredded Wheat cereal (2/3 cup).
6. Cheese toast — 1 slice reduced-calorie bread + 1 ounce mozzarella cheese.
7. Celery and cheese — 3 celery sticks + 1 ounce skim ricotta cheese filling.
8. Cheesy popcorn — 2 cups air-popped popcorn + 2 tablespoons parmesan cheese.
9. Buttered popcorn — 2 cups air-popped popcorn + butter flavored granules (Butter Buds).
   TIP: To make seasonings stick to air-popped popcorn, spray popper with non-stick cooking spray and add seasonings. Then add and pop popcorn.
10. Herbed popcorn — combine 1/2 teaspoon each marjoram, oregano, basil, onion powder and garlic powder; shake on popcorn.
11. Nacho popcorn — shake nacho or taco seasoning mix on popcorn.
12. Cheesy potato — 1 small baked potato + 1 ounce nonfat or low-fat cheese.
13. French fries — broil red potato slices; sprinkle with parmesan cheese.
14. Mexican potato — 1 small baked potato + picante sauce.
15. Chinese potato — 1 small baked potato + "lite" (low-sodium) soy sauce.
16. Italian potato — 1 small baked potato + 3 tablespoons spaghetti sauce.
17. Greek potato — 1 small baked potato + 1 tablespoon crumbled feta cheese + 1 tablespoon nonfat yogurt.
18. Yogurt potato — 1 small baked potato + low-fat yogurt + low-fat mozzarella cheese.
19. Mini pizza — 1 tortilla or English muffin half + 2 tablespoons tomato sauce + 1 tablespoon grated cheese + 2 tablespoons green pepper.
20. Lasagna — use chicken or make a vegetarian lasagna.
21. Stir-fry vegetables in fat-free broth, water or wine instead of oil until just crisp-tender.
22. Cereal and milk — 1/2 cup cereal + 1/2 cup non-fat milk.
23. Fruit and yogurt — 1/2 cup mixed fruit topped with 1/2 cup plain yogurt.
24. Milkshakes — blenderize 1 cup skim milk + fresh fruit (frozen) + flavor extract + cinnamon + ice. (A refreshing dessert without excess sugar and fat calories.)
25. Chocolate treat — 1/2 cup plain yogurt + 1/2 packet sugar-free cocoa drink mix.

VEGETABLE IDEAS

Are you eating vegetables every day? Balance your act with more veggie ideas!!!

1. To spaghetti, meat or pizza sauce, add grated carrots, onions, mushrooms and green peppers.

2. To lasagna, add a layer of broccoli or spinach.

3. To casseroles, add green peas, carrots, celery, onion, green pepper and mushrooms for color and flavor.

4. To baked beans, chili, Mexican bean dishes and meatloaf, add extra tomato sauce, canned tomatoes and carrots (grated or diced).

5. To potato salad, add carrots, peas, and celery.

6. To soups: add mixed vegetables, potatoes, corn and beans.

7. Blend vegetables into potato soup. The soup looks like a creamed soup without vegetables.

8. Stuff a baked potato with:
   - spinach + low-fat or nonfat cheese + nonfat yogurt
   - broccoli + mushrooms + low-fat or nonfat cheese
   - low-fat cheese + nonfat yogurt + canned tomatoes
   - spaghetti sauce + low-fat or nonfat cottage cheese or ricotta
   - fat-free sour cream and picante sauce

9. Make spinach or broccoli dips, using nonfat yogurt or cottage cheese as a base.

10. Eat stir-fried vegetable dishes. "Stir-fry" with broth, or cook mushrooms first and use their "juice" for "stir-frying".

11. Make a vegetarian pizza with lots of tomato, zucchini, green or red pepper, onion, mushroom, olives and carrots.

12. Melt low-fat cheese on vegetables, or use fat-free "butter" granules.

13. Stuff vegetables, such as stuffed squash, tomatoes, peppers. For stuffing, use rice and ground turkey or tuna salad, or beans/rice mixture.

14. Stuff a pita pocket with mixed vegetables or salad.

15. Try succotash (corn + lima bean mixture).

16. Have zucchini or carrot muffins and bread.

17. Make a shish-ka-bob of vegetables and add more vegetables to meat shish-ka-bobs.

18. Fill tortillas with spinach, cottage cheese, parmesan cheese and heat.

19. Buy baby carrots, already washed, peeled, and ready to eat.

20. Eat more beans: black beans, navy beans, etc. — add to rice, spaghetti sauces, tortillas, soups. Blend beans with picante sauce for bean spread.

21. Try vegetables raw and chilled:

   a. raw vegetables with a yogurt-based dip, salsa, hot sauce, Ranch dressing
   b. big tossed salads with a wide variety of vegetables
   c. cold green bean, 3 bean or green pea salads
   d. carrot-raisin salad
   e. Waldorf salad (apples, celery, cheese, nuts, green pepper)
   f. fruit salads with sliced carrots and celery
   g. jello salad with grated carrots in place of fruit
   h. spinach salads with added fruit (oranges, etc.)
   i. coleslaw with fruit (raisins, pineapple, apple) for sweeteners
   j. marinated vegetables (sliced carrots, celery, cherry tomatoes, mushrooms, broccoli, yellow squash, zucchini combined with vinaigrette dressing)
   k. pickled vegetables

22. Eat more beans (rich in all vegetable nutrients):

   a. bean soup
   b. bean chili
   c. bean tacos, enchiladas and Mexican dishes
   d. beans on salads

23   Sweet potato pie for dessert!

24. Popcorn for snacks!

25. Tomato or carrot juice for beverages.

REMEMBER:

The 4 most nutrient-rich vegetables are —

Potatoes, Beans, Broccoli, Carrots!

V
REDUCING FOOD CUES AND FOOD FATS

HABIT FOCUS

1. "Eliminate Food Cues" that trigger eating (135-136).
2. Identify your cues and solutions (137).

NUTRITION FOCUS

1. Decrease "Fats-Cholesterol" to reduce weight and risk of atherosclerosis (138-139).
2. Compare "Fats-Cholesterol List" of foods (141).
3. Choose more foods with low to medium "Percent Fat Calories" (142).
4, Determine "15 ways to eat less fat" (143).
5. Select "Cheeses" wisely (144-145).

EXERCISE FOCUS

Keep exercising 3-5 times a week!

RECORDS

Don't forget! Records keep you on your toes!

GOALS
HABIT:	Avoid or remove food cues from your environment
FOOD:	Eat 10 poultry or fish meats this week
EXERCISE:	Exercise 5 times this week
RECORDS:	Food, exercise, weight - count poultry and fish meals eaten

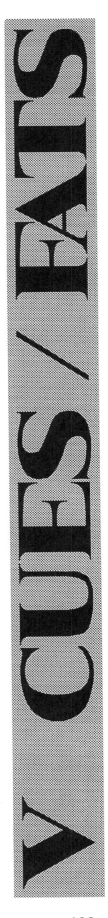

V CUES/FATS

ELIMINATE FOOD CUES!

DO YOU MINIMIZE FOOD CONTACT? DO YOU KNOW WHAT TRIGGERS OVER-EATING FOR YOU? Food cues are signals that lead you to eat, even when you are not hungry. Cue elimination is getting rid of those signals that say "Time to eat" such as vending machines, bakeries, restaurants, ice cream shops, T.V., movies, afternoons, ads, coupons, "specials", etc. You can either avoid or remove "cues" or change your response to them.

Can you think of any **environmental cues** that provoke hunger for a meal or snack?

1.   4.
2.   5.
3.   6.

Look at the following situations that provide food exposure. What can you do to minimize your food contact and vulnerability with each situation?

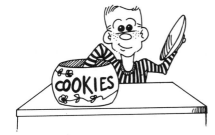

Storing Food

1. Store food out of sight and in inconvenient places. "Out of sight, out of mind."
2. Remove food from all places in the house other than appropriate storage areas such as candy jar on top of the T.V., nuts in the living room, etc.
3. Store problem foods in opaque containers that you cannot see through.
4. Rearrange the refrigerator and cupboards by "hiding" problem foods in the back. Put less tempting or low-calorie foods in front.
5. Keep natural wrappers on foods until ready to use them.
6. **Encourage** all non-overweight family members to keep problem foods (candy, etc.) out of sight.

Serving Food

1. Serve from the **stove** in allotted portions.
2. Avoid serving dishes on the table. This encourages seconds.
3. Let someone else serve your plate.
4. If serving dishes are on the table, place them away from you and ask that others not pass them your way.

Cleaning Up

1. Clean up immediately and have someone else scrape the dishes.
2. Put away leftovers immediately to avoid the temptation to finish them. (Maybe have someone else put them away.)
3. Don't ruin your day by eating leftovers or any food on another's plate.
4. Soak cooking utensils and dishes while you eat.

After-Dinner Activities

1. Leave the table immediately and involve yourself in activities.
2. If you plan to remain at the table and converse, remove the plates and serving dishes. Sip on water, coffee or tea, if anything.
3. Eat a sugar-free mint or brush your teeth immediately after a meal as a signal that the meal is over.
4. Clean up immediately.
5. Serve after-dinner coffee or tea, or calorie-free beverage in another area to change the setting and the habit.

Where Do You Eat?

If you eat in many different places at home, you may develop expectations to eat when in that area — at the kitchen sink, in the T.V. room, in your favorite chair, in the bedroom, etc. Learn to control your eating environment.

1. Designate an appropriate eating place for all meals and snacks, such as dining room table, restaurant table, etc.
2. Make this place attractive and inviting.
3. If you are already eating at the table, change your place at the table to increase your eating awareness.
4. Sit down whenever you eat anything. This helps you control "extra" unconscious eating while lying down or standing to prepare food or grabbing food from the refrigerator.
5. Avoid places where you tend to overeat, such as restaurants, buffets, etc.
6. Avoid activities such as talking on the phone, visiting with friends, writing letters, reading in the kitchen, whenever possible.

What Do You Do While Eating?

1. When you are eating, only eat!
2. Eliminate distractions so that you can concentrate on enjoying your food and the company with you.
3. Taste your food, feel the texture, and savor each bite.
4. Don't let reading, writing, watching T.V. make you oblivious to a delicious meal.
5. Identify emotion-related eating: boredom, fatigue, anger, guilt, stress, loneliness. Alter your response to these circumstances. (Refer to the "Pleasure Activities" list on p. 30.)
6. Make a list of alternative activities to replace over-eating: necessities, hobbies, exercises, relaxation, etc.

1.	3.	5.
2.	4.	6.

ELIMINATE FOOD CUES!

Complete Your Worksheet:

	FOOD CUES	YOUR RESPONSE	SOLUTIONS	RESULTS
1.	Donuts at office Why? visibility, social.	Not hungry. Eat because convenient and social activity.	Sip non-caloric drink while socializing. Keep distance from food. Talk, talk, talk.	Entered room with coffee. Was late to minimize food exposure.
2.	Popcorn at movies Why? aroma, association.	Buy popcorn even if not hungry.	Avoid popcorn area and inviting lines. Take sugar-free drink and gum.	Enjoy own snacks and sense of control.
3.	Alcohol at social events. Why? Social expectation. **ADD YOUR OWN BELOW:**	Keep drink in hand throughout event.	Arrive late to drink less. Limit to 1 caloric drink only. Keep non-caloric drink in hand, club soda, mineral water, etc.	No peer pressure to drink. Did not miss alcohol. Enjoyed friends more.
4.				
5.				
6.				

FATS - CHOLESTEROL

- Diet is one of many factors associated with heart disease, particularly the development of atherosclerosis.

- Atherosclerosis, or "hardening of the arteries", is the disease process that underlies the most serious and common cardiovascular disorders. It is the result of elevated blood fats that deposit on artery walls and harden. This narrows blood vessels impairing blood flow and leads to heart attacks and strokes.

- You can limit the progression of atherosclerosis or even reverse it with appropriate eating, exercise, and a healthy weight.

HOW TO DECREASE YOUR RISK OF DEVELOPING ATHEROSCLEROSIS

1. Eat a nutritious, balanced diet, low in fat, high in fiber.
2. Attain and maintain a desirable weight.
3. Minimize the amount of cholesterol, total fat, and saturated fat you eat.
4. Modify the type of fat in your diet: eat more unsaturated (vegetable) fats and less saturated (animal) fats. Unsaturated fats are polyunsaturated or monounsaturated.
5. Eat more complex carbohydrates such as fresh fruits, vegetables, peas, beans, potatoes, corn and wholegrained or enriched grains such as breads, cereals, brown rice, oats and pasta. These are nutritious, high-fiber and free of cholesterol and fat.
6. Eat less protein - 4-6 oz./day of lean meat, fish, poultry; and no more than 3 eggs per week.
7. Do not smoke.
8. Exercise aerobically 3-5 times a week. Get fit!
9. Keep blood cholesterol and triglyceride levels normal (see pg. 140).
10. Keep your blood pressure and blood sugar normal.
11. Eat seafood 2-3 times a week because the omega-3 fatty acids in fish will lower cholesterol and triglycerides.
12. Eat more soluble fiber in oatmeal and beans (1/2 - 1 cup daily) to lower cholesterol.

FATS IN OUR FOODS

Dietary cholesterol
- fat-type substance in animal sources only
- contributes to elevated blood cholesterol
- Sources
  o egg yolks, liver and organ meats, lard, such as meat fat
  o whole milk and dairy products, such as butter, cream, cheese, ice cream
  o meat and meat products, such as sausage, cold cuts, beef, ham, pork, lamb, bacon
- "Cholesterol-free" foods
  o foods of **plant** origin - fruit, vegetables, grains, beans, peas
  o skim milk and yogurt
  o polyunsaturated oils and margarine; monounsaturated fats
  o cholesterol-free cheeses, egg substitutes, etc.
- Eat no more than 100-300 mg. cholesterol daily (150 mg are in 6 oz. poultry/fish/meat).

© 1993, *The Balancing Act Nutrition and Weight Guide*, G. Kostas, M.P.H., R.D., Dallas, Texas

Saturated fats

- fats of **animal** origin usually
- contribute to elevated blood cholesterol and triglycerides
- Sources
    - visible or "hidden" fat in meat (beef, lamb, pork, sausage, bacon, hot dogs, etc.)
    - dairy products made from whole milk or cream (butter, whole milk, cheese, cream, sour cream, ice cream)
    - coconut and palm (kernel) oils
    - cocoa butter (in chocolate)
    - "hydrogenated" or "hardened" vegetable oils (in peanut butter, stick margarine, crackers, commercial bakery products, etc.)

Polyunsaturated fats

- fats of **plant** origin usually
- help to lower blood cholesterol
- Sources
    - safflower, corn, sunflower, soybean, cottonseed oils
    - soft tub margarines made from these oils, with "liquid oil" listed as first ingredient
    - unhydrogenated ("natural") peanut butter, where oil separates out
    - seafood

Monounsaturated fats

- fats of **plant** origin
- help to lower blood cholesterol
- Sources
    - olive oil, olives
    - peanuts, peanut oil
    - canola oil

Total fats

- women: eat 20-30 grams fat daily for weight loss; 50 grams for maintenance
- men: eat 30-60 grams fat daily for weight loss; 70 grams for maintenance
- easy way to achieve this daily:

eat 4-6 oz./day of lean meat/fish/poultry	=	4-18 grams fat
eat 3-6 tsp./day of unsaturated fats	=	15-30 grams fat
eat fruit, vegetables, grains, beans	=	0-10 grams fat
	Daily total	**19-58 grams fat**

KEY TIPS

- **Eat the right amount and type of fat daily and you will lose weight more quickly and keep it off, lower your blood cholesterol and triglyceride levels, and reduce your risk of heart disease.**

- **Lose 10 pounds, and cholesterol drops 25 points!**

FATS IN BLOOD

Serum cholesterol

- fat-type substance
- excessive amounts deposit in arterial walls
- HDL is "good" cholesterol that prevents fat deposits
- LDL is "bad" cholesterol that cuases fat deposits
- total cholesterol to HDL ratio is a key predictor of heart health
- To **lower** LDL and total cholesterol:
  - limit foods rich in cholesterol, saturated fat and total fat
  - eat more polyunsaturated and monounsaturated fats in place of saturated fats
  - attain recommended body weight
  - exercise aerobically 3-5 days per week
- To **raise** HDL:
  - exercise aerobically the equivalent workout of walking/jogging 11-15 miles per week
  - do not smoke
  - lose weight

Serum triglycerides

- type of fat
- elevated levels may promote heart disease
- To **lower** triglyceride levels:
  - attain your recommended body weight
  - reduce your intake of animal fats
  - reduce alcohol, sugar and sugar-rich foods, such as soft drinks, candy, honey, desserts, etc.
  - exercise aerobically

Desired Levels

Total cholesterol	less than	200
HDL cholesterol		45-55
LDL cholesterol	less than	130
cholesterol to HDL ratio	less than	4.0 (men)
	less than	3.0 (women)
triglycerides	less than	120

FAT - CHOLESTEROL LIST

Use this guide to eat less total fat, saturated fat, and cholesterol.

Daily Goals: 20-30 grams fat (women) or 30-60 grams fat (men) — for weight loss
50 grams fat (women) or 70 grams fat (men) — for weight maintenance
100-300 mg cholesterol
10-15 grams saturated fat
or, the advise of your physician or registered dietitian.

FOOD	SERVING SIZE	CHOLES-TEROL (milligrams)	SATURATED FAT (grams)	TOTAL FAT (grams)
Egg	1	213	1.5	6
Liver, beef	3 ounce	370	3.5	9
Beef, pork, lamb (lean)	3 ounce	75	3.5	8
Veal, lean	3 ounce	90	2.5	5
Chicken, Turkey (light meat without skin)	3 ounce	60	1.3	3
Fish	3 ounce	45	.1	2.5
Oysters, clams, crab	3 ounce	120	.1	2.1
Shrimp (15 medium), lobster	3 ounce	95	.2	1.0
Frankfurter, all beef	1	32	6.5	17
Cold cuts	3 ounce	75	6.5	21
Cheese, American or cheddar	1 ounce	25	6.0	10
Cheese, mozzarella (part skim)	1 ounce	15	3.0	5
Cheese, cottage (1 percent fat)	1 cup	5	1.5	2.5
Cheese, ricotta (part skim)	1 cup	40	6.0	10
Cream cheese (2 tablespoons)	1 ounce	30	5.0	10
Milk, whole	1 cup	35	5.0	8
Milk, skim	1 cup	5	0	2.5
Yogurt, low-fat	8 ounce	15	2.5	6
Yogurt, nonfat	8 ounce	5	0.0	0
Ice cream	1 cup	55	8.0	18
Ice milk	1 cup	15	3.0	6
Butter	1 tablespoon	35	7.0	14
Margarine, tub	1 tablespoon	0	2.0	11
Oil, vegetable	1 tablespoon	0	0.0	14

NOTE: Not all foods are high in both cholesterol and saturated fat. Cut down on foods containing large amounts of **either**.

PERCENT FAT CALORIES IN FOODS

LOW-FAT (< 15%)

Fruit
Vegetables
Grains (bread, cereal, pasta, rice, oatmeal, tortillas, melba toast, popcorn)
Beans and peas (legumes) cooked without bacon, salt pork, ham
Skim milk
Seafood (cod, sole, perch, trout, shrimp, halibut, flounder, etc.)
Canned tuna in water

MEDIUM-FAT (25-45%)

2% fat milk, low-fat yogurt, ice milk
Skim milk (diet) cheeses, i.e., Weight Watcher's, Borden's, Lite Line, 1% fat cottage cheese, skim ricotta, Laughing Cow reduced-calorie.
Chicken, turkey, poultry without skin
Granola

HIGH-FAT (50-75%)

Low-fat cheeses (mozzarella, parmesan, bonbel, fondue)
Chicken, turkey, poultry with skin
Lean meat with fat removed before cooking (flank, tenderloin, top sirloin)
Party crackers
Chocolate

VERY HIGH-FAT (80-100%)

Whole milk
Most cheeses (American, colby, cheddar, Swiss, co-jack, etc.)
Cream soups, cream cheese
Cream (sweet or sour)
Ice cream
Dips

Meat without fat removed or trimmed
Prime rib, brisket, spare ribs
Sausage, bacon, hot dogs
Cold cuts, hamburger meat

Salad dressing
Mayonnaise
Margarine

Nuts, seeds
Olives, avocado
Peanut butter
Chips
Desserts

15 WAYS TO HELP YOU EAT LESS FAT

1. Eat less protein: 4-6 oz./day TOTAL of lean meat, poultry, seafood, cheese.

2. Add less fat to foods: 3-6 tsp. (or 1-2 tbsp) daily of margarine, butter, mayonnaise, salad dressings, sauces, gravies, cream.

3. Eat more (at least 10) complex carbohydrate foods/day (fruit, vegetables, bread, cereal, grains, starches, beans). These are fat-free, high in fiber, and very "filling" . . . ideal for weight control.

4. Let 3/4 of your plate contain plant foods (vegetables, starches, beans) and 1/4 of your plate contain protein (entree).

5. Eat fewer high-fat foods (meat, ground beef, cheese, hot dogs, sausage, ice cream, whole milk, fried foods, greasy foods, donuts, sweet rolls, candy bars, desserts, crackers, fast food, mayonnaise, salad dressings, creamy or cheese toppings).

6. Cook with less fat. Broil, bake, grill, steam, boil, stir-fry. Use vegetable sprays and butter substitutes (i.e., Molly McButter). Keep It Simple and Sensible (KISS principle).

7. Read food labels. Select foods with 0-3 grams fat per 100 calories.

8. Eat out selectively. Split entrees. Get dressings and sauces on the side to add conservatively. Order grilled, baked, broiled, boiled, steamed foods.

9. Collect 8-10 great lowfat recipes you enjoy. Buy a lowfat cookbook. Keep recipes simple, with 5-6 ingredients at most. Choose easy, convenient, quick recipes.

10. Eat spicy foods — you won't miss fattening sauces. Add picante sauce, ginger, Italian spice blends, etc.

11. Eat more all-vegetable meals (salads, soups, baked potatoes, pasta, vegetables, beans).

12. Vary protein sources: 3-4 chicken, 3-4 fish, 3-4 lean meat,
                               3-4 all-vegetables meals/week.

13. Choose specialty, lowfat products . . .reduced-calorie margarines, lowfat and fat-free salad dressings and mayonnaise, nonfat yogurt, skim milk, nonfat and lowfat cheeses, tuna in water, "lite" frozen dinners, butter-flavored sprinkles.

14. With beef, choose lean cuts (filet, tenderloin, flank, top round, top sirloin) of "select" grade. Eat 3-4 oz. portions; cook without added fats.

15. Choose lowfat treats and toppings . . .
    *   yogurt, cottage cheese, picante sauce, butter sprinkles on baked potatoes
    *   cottage cheese, picante sauce, wine vinegar, lemon on salads
    *   bagels, fruit, "lite" popcorn, pretzels, popsicles, frozen nonfat yogurt or ice milk, Cheerios

CHEESES

Cheese is a nutritious food, unless eaten in excess. Eat cheese for calcium, Vitamin A, quality protein and other nutrients. Since most cheeses are high in total fat, saturated fat, cholesterol, calories and sodium, select cheeses wisely. Choose **fat-free, low-fat, medium-fat** (reduced-fat) or **cholesterol-free** cheeses. Avoid **high-fat** cheeses completely, or eat them only occasionally. Popular high-fat cheeses contain 1 tablespoon of butterfat per 1 ounce (1 oz.) cheese — usually one slice. Eight slices of traditional cheese contain 8 tablespoons of butterfat...equal to one stick of butter!

READ FOOD LABELS BEFORE BUYING CHEESE. Select cheeses with 5 or less grams of fat per ounce.

CHOLESTEROL-FREE CHEESES: (vary in fat and calories)
Butterfat is replaced with skim milk and/or corn oil. Example: Golden Image Cheese (Kraft).

FAT-FREE CHEESES (no fat): Contain a trace amount of fat and 30-50 cal. per oz. cheese

Alpine Lace Free 'n Lean cheeses —
  slices, cream cheese, cheesespreads
Borden's fat-free cheese and singles
Borden's fat-free cottage cheese
Frigo fat-free ricotta cheese
Guiltless Gourmet Nacho Cheesespread

Healthy Choice cheeses
Kraft Free Singles-American, cheddar
Kraft Healthy Favorites
Lifetime fat-free cheeses
Philly-free cream cheese
Smart Beat fat-free slices

LOW-FAT CHEESES (25% FAT): Contain 1-3 gm fat and 40-70 cal. per oz. cheese

Borden Lifeline slices (1-1/2 slices = 1 oz.)
  (1 slice = 35 calories)
Cheddar, skim
Cottage Cheese (dry, 1-2% fat)
Farmers (skim milk)
Gammelost
Hoop or Pot
Kraft Light 'N Lively slices (1-1/3 slices = 1 oz.)
  (1 slice = 35 calories)
Kraft Light Singles
Laughing Cow (skim milk) gruyere cheese
  wedges or mini-bonbel rounds

Le Maigrelait
Philadelphia Light Cream Cheese
Ricotta (part skim)
Sargento Moo Town Snackers Light String
  Cheese
Sargento Preferred Light Mozzarella
Smart Beat American Sandwich Slices
Tofu (from soybeans — cholesterol-free)
Weight Watcher's American or Mozzarella
  slices (1 slice = 1 ounce)
  (1 slice = 50 calories)

(continued on page 145)

REDUCED-FAT CHEESES (50% fat): Contain 4-7 gm fat and 70-90 cal. per oz. cheese
(These are medium-fat cheeses)

Alpine Lace Monti-Jack Lo
Bonbel
Borden Light American
Brie (low-fat milk)
Camembert (Domestic)
Edam
Feta
Fondue cheese
Formagg
Kraft Cracker Barrel Light
Kraft Light Naturals — Sharp Cheddar,
   Monterrey Jack, Mozzarella, Swiss, Colby

Mozzarella
Neufchatel (to replace cream cheese)
Nutrend (Merrywood Farms) — Hot Pepper,
   Smokey, Yellow American, Longhorn
Parmesan
Pizza cheese (Mozzarella)
Port du Salut (low-fat)
Rondele — Lite Soft Spreadable Cheese
Sargento Light — Cheddar, Swiss, Mozzarella
String Cheese (Mozzarella)
Velveeta Light Singles (Kraft)
   (1-1/3 slices = 1 oz.) (1 slice = 35 cal.)
Weight Watcher's Cheddar

HIGH-FAT CHEESES (90% fat): Contain 8-10 gm fat per 1 oz. cheese (100-110 cal. per oz.)

American (including slices)
Bleu cheese
Boursin
Brick
Brie
Cheddar — natural or processed
Colby
Co-Jack
Cracker Barrel (Kraft) — all types
Cream cheese
Fontina
Gjetost
Golden Image (Kraft)
Gouda
Gruyere

Havarti
Jarlsberg
Limburger
Longhorn
Monterrey Jack
Muenster
Parmesan
Port
Port du Salut
Provolone
Queso blanco white cheese
Romano
Roquefort
Scandic (mini-cholesterol)
Stilton
Swiss

PLEASE NOTE:
1. Sodium content of cheeses:
    1 ounce processed cheese = 400 milligrams sodium
    1 ounce natural cheese = 200 milligrams sodium
    1 ounce natural Swiss, gruyere, ricotta = 100 milligrams sodium
    Special "low-sodium" cheeses are now available: cheddar, colby, gouda, jack, muenster, cottage, etc.
2. 1 ounce of low-fat cheese = 1 ounce "lean meat" based on protein, calories and fat.
3. 1 ounce of low-fat cheese = 3/4 ounce of high-fat cheese, based on calories and fat.

VI
MIND YOUR P's and S's

HABIT FOCUS

1. **P** — "Planning" ahead prevents impulse eating (149). Use forms for "Meal Plans" (151-152) and plan 1-7 days in advance, referring to "sample" given.

2. **P** — "Portions Count" — measure portions for weight control (153).

3. **P** — "Pace" yourself (154).

NUTRITION FOCUS

1. **S** — "Sugar" — What? Where? Why? (155).

   Know your "Cereals" (161) — How Sweet It Is!

2. **S** — "Sodium" — sources, alternatives, comparisons (162-165).

3. Eat a pre-planned meal. Enjoy feeling "in charge" of what you eat.

RECORDS

How are those records coming?

GOALS

HABIT: practice portion control and pace yourself when eating (allow 20 minutes per meal). Plan meals in advance.

FOOD: decrease high-sugar, high-sodium foods - find alternatives.

EXERCISE: 30 minutes at least per workout, 5 days this week.

RECORDS: food, exercise, weight
Count high-sugar, high-sodium foods you eat.

Complete "End of Month progress Check" (Appendix A).

PLANNING

TO FAIL TO PLAN IS TO PLAN TO FAIL!!!

PLANNING prevents the day's circumstances, your moods, your environment, etc. from interfering with your good intentions.

Planning keeps you aware of your eating and prevents automatic or unconscious eating that may lead to compulsive eating.

THINK: "Is this food allowed on my plan?" "How much?" "Am I really hungry?"

PRIOR THOUGHT prevents impulse eating — and provides a lifetime of weight control.

MEALS

- A pre-thought plan for meals frees you from **thinking food** all day.

- **PLAN** your meals and snacks based on your eating pattern **before you eat,** not after you eat. **Write a day's menu a day or morning in advance** (or a week's menu for shopping efficiency) as this is the easiest, surest way to follow your pattern regularly and consistently.

- **Distribute your food** into 3 meals, spaced as evenly as possible. If you wish to **include a snack, PLAN** for it also.

- **PACK** a lunch — now you are in control of this meal!

- Write down several **VARIED** breakfast and lunch menus. Keep these meals **FUN!**

FOOD PREPARATION

- **MODIFY** recipes, substituting low-calorie ingredients for high-calorie ones.

- **SELECT** foods that require time to prepare. These allow you to think before you eat, whereas convenient foods do not (i.e., fruit salads, vegetable salads, milkshake, popcorn, tuna salad, fresh vegetables, etc.)

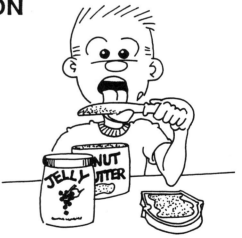

- **DO NOT LICK** utensils as you prepare foods or clean up. Those extra calories add up!

- **NO NIBBLING.** Sip on a low-calorie beverage or munch on a raw carrot.

- **SAMPLE AS LITTLE AS POSSIBLE.** Use a 1/4 tsp. measure for tasting.

BINGES

- Avoid foods in the house you are most likely to **BINGE** on.

- Follow a binge with a **CONSTRUCTIVE ACTIVITY** such as taking a walk, writing a letter or doing a chore. **DON'T FEEL GUILTY.** Decide how to prevent the situation in the future.

- Resolve to cut back on foods at the next meal or next day.

PROBLEM FOODS

- **DO NOT BUY THEM!**
- If they are in the house, make sure they are **concealed** and stored properly.
- Make a list of satisfying, low-calorie **food substitutes** for **problem foods**.
- Make a list of satisfying **alternative activities** to do in place of snacking: hobbies, music, reading, needlework, sewing, sports, walking, sleeping, relaxation, carpentry, necessary activities such as errands, house projects, phone calls, bills, letters, etc.
- If this food is impossible to avoid, include **one small serving** of it in your daily eating plan and omit its caloric equivalence in foods.
- **Delay** eating this food for 10 minutes. Chances are, you won't want it.

SNACKS

- It is okay to snack, but **snack sensibly** and plan it as a part of your meal plan. Keep the snacks low-calorie and portions small.
- Limit **empty calorie** snacks — those that supply calories but contain very few nutrients. These should be no more than 10 percent of your calorie intake.
  Example: On a 1500 calorie diet allow no more than 150 calories (1500 X 10 percent) for a snack; such as angel food cake (121 calories), 6 vanilla wafers (110 calories), 1/2 cup frozen yogurt (110 calories), etc.
- Keep **low-calorie snacks and free foods** convenient:
  - fresh fruits or vegetables
  - low-fat or skim cheeses
  - bread sticks or "thin" bread
  - melba toast or graham crackers
  - popcorn or pretzels (unsalted)
  - shredded wheat biscuits
  - skim or 2 percent milk
  - plain yogurt (may add fruit to it for "fruited yogurt")
  - low-cal milkshake or low-cal hot cocoa
  - vegetable or chicken noodle soup
  - angel food cake or vanilla wafers or popsicle
- Choose **crunchy, chewy** foods which are more satisfying.
- **Liquids** can fill an empty feeling, especially warm beverages.
- Foods high in **water** or **fiber** content or both are low in calories, such as popcorn, fruit, vegetables, shredded wheat, baked potato, etc.
- **Do not keep high-calorie snacks available.**
- Snack only in your designated **eating place**.
- Avoid excessive **evening** snacking. Plan the time you will snack and the amount.

MEAL PLANS

___ MILK	___ VEG.	___ FRUIT
___ STARCH	___ MEAT	___ FAT

SHOPPING LIST

	MONDAY SAMPLE	TUESDAY	WEDNESDAY	THURSDAY	FRIDAY	SATURDAY	SUNDAY
BREAKFAST							
Milk	1 cup skim milk						
Veg.							
Fruit	1 orange						
Starch	2 English muffin halves						
Meat							
Fat	1 tsp margarine						
Free							
LUNCH							
Milk							
Veg.							
Fruit	1 apple						
Starch	2 wholewheat bread slices						
Meat	2 oz. turkey						
Fat	1 tsp. mayon.						
Free	1 tsp. mustard lettuce, tomato slices						
SUPPER							
Milk							
Veg.	Salad ½ c. carrots ½ c. broccoli						
Fruit							
Starch	½ cup brown rice 1 roll						
Meat	3 oz. chicken, broiled						
Fat	1 Tbsp. Ranch dressing						
Free							
SNACKS	8 oz. fat-free yogurt 1 cup grapes						

TOTAL DAILY

	Monday SAMPLE	TUESDAY	WEDNESDAY	THURSDAY	FRIDAY	SATURDAY	SUNDAY
Milk	☒ ☒	☐ ☐	☐ ☐	☐ ☐	☐ ☐	☐ ☐	☐ ☐
Fruit	☒ ☒	☐ ☐ ☐	☐ ☐ ☐	☐ ☐ ☐	☐ ☐ ☐	☐ ☐ ☐	☐ ☐ ☐
Veg.	☒ ☒	☐ ☐ ☐	☐ ☐ ☐	☐ ☐ ☐	☐ ☐ ☐	☐ ☐ ☐	☐ ☐ ☐
Starch	☒ ☒ ☒ ☒	☐ ☐ ☐ ☐	☐ ☐ ☐ ☐	☐ ☐ ☐ ☐	☐ ☐ ☐ ☐	☐ ☐ ☐ ☐	☐ ☐ ☐ ☐
Meat	☒ ☒ ☒	☐ ☐ ☐ ☐	☐ ☐ ☐ ☐	☐ ☐ ☐ ☐	☐ ☐ ☐ ☐	☐ ☐ ☐ ☐	☐ ☐ ☐ ☐
Fat	☒ ☒ ☒	☐ ☐ ☐	☐ ☐ ☐	☐ ☐ ☐	☐ ☐ ☐	☐ ☐ ☐	☐ ☐ ☐

© 1993, *The Balancing Act Nutrition and Weight Guide*, G. Kostas, M.P.H., R.D., Dallas, Texas

151

MEAL PLANS

	MILK	VEG.	FRUIT
	STARCH	MEAT	FAT

SHOPPING LIST

	MONDAY	TUESDAY	WEDNESDAY	THURSDAY	FRIDAY	SATURDAY	SUNDAY
BREAKFAST							
Milk							
Veg.							
Fruit							
Starch							
Meat							
Fat							
Free							
LUNCH							
Milk							
Veg.							
Fruit							
Starch							
Meat							
Fat							
Free							
SUPPER							
Milk							
Veg.							
Fruit							
Starch							
Meat							
Fat							
Free							
SNACKS							
TOTAL DAILY	Milk ☐ ☐	Milk ☐ ☐	Milk ☐ ☐	Milk ☐ ☐	Milk ☐ ☐	Milk ☐ ☐	Milk ☐ ☐
	Fruit ☐ ☐ ☐	Fruit ☐ ☐ ☐	Fruit ☐ ☐ ☐	Fruit ☐ ☐ ☐	Fruit ☐ ☐ ☐	Fruit ☐ ☐ ☐	Fruit ☐ ☐ ☐
	Veg. ☐ ☐ ☐	Veg. ☐ ☐ ☐	Veg. ☐	Veg. ☐ ☐ ☐	Veg. ☐ ☐ ☐	Veg. ☐ ☐ ☐	Veg. ☐ ☐ ☐
	Starch ☐ ☐ ☐	Starch ☐ ☐ ☐	Starch ☐ ☐ ☐	Starch ☐ ☐ ☐	Starch ☐ ☐ ☐	Starch ☐ ☐ ☐	Starch ☐ ☐ ☐
	Meat ☐ ☐ ☐	Meat ☐ ☐ ☐	Meat ☐ ☐ ☐	Meat ☐ ☐ ☐	Meat ☐ ☐ ☐	Meat ☐ ☐ ☐	Meat ☐ ☐ ☐
	Fat ☐ ☐ ☐	Fat ☐ ☐ ☐	Fat ☐ ☐ ☐	Fat ☐ ☐ ☐	Fat ☐ ☐ ☐	Fat ☐ ☐ ☐	Fat ☐ ☐ ☐

PORTIONS COUNT

WHAT DO YOU DO TO PRACTICE PORTION CONTROL?

You must become aware of portion sizes to lose weight! Many persons eat an excellent, nutritious diet with all the right foods. Without **portion** control, however, too much of even the right food can make you gain weight!

Try these portion control ideas:

1. Serve yourself measured portions. Use measuring cups and spoons, scales to weigh meats and cheeses.

2. Avoid seconds. Relax and think. Let 20 minutes pass before going for the second helping. Chances are, you won't want seconds!

3. Use a smaller dinner plate or dish to satisfy your psychological need to see a **full** plate. Spread food to cover the plate.

4. Set some food such as a crust on the side of your plate and leave it behind. Break away from the "clean plate syndrome," the compulsion to eat everything on the plate.

5. Cut food into smaller pieces. It seems like more and the meal lasts longer.

6. Measure cheese and meat to become familiar with 1 oz. and 3 oz.portions, respectively. Measure salad dressings, mayonnaise, peanut butter, and margarine in tablespoons to see how much you usually eat and how to "guestimate". Strive to use 1 tablespoon at most.

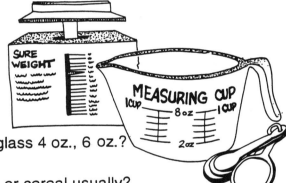

7. Measure your glass sizes at home. Is your juice glass 4 oz., 6 oz.? Is your milk glass 8 oz., 10 oz., 12 oz., 16 oz.?

8. Do you eat 1/2 cup, 1 cup, or 2 cups rice or pasta or cereal usually?

9. As time goes on, you need not measure everything. You'll be a good judge after practicing the first week or two. "Spot check" yourself now & then.

10. Have the deli attendant slice cheeses and cold cuts in 1 oz. slices (8 slices = 8 oz.) for your convenience.

11. Buy 3 oz. boneless, skinless chicken breasts, etc.

12. Purchase individually wrapped, portion-controlled servings (such as cheese slice "singles" or wedges or frozen dessert bars).

13. Split an entre when eating out. Most are 6-8 oz. You want 3-4 oz. at a meal.

14. Always slice fresh fruit and eat. Slices are more filling than one whole fruit.

PACE

HOW FAST DO YOU EAT?

1. Eating fast, without pausing or slowing down, leads to excessive eating. It takes approximately 20 minutes after eating to feel full.
2. Eat and chew slowly taking 20-30 minutes for meals and 10 minutes for snacks.
3. Make it your goal to be the last one to finish eating at the table.
4. Lay down your utensil between bites. Sip on beverage between bites.
5. Swallow each bite before taking the next bite.
6. Take a few brief breaks during the meal to sip water, talk with people at the table and enjoy the atmosphere.
7. Take smaller bites.
8. Serve food in courses — salad before entree. Courses slow you down!
9. **Eat "slow" foods** — foods with "crunch" such as popcorn, pretzels, hard rolls, fresh fruit, raw vegetables, toasted bread for sandwiches, baked potatoes not mashed, corn-on-the-cob or hot liquids such as soup, broth, hot tea, low-calorie hot cocoa.
10. **Enjoy** your eating environment. Serve food attractively. Play soft music. Keep surroundings relaxed, pleasant and attractive.
11. Converse with each person at the table. **Talk** so that you'll slow down!

SLOW AND STEADY WINS THE RACE!

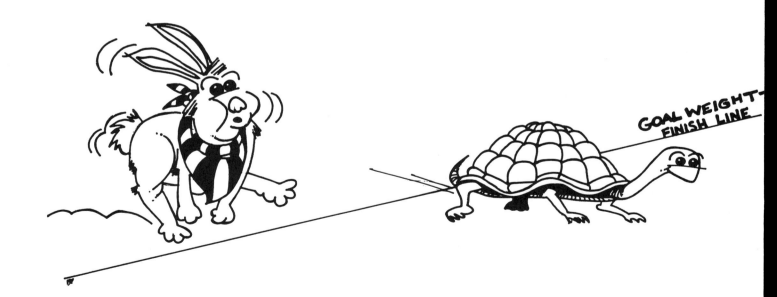

GOAL WEIGHT FINISH LINE

SUGAR

Excessive sugar inevitably leads to weight gain and poor health and fitness. It's easy to overconsume sugar, even unaware. Be informed.

WHAT IS SUGAR?

1. **Sucrose**, the technical term for **sugar**, occurs naturally in sugar cane or sugar beets. It is a "simple carbohydrate", easily absorbed by the body.

2. It is the most popular food additive. It adds taste, sweetening, texture, appearance, color, thickening and firmness and acts as a preservative.

3. Some forms of "sugar" are indicated by words ending in **"-ose"**:

sucrose	galactose	fructose	glucose
lactose	maltose	dextrose	mannose

   Other forms of "sugar" include -
corn syrup	dextrin	brown sugar maple syrup
sorghum	honey	molasses table sugar

   sugar alcohols (sorbitol, mannitol, dulcitol, zylitol)

4. One teaspoon of sugar (all forms) = 15 calories. These are "empty" calories that do not provide vitamins, minerals or fiber.

5. Refined sugar increases blood sugar levels within 15 minutes, resulting in "quick energy". This lasts only a few minutes because insulin reacts immediately to lower blood sugar. This rapid drop may make you feel less energetic and crave more sugar. Complex carbohydrates such as fruits, vegetables, starches and wholegrains are broken down slowly by your body, allowing a more constant blood sugar level which gives longer lasting energy. Eat more complex carbohydrates and you'll find you want less sugar, you'll have more energy, and you'll have more control over your "sweet tooth" and appetite.

WHERE IS SUGAR?

- Sugar is added to a great variety of foods, prepared commercially and at home:

soft drinks	cereal	ketchup
cakes, pies	canned fruit	salad dressing
cookies, candy	fruit yogurt	peanut butter
jam, jelly	soups	pudding
spaghetti sauce	ice cream	non-dairy coffee creamers

- Read labels when you shop and look for "sugar" and its other names.

- Ingredients on the label are listed from greatest quantity to least. So, if some form of sugar is one of the first three ingredients, or if various forms of sugar are listed separately throughout the ingredient list, then the product is most likely high in sugar content. Find a lower-sugar product if possible. Or, choose a very small portion of the sugar-rich food. Ask yourself if this food is really worth its calories. If not, move on.

WHY LIMIT SUGAR?

EXCESS SUGAR MAY LEAD TO THESE HEALTH PROBLEMS:

Tooth Decay Bacteria thrives on sugar and destroys tooth enamel, causing cavities.

Extra pounds Sweets compact **a lot** of calories into a **small** amount of food. Excess sweets lead to excess calories that are stored as body fat.

Diabetes Excess sugar calories may lead to excess weight, which requires more insulin than the body can supply; diabetes may result.

Hypo-glycemia Although sugar does not cause hypoglycemia, persons with hypoglycemia should avoid sugar to prevent unpleasant symptoms such as shakiness, headaches, weakness, fatigue, confusion and to help maintain constant blood sugar levels.

Heart Disease Excess sugar promotes insulin production which converts blood glucose to fatty acids and triglycerides, which may deposit in arteries and lead to atherosclerosis.

Triglycer-ides Excess sugar may elevate triglycerides (fats) in the blood, increasing one's risk of heart disease.

15 WAYS TO EAT LESS SUGAR

1. Cut back - the less sugar you eat, the less sugar you want. The more you eat, the more you want. Sugar can be addictive, or trigger a craving for more sweets or more food. If sugar leads to compulsive over-eating or binging, avoid it. Otherwise, eat it with limits.

2. Choose sugar-free products. Substitute unsweetened fruit juice or plain water for regular soft drinks, punches and fruit drinks which contain large amounts of sugar.

3. Buy unsweetened cereals such as shredded wheat, puffed wheat, puffed rice, etc.

4. Eat fewer and smaller desserts such as pie, cake, cookies, candies, desserts, etc.

5. Reduce sugar in recipes. Use concentrated fruit juice, cinnamon, nutmeg or flavor extracts such as vanilla and almond for added flavor. Replace 1/4 cup of sugar with a mashed banana in cookies.

6. Make it a habit to not buy sweets. Buy and eat fresh fruits instead.

7. Don't use sweets as rewards. Buy a new musical C.D. or tape, call a friend, etc.

8. Drink coffee or tea without sugar. Drink flavored, unsweetened coffee or tea.

9. Sweeten cereal by adding fruit, raisins, vanilla extract or cinnamon instead of sugar.

10. Read labels for "sugars". Know what you are eating.

11. Eat sugar-free, nonfat frozen yogurt as a "treat".

12. Split a dessert with 2-4 other persons if you really want it. Eat it slowly and enjoy!

13. Learn fun alternatives for sweets - choose a bagel rather than a donut; add a teaspoon of jam (15 calories) to bread as a "sweet snack".

14. Select miniature "fun size" candy portions, not large ones. Most miniatures are 75 calories.

15. Set a limit - 100 to 150 "sweet calories" daily (i.e. a small yogurt or 12 oz. soda).

DIET AND DENTAL HEALTH

- Dental disease is the most prevalent disease known to man; yet it is preventable.
- Proper nutrition and dental care are our best defenses against dental decay and periodontal disease, which weakens teeth and gums.
- Poor dental health interferes with good nutrition. Poor nutrition interferes with good dental health.
- You can strengthen your teeth and gums, and resist dental decay.

PROPER DENTAL CARE:

1. Brush teeth thoroughly after meals or after eating a "sugar-rich" food.
2. Floss once a day.
3. Brush tongue and gums.
4. Do not open bottles or packages with your teeth.
5. Have regular dental check-ups (twice a year) and fluoride treatments as needed.
   Steps 1, 2, and 3 above remove or reduce oral bacteria which produce acids from food sugar that decay (demineralize) tooth enamel. Plaque formation can lead to gum problems.
6. Rinse your mouth after meals and snacks. Drink a glass of water.

PROPER NUTRITIONAL CARE:

1. Eat a well-balanced, healthy diet.
2. Avoid simple sugars (sucrose) such as sugar, jams, honey, candies, candied apples, soft drinks, desserts, chewing gum, sugar-coated cereals, fruit canned in heavy syrup or sweetened fruit juices, pastries, pies, cakes, cookies, etc. Choose sugar-free foods.
3. Read food labels. Look for **sugar** as: sugar, corn syrup, corn sweetener, molasses, honey, maple syrup, brown sugar, sucrose, lactose, dextrose, mannose and glucose. These are all forms of simple sugars to avoid. Look for sugar alcohols, too - sorbitol, mannitol, etc.
4. If you must eat sweetened foods, eat them **with** meals, not between meals.
5. Avoid frequent snacking of sugar-containing foods or beverages.
6. Choose unsweetened between-meal snacks: fresh fruits and vegetables, milk, cheese, sugar-free yogurt, bagels, peanut butter, wholegrained breads and crackers, cooked or dry cereal, popcorn, nuts, seeds, sugarless drinks and chewing gum.
7. Chew high-fiber foods for healthy gums, teeth and jaw muscles - bran cereals, nuts, apples, carrots, celery, seeds, popcorn, bagels.
8. Avoid "sticky" sweets - caramels, peanut butter, candy bars, raisins, etc.
9. Include calcium for strong bones and teeth. Dairy products such as skim milk, cottage cheese, low-fat cheese or low-fat yogurt, as well as tuna, salmon and green leafy vegetables are best sources of calcium.
10. Include a source of Vitamin C daily for healthy gums. Good sources are: citrus fruit and juices, tomatoes, broccoli, potatoes, green leafy vegetables, strawberries and melon.
11. Never eat extremely hot or extremely cold beverages and foods. Thermal irritation can crack teeth!
12. Never chew on ice. This breaks down the enamel.
13. Avoid comforting a baby with a bedtime milk or juice bottle as the child goes to sleep. The result is "nursing bottle mouth", where teeth are destroyed by decay.

14. It's not just the **amount** of sugar you eat that is important. Other factors that contribute to cavities (tooth enamel decay) are:

> FREQUENCY- the more often you eat sugar-rich foods, the more often acids form on teeth, and erode tooth enamel.
>
> LENGTH OF TIME- the longer sugar is in your mouth (from cough drops, lifesavers, candies, etc.), the longer acid attack continues.
>
> PHYSICAL FORM- soft, sticky sweets such as caramels, toffees, mints, peanut butter cracker sandwiches, candied applies, etc. are difficult to clean from teeth.

IT IS UP TO YOU! ONLY YOU CAN PREVENT DECAY AND DISEASE AND LOSS OF YOUR TEETH!!! Take care of your teeth and gums - and they will last a lifetime!

KEY NUTRIENTS FOR DENTAL HEALTH

CALCIUM, PHOSPHORUS, VITAMIN D - for tooth formation and strength

> **Sources:** low-fat milk products, green leafy vegetables, canned salmon and sardines with bones, egg yolk and liver

VITAMIN A - tooth enamel

> **Sources:** carrots, cantaloupe, tomatoes, dark green vegetables, yellow, orange and red vegetables and fruits, fortified low-fat milk and cheese

VITAMIN C - for healthy mouth tissues and gums

> **Sources:** citrus fruit, strawberries, broccoli, potatoes, tomatoes, dark green vegetables

PROTEIN - for enamel and dentin

> **Sources:** lean meat, fish, poultry, milk products, beans

B-COMPLEX VITAMINS - for strong oral tissue and repair

> **Sources:** wholegrains, dark green vegetables, beans, red meat, poultry, fish

FLUORIDE - to prevent tooth decay

> **Sources:** fluoridated water or toothpaste

FIBER - for strong gums and clean tooth surfaces

> **Sources:** wholegrains, beans, fruit, vegetables, popcorn, nuts and seeds

OVERALL BALANCED NUTRITION - for overall body health and oral health

> **Sources:** all food types in balance, moderation and variety

HIDDEN SUGARS

Food Item	Size Portion	Approx. Sugar Content in Teaspoonsful of Granulated Sugar
BEVERAGES		
Cola drinks	8 ounces	6
Ginger ale	8 ounces	4 1/2
Orange-ade	8 ounces	5
Root beer	8 ounces	3 1/2
Seven-Up	8 ounces	6
Soda pop	8 ounces	5
Sweet cider	8 ounces	4 1/2
JAMS and JELLIES		
Apple butter	1 tablespoon	1
Jelly, Jam	1 tablespoon	4-6
CANDIES		
Chocolate milk bar (e.g. Hershey)	1 (1 1/2 ounces)	2 1/2
Chewing gum	1 stick	1/2
Choc cream	1 piece	2
Choc mints	1 piece	2
Fudge	1 ounce square	4 1/2
Gum drop	1	2
Hard candy	4 ounces	20
Lifesavers	1	1/3
Peanut brittle	1 ounce	3 1/2
Marshmallow	1	1 1/2
FRUIT and CANNED JUICES		
Raisins	1/2 cup	4
Currants, dried	1 tablespoon	4
Prunes, dried	3-4 medium	4
Apricots, dried	4-6 halves	4
Applesauce (unsweetened)	1/2 cup scant	2
Prunes, stewed (sweetened)	4-5 medium and 2 tablespoons juice	8
Canned peaches	2 halves and 1 tablespoon syrup	3 1/2
Fruit salad	1/2 cup	3 1/2
Fruit syrup	2 tablespoons	2 1/2
Orange juice	1/2 cup scant	2
Pineapple juice (unsweetened)	1/2 cup scant	2 3/5
Grape juice (commercial)	1/2 cup scant	3 2/5
Canned fruit juices (sweetened)	1/2 cup	2

Food Item	Size Portion	Approx. Sugar Content in Teaspoonsful of Granulated Sugar
BREADS and CEREALS		
Bread, regular	1 slice	1/2
Corn Flakes, Wheaties, Rice Krispies	1 bowl and 1 tablespoon sugar	4-8
Hamburger or hot dog bun	1	3
CAKES and COOKIES		
Angel food cake	1 (4 ounce piece)	7
Applesauce cake	1 (4 ounce piece)	5 1/2
Banana cake	1 (2 ounce piece)	2
Cheese cake	1 (4 ounce piece)	2
Chocolate cake (plain)	1 (4 ounce piece)	6
Chocolate cake (iced)	1 (4 ounce piece)	10
Coffee cake	1	4 1/2
Cup cake (iced)	1	6
Fruit cake	1 (4 ounce piece)	5
Jelly roll	1 (2 ounce piece)	2 1/2
Pound cake	1 (4 ounce piece)	5
Sponge cake	1 (1 ounce piece)	2
Strawberry shortcake	1 serving	4
Brownies (unfrosted)	3/4 ounce square	3
Molasses cookies	1	2
Chocolate cookies	1	1 1/2
Fig newtons	1	5
Ginger snaps	1	3
Macaroons	1	6
Nut cookies	1	1 1/2
Oatmeal cookies	1	2
Sugar cookies	1	1 1/2
Chocolate eclair	1	7
Cream puff	1	2
Donut (plain)	1	3
Donut (glazed)	1	6
DAIRY PRODUCTS		
Ice cream	1/3 pint (3 1/2 ounces)	3 1/2
Ice cream bar	1 (depending on size)	1-7
Ice cream cone	1	5 1/2
Eggnog, all milk	(8 ounces)	4 1/2
Ice cream soda	1	5

Food Item	Size Portion	Approx. Sugar Content in Teaspoonful of Granulated Sugar	Food Item	Size Portion	Approx. Sugar Content in Teaspoonful of Granulated Sugar
DAIRY (cont'd)			**DESSERTS** (cont'd)		
Cocoa, all milk	1 cup (5 ounce milk)	4	Raisin pie	1 slice	13
Ice cream sundae	1	7	Banana pudding	1/2 cup	2
Chocolate, all milk	1 cup (5 ounce milk)	6	Bread pudding	1/2 cup	1 1/2
Malted milk shake	10 ounces	5	Chocolate pudding	1/2 cup	4
Sherbet	1/2 cup	9	Plum pudding	1/2 cup	4
DESSERTS			Rice pudding	1/2 cup	5
Apple cobbler	1/2 cup	3	Tapioca pudding	1/2 cup	3
Custard	1/2 cup	2	Brown Betty	1/2 cup	3
French pastry	1 (4 ounce piece)	5	Plain pastry	1 (4 oz piece)	3
Jello	1/2 cup	4 1/2			
Apple pie	1 slice (average)	7	**SUGARS & SYRUPS**		
Cherry pie	1 slice	10	Brown sugar	1 tablespoon	3*
Cream pie	1 slice	4	Granulated sugar	1 tablespoon	3*
Custard pie	1 slice	10	Corn syrup	1 tablespoon	3*
Coconut pie	1 slice	10	Karo syrup	1 tablespoon	3*
Lemon pie	1 slice	7	Honey	1 tablespoon	3*
Peach pie	1 slice	7	Molasses	1 tablespoon	3*
Pumpkin pie	1 slice	5	Chocolate sauce	1 tablespoon	3*
Rhubarb pie	1 slice	4			

*actual sugar content

- HOW MUCH HIDDEN SUGAR DO YOU EAT DAILY?

- DID YOU REALIZE A 12 OZ. SOFT DRINK CONTAINS 9-10 TEASPOONS OF SUGAR?

CEREALS - TOP CHOICES

Select high-fiber cereals (predominantly wholegrains) that are low in sugar. Choose those with at least 4 grams of fiber, and no more than 7 grams sugar, 2 grams fat and 300 mg. sodium per serving. All of the following cereals meet these criteria.

[√] are best choices:

	Cereals	Serving Size (1 ounce)	Calories	Sugar (grams)	Fiber (grams)	Fat (grams)	Sodium (mg)
√	All-Bran (Kellog's)	1/3 c	70	5	9	1	260
√	All-Bran w/ Extra Fiber Kellogg's)	1/2 c	50	0	14	0	140
	Alpen	1/4 c	110	5	3	2	61
	Bran Buds	1/3 c	70	8	11	1	200
√	Bran Chex	2/3 c	90	5	5	0	200
√	Complete Bran Flakes (Kellogg's)	2/3 c	90	5	5	0	220
√	Bran Flakes (Post)	2/3 c	90	5	5	0	210
	Cheerios (regular)	1 1/4 c	110	1	2	2	290
	Corn Flakes	1 c	100	2	1	0	290
√	Fiber One	1/2 c	60	0	13	1	140
√	Fiberwise (Kellogg's)	2/3 c	90	5	5	1	140
√	Grape Nut Flakes	7/8 c	100	5	3	1	140
	Grape Nuts	1/4 c	110	3	3	0	170
√	Heartwise	2/3 c	90	5	5	1	140
	Low Fat Granola (Kellogg's)	1/3 c	120	7	2	2	60
√	Multi-Bran Chex	2/3 c	90	6	4	1	120
	Muselix Crispy Blend (Kellogg's)	2/3 c	160	6	3	2	150
√	Nutrigrain Raisin Bran	1 c	140	9*	5	1	200
√	Oat Bran Cereal	3/4 c	100	5	4	2	105
	Puffed Kashi (other puffed cereals have <1g fiber)	1 1/3 c	90	0	3	0	0
√	Raisin Bran (Skinner)	1/2 c	110	6	4	2	45
√	Shredded Wheat (Nabisco)	1 lg. biscuit	90	0	4	1	0
	Shredded Wheat (spoon size)	2/3 c	90	0	3	1	0
√	Shredded Wheat 'n Bran (Nabisco)	1 lg. biscuit	90	0	4	1	0
	Total	1 c	100	3	3	1	200
√	Uncle Sam Cereal	1/2 c	110	0	7	1	65
	Wheaties	1 c	100	3	3	1	200
	Whole Grain Wheat Chex	2/3 c	100	3	3	1	190

*naturally occurring, no added sugar

LIMIT YOUR SODIUM!

- **Sodium** is a mineral which occurs in some amount in everything you eat.
- The chief source of **sodium** in your diet is table salt (sodium chloride).
- Even if you never added salt to your food, you would eat enough **sodium** to meet your body's needs.
- We recommend that everyone limit **sodium** to prevent hypertension.
- Eat 2,000 - 4,000 mg. sodium daily (rather than the typical 5,000+ mg. daily that most Americans eat). Here's how to do it without counting.

HOW TO SENSIBLY CUT BACK ON SODIUM:
1. Do not add salt to food during cooking.
2. Limit these high-sodium foods:
   - salty and smoked meats: ham, bacon, luncheon meats, hot dogs, sausage, chipped or corned beef, salt pork, kosher meat
   - salty and smoked fish: anchovies, caviar, herring, sardines. (Choose tuna packed in water or "reduced sodium" brands.)
   - processed cheeses and cheese products (instead, use "natural cheese" and "low sodium" cheeses. Read labels.)
   - bouillon cubes*, consommé, canned soups*, and dried soup mixes
   - canned vegetables*, tomato juice*, sauerkraut, pork and beans
   - snack foods: potato chips*, pretzels*, salted nuts*, salted popcorn*, snack crackers, party dips and spreads
   - crackers* with salted toppings
   - olives, pickles*, relishes, horseradish, bottled salad dressings*
   - meat extracts and meat tenderizers
   - prepared sauces: barbecue, chili, steak, soy*, tomato*, tartar, Worcestershire, mustard*, catsup*, Kitchen Bouquet
   - condiments: salt and spices containing salt or MSG (as mono-sodium glutamate or hydrolyzed vegetable protein); lemon pepper
   - other: frozen dinners, instant cereal packets, instant pudding mixes, pizza (unless homemade), fast foods, pot pies
   - breakfast cereals*: cornflakes, bran flakes, Grapenuts, granola
3. Eat wholesome foods - the more natural and less processed, the better.
4. If you must add salt, add a little at the table - not in the cooking - for a stronger taste.
5. Try salt-free seasonings or salt substitutes in place of salt.
6. Check your medicine. Often it contains salt (i.e., Alka-Seltzer, antacids, Rolaids, Metamucil instant mix, Vick's cough medicines, laxatives, pain relievers, sedatives).
7. *Select low-sodium cereals: **lowest** in sodium: shredded wheat, puffed wheat, puffed rice, low-sodium corn flakes and low-sodium rice krispies.

SEASONING WITHOUT SALT

HERB AND SPICE BLENDS

PREPARE YOUR OWN **HERB** BLEND to use in cooking and in the salt shaker at the table:

1. **Season-All** (mix for meats and vegetables)

   1 teaspoon basil

   1 teaspoon marjoram

   1 teaspoon thyme

   1 teaspoon oregano

   1 teaspoon parsley

   1 teaspoon savory

   1 teaspoon mace

   1 teaspoon ground cloves

   1/4 teaspoon nutmeg

   1 teaspoon black pepper

   1/4 teaspoon cayenne

2. **All-Purpose Spice Blend**

   5 teaspoons onion power

   2 1/2 teaspoons paprika

   1 1/4 teaspoons thyme

   1/4 teaspoon celery seed

   2 1/2 teaspoons garlic powder

   2 1/2 teaspoons mustard powder

   1/2 teaspoon ground white pepper

3. **Herbed Seasoning Blend**

   2 tablespoons dill weed or basil

   1 teaspoon oregano leaves, crushed

   2 tablespoons onion powder

   1/4 teaspoon grated lemon peel (dried)

   1 teaspoon celery seed

   1/16 teaspoon black pepper

4. **Spicy Flavor Blend**

   2 tablespoons savory, crushed

   2 1/2 teaspoons onion powder

   1 3/8 teaspoons curry powder

   1 1/4 teaspoons cumin

   1 tablespoon powdered mustard

   1 1/4 teaspoons ground white pepper

   1/2 teaspoons garlic

COMMERCIAL PRODUCTS

Bakon Seasonings
(6 different blends)
Bakon Yeast Inc.
P.O. Box 19203
Portland, Oregon 97219

Chef's Selection
Products, Inc.
2601 Colorado Ave.
Santa Monica, CA 90404

Mrs. Dash Salt-Free
Alberto-Culver Co.
2525 Armitage Ave.
Melrose Park, IL 60160

New Vegit
Modern Products Inc.
P.O. Box 09398
Milwaukee, WI 53209

No Nak Pleasoning
Frank J. Italiano Inc.
P.O. Box 2701
LaCrosse, WI 54601

Parsley Patch Seasonings (6 blends)
Dia-Mel Salt-it
Low Sodium Baking Powder
Adolph's Unsalted 100% Natural Tenderizer

DO NOT USE:

- Lite Salt — it contains sodium in 1/2 the amount of regular salt!
- Sea Salt — 1 gram of sea salt = 780 milligrams salt
  1 teaspoon of sea salt = 1,716 milligrams sodium

HOW TO COOK WITH HERBS AND SPICES

FOOD	SEASON WITH ...
Beef	allspice, bay leaf, caraway seed, garlic, marjoram, dry mustard, nutmeg, onion, broiled peaches, pepper, green pepper, thyme
Fish	bay leaf, curry, marjoram, dry mustard, lemon, parsley, margarine, lemon juice, green pepper, tomatoes
Lamb	basil, curry, garlic powder, mint, rosemary, thyme
Poultry	cranberries, parsley, paprika, rosemary, sage, thyme
Veal	bay leaf, curry, ginger, marjoram, oregano, rosemary, thyme
Eggs	curry, dry mustard, onion, paprika, parsley, thyme, green pepper, tomatoes
Asparagus	caraway seed, lemon juice, mustard seed, sesame seed, tarragon
Beans	basil, dill seed, unsalted French dressing, lemon juice, marjoram, mint, mustard seed, nutmeg, oregano, sage, savory, tarragon, thyme
Beets	allspice, bay leaves, caraway seed, cloves, dill seed, mustard seed, tarragon
Broccoli	caraway seed, dill seed, mustard seed, oregano, tarragon
Cabbage	caraway seed, dill seed, mint, mustard seed, dry mustard, nutmeg, poppy seed, savory, thyme, vinegar
Cauliflower	caraway seed, chives, dill seed, lemon juice, mace, nutmeg, parsley, rosemary, tarragon
Corn	curry, green peppers
Cucumbers	basil, dill seed, lemon juice, mint, tarragon, nutmeg
Eggplant	chives, grated onion or garlic, marjoram, oregano, chopped parsley, tarragon
Lettuce salad	basil, caraway seed, chives, dill, garlic, lemon, onion, tarragon, thyme, vinegar
Onions	caraway seed, mustard seed, nutmeg, oregano, pepper, sage, thyme
Peas	basil, dill, marjoram, mint, oregano, lemon, parsley, green pepper, poppy seed, rosemary, sage, savory, thyme
Potatoes	basil, bay leaves, caraway seed, chives, dill seed, mace, mustard seed, onion, oregano, paprika, parsley, green pepper, poppy seed, rosemary, thyme
Spinach	basil, mace, marjoram, nutmeg, oregano
Squash	allspice, basil, cinnamon, chives, cloves, fennel, ginger, mace, mustard seed, nutmeg, onion, rosemary
Sweet potatoes	allspice, cardamon, cinnamon, cloves, nutmeg
Tomatoes	allspice, basil, bay leaf, curry, marjoram, onion, sage, thyme

SODIUM COMPARISONS

NOTE: Sodium content increases as food processing increases.

AS FOODS	Sodium (mg)	ARE PROCESSED...	Sodium (mg)	SODIUM INCREASES	Sodium (mg)
APPLE 1 medium	1	**APPLESAUCE** 1 cup	6	**APPLE PIE** 1/8, frozen	482
BREAD 1 slice	130	**HOMEMADE BISCUIT** 1 biscuit	175	**CANNED BISCUIT** 1 biscuit	270
BUTTER 1 tablespoon, unsalted	2	**BUTTER** 1 tablespoon, salted	120	**MARGARINE** 1 tablespoon	150
CABBAGE 1 cup	22	**COLE SLAW** 1 cup	150	**SAUERKRAUT** 1 cup, canned	1,760
CHICKEN 3 ounces, baked	86	**FAST FOOD CHICKEN** 3 ounces, fried	500	**CHICKEN PIE** 1 frozen pie	863
CORN 1 ear	1	**CORN FLAKES** 1 cup	325	**CANNED KERNELS** 1 cup	400
GRAPES 10 seedless	1	**GRAPE JELLY** 1 tablespoon	3	**WHITE WINE** 4 ounces, domestic	20
LEMON 1 lemon	3	**SOY SAUCE** 1 tablespoon	1,330	**SALT** 1 teaspoon	2,300
PEANUTS (NO SALT) 1 ounce (30 nuts)	1	**PEANUT BUTTER** 1 tablespoon	95	**PEANUT BUTTER COOKIES** 3 cookies	150
CHEESE, CHEDDAR 1 ounce	175	**CHEESE SPREAD** 1 ounce	380	**CHEESE SOUP** 1 cup, canned	1,020
POTATO - BAKED 1 ounce	5	**FRENCH FRIES** 1/2 cup (18 fries)	120	**POTATO CHIPS** 1/2 cup (10 chips)	200
TOMATO 1 medium	4	**TOMATO JUICE** 1 cup	500	**TOMATO SOUP** 1 cup (Del Monte)	900
TOMATO PASTE 1 cup (Del Monte)	60	**TOMATO SAUCE** 1 cup (Del Monte)	1,300	**SPAGHETTI SAUCE** 1 cup	2,000
TUNA IN WATER 3 ounces	372	**TUNA IN OIL** 3 ounces	442	**TUNA NOODLE CASSEROLE** 1 cup	715
WATER 12 ounces tap	4	**SOFT DRINK** 12 ounces	50	**CLUB SODA** 12 ounces	90

VII
EATING OUT AND SPECIAL OCCASIONS

HABITS FOCUS

1. Develop strategies to "Manage Special Occasions" — parties, eating out, alcohol, fast foods, restaurant meal comparisons, salad bars, traveling, vacations, weekends, holidays (169-172). Find your favorite restaurant on pages 175-177.

NUTRITION FOCUS

1. Need a boost? Try exciting new 500 calorie meals out (178)!
2. Be alert to calorie excesses and exercise your options.

EXERCISE FOCUS

Continue exercising — even when special occasions arise. Plan exercise so you do not disrupt your regular program.

RECORDS

These records are helping you to achieve your goals. Keep them up! You may wish to keep a journal as well.

GOALS

HABIT: practice three new eating out skills or strategies

FOOD: be selective when ordering foods out - choose wisely

EXERCISE: go that "extra mile" to burn off extra calories eaten on those special occasions.

RECORDS: food, exercise, weight - review meals out, how did you do?

168　© 1993, *The Balancing Act Nutrition and Weight Guide*, G. Kostas, M.P.H., R.D., Dallas, Texas

MANAGING SPECIAL OCCASIONS

DO YOU FOREGO YOUR EATING GOALS AND EAT "EVERYTHING" WHEN EATING OUT?

Special situations easily trigger eating and may disrupt your good eating goals. How do you handle eating in restaurants, entertaining friends or relatives, parties, traveling, vacations, holidays, weekends, binges, snacks, celebrations?

DEVELOP STRATEGIES FOR HANDLING THOSE SPECIAL OCCASIONS!

- **ANTICIPATE** an eating situation and how you will take control of it. Rehearse an imagined scene. Be optimistic and picture yourself successfully eating in a planned manner and enjoying it!! Re-enact your "preview". Enjoy your success.

- **PLAN ALTERNATIVE ACTIVITIES** — always keep in mind alternative activities you can do in various eating situations to avoid overeating. Imagine these in advance, then practice them. Examples: drink more water before eating; take a before-dinner walk; plan a dinner conversation.

- **LEARN TO RELAX** — practice relaxation techniques such as imagery, or exercise before eating or enjoy other activities that calm you and help you control your eating urges. A walk or shower, music or manicure may relax you.

- **PRE-PLAN MEALS AND SNACKS ...** and follow your decision.

ENTERTAINING & PARTIES

Re-think entertaining and parties as a time for <u>people</u> — not just food and drink.

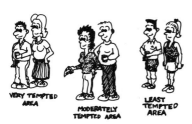

TEMPTATIONS

VERY TEMPTED AREA   MODERATELY TEMPTED AREA   LEAST TEMPTED AREA

AS A HOSTESS OR HOST

1. Present food creatively and decorate the table festively. Its **APPEARANCE** and **PRESENTATION** is more appealing than its calorie content.

2. Prepare **LOW-CALORIE FOODS,** such as raw vegetables and fresh fruits with an optional cottage cheese or yogurt dip, salads, baked or broiled meats, sauces on the side. Guests appreciate your health-consciousness and being able to choose to use or avoid the extras. You don't have to serve only "diet foods". Serve smaller portions of your favorite rich foods and larger portions of lighter foods.

3. Cut desserts into different size portions. Let your guests control their portions.

4. Prepare the least tempting foods first and the most tempting last. You will have less time to snack on your favorite things.

5. Have everything ready early so you can relax and get ready at a leisurely pace.

6. Give away leftovers.

7. If you receive food gifts, wrap them up and freeze them to serve to future guests.

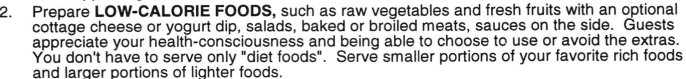

AS A GUEST —

1. Never go to a party hungry. Eat a small, healthy snack (i.e. apple) before going. Don't leave yourself with the excuse "I've starved all day!"

2. Go to a party to enjoy the people more than the foods. Talk more and eat less. Make it a point to talk with at least 10 persons individually. **TALK...TALK...TALK!**

3. Take something with you to eat — a raw vegetable plate, fruit plate, popcorn, low-fat cheese, crackers, pretzels, etc. Your hosts or hostess will appreciate your gesture and you will be sure to have something you want to eat.

4. Set ground rules before you eat out. Decide to eat one serving of everything or decide to decline certain foods such as rolls and butter, "loaded" potatoes, olives, nuts, etc. **HAVE A "MIND SET"!**

5. Drink club soda, water, low-calorie beverages. Always having something in your hand at a party, for example, a drink, seems to be comfortable for a lot of people, and keeps a hand too occupied to reach for more food! **AVOID** high-calorie drinks and alcohol which are those "extra, empty" calories.

6. Minimize your food contact. Move food dishes to an unreachable distance from you or move yourself from the foods. Never stand near a food table to talk.

7. At a buffet, look at the whole table and decide what you want. Then fill a plate one time and no seconds! Move away from the food table. Sit at a distance.

8. Serve yourself. Do not accept food from others.

9. Eat slowly. The quicker you finish, the more your host may tempt you with second helpings. In 20 minutes, more food seems less appealing.

10. Plan responses to insistent hosts and hostesses. For example, "No, thank you. I've had enough," or "Everything has been delicious, but I can't eat another bite," or "No, thank you. But I would enjoy a glass of water."

11. Remind yourself that eating and overeating do not say "I like you", and refusing food does not mean rejection. Praise the host or hostess for the good food and evening.

12. Don't tell anyone that you are "dieting". You might be encouraged to "Forget the diet, it is a special occasion!" Besides, no one really notices if you skip rich dishes.

13. Request a small serving or 1/2 a serving. When you verbalize your commitment, you will not back down!

Eating Out

1. Choose restaurants with a widely varied menu so that you can select foods included in your eating program.

2. Don't starve yourself all day if going out for dinner. Have a light breakfast and lunch to avoid overindulging at the restaurant.

3. Learn to enjoy the company more than the food on your plate.

4. Decide ahead of time what you will order. This prevents temptation.

5. Order from the menu with your meal plan in mind.

6. Find buffets and cafeterias that allow you to make lower-calorie selections.

7. Frequent the same restaurant, when possible. A regular customer knows the menu and knows what foods can be prepared in special ways to avoid extra calories.

8. Don't hesitate to ask how foods on the menu are prepared. Ask for certain foods that may be available but not listed on the menu (margarine, baked fish or chicken, skim milk, baked potato instead of soup, clear soup instead of a creamy one, onion soup without the bread and cheese topping, a steamed vegetable plate).

9. Start your meals with volume — water, diet drinks, salads, raw vegetables, clear soup. (Or start with a snack like this at home.)

10. Avoid menu items that are fried or creamed, with thick gravies, cheese sauces, or sugar glazes. If you have no choice, remove the crust or push the sauce aside and eat the food underneath.

11. Order meat broiled or baked; choose poultry (no skin), veal, fish (lowest-calorie) or lean cuts of beef (filet, top sirloin, flank, London broil, shishkabob).

12. Ask that food you don't want be left off the plate (potato chips, fries, etc.).

13. Ask that bread and butter, chips, crackers be removed from the table. Or, if with company, move the before meal snack to the far end of the table, away from you to avoid temptation.

14. Order water, tea, diet drink, club soda or coffee as a beverage.

15. Salad dressing — take your own low-calorie brand from home (you can buy individual packets); or ask for a low-calorie dressing; or ask for oil and vinegar (herb or wine vinegar), lemon, or hot sauce. **Always ask that salad dressing be brought on the side** so that you control the amount added!

16. Salad bars -
    - **CHOOSE** lettuce greens, cucumbers, radishes, carrots, green pepper, onions, beets, mushrooms, bean sprouts, cauliflower, tomatoes, beans, peas, broccoli — these are low-calorie ingredients (you may use juice from a 3-bean salad as dressing.
    - **AVOID** thick, creamy salad dressings, croutons, cheese toppings, seeds, nuts, olives, avocado, bacon bits, creamed items — those high-calorie ingredients.
    - **LIMIT** prepared salads — pasta, potato, cole slaw, chicken or tuna salad, marinated vegetables, etc.

17. Assume butter sauce is added to broiled fish or chicken. Ask for **unbuttered** broiled fish or chicken with butter sauce **on the side!**

18. Ask for small servings; for example: a **small** potato.

19. Eat half of an oversized portion. Share an order with another person.

20. Measure food at home so you will be familiar with the portion sizes.

21. Eat the amount of food specified by your eating plan — leave the rest on your plate. You don't have to clean your plate! Ask for foil with your order and immediately set aside a take-home portion.

22. Remove the top slice of bread or bun from a sandwich if the sandwich is big.

23. Order a hamburger with tomato, lettuce, mustard, onion, pickle; and without cheese, mayonnaise, catsup, "secret sauce", sweet relish or chili.

24. Sip slowly on beverages throughout the meal.

25. Decide ahead of time to pass up dessert, despite what others do. Sip on water, coffee or tea.

26. Practice your cue elimination techniques and your meal eating techniques such as sitting, eating slowly, etc.

27. If you are having a hard time with the waiter meeting a certain request, say that you are allergic to that high-calorie food and cannot eat it!

28. Be **ASSERTIVE** and ask for what you want; for example: margarine instead of butter.

29. If you overeat, have your own compensating strategy for the next day: an "all vegetable" day, "more exercise" day, "mini-meal" day or a "two meal" day.

ALCOHOL

JUST SAY NO!

1. This is a **drug** with many calories but few nutrients! Avoid or limit it.
2. Do not be pressured into something you don't want or need.
3. You can order a diet soft drink, club soda with a twist of lime, tomato juice, V-8 juice, fruit juice, iced tea, bottled water, flavored waters, sugar-free fruit-flavored seltzers, or other low-calorie drinks. Try mixing club soda and juice!
4. Know the calories you are drinking:

$$\text{Alcohol Calories} = (\text{number of ounces}) \times (\text{the proof}) \times (.8)$$

BEVERAGE	SERVING SIZE	CALORIES
Alcohol-free beer	1 12-ounce can	65
Beer	1 12-ounce can	150
Beer, light	1 12-ounce can	100
Bloody Mary	5-ounce cocktail	125
Bourbon + Coke	8-ounce cocktail	195
Champagne	4 ounces	85
Daiquiri	3 1/2-ounce cocktail	125
Egg Nog	4 ounces	335
Gin and Tonic	8-ounce cocktail	155
Grasshopper	3 1/2-ounce cocktail	175
Manhattan	3 1/2-ounce cocktail	165
Margarita	8-ounce cocktail	300
Martini	3 1/2-ounce cocktail	140
Whiskey sour	3 1/2-ounce cocktail	200
Wine, table	3 1/2-ounces (12 percent alcohol)	85
Wine, dessert	3 1/2-ounces (18 percent alcohol)	140

5. A safe limit is, at most, 100 calories from alcoholic beverages daily (100 calories = 4 oz. wine, 1 1/2 oz. liquor, 12 oz. "light" (reduced-calorie) beer, 8 oz. regular beer).
6. Alcohol converts to fat when metabolized by the body and can cause high triglycerides, a coronary risk factor. Alcohol also raises blood pressure, another coronary risk factor. Alcohol adds extra calories and weight, a third coronary risk factor. Recent studies show that alcohol causes the body to burn less fat — so fat-burning and weight loss slow down. Beyond these risks, alcohol in any amount can lead to alcoholism, if you are susceptible. **Compulsive eaters, beware!** Over-eating can also lead to over-drinking and over-eating can replace over-drinking. Liver damage and other major health and life problems can result from alcohol. Seek professional assistance if you must drink daily.

EATING OUT TIPS

FOOD	CHOOSE	LIMIT
APPETIZERS	Broth, bouillon, consommé, gazpacho, tomato juice, V-8 juice, fruit, fruit cup, fruit juice, raw vegetables, shrimp or crab cocktail, oysters on the half shell	Cream soups, chowders, fried foods, nachos, potato skins
SALADS	Fresh fruit, vegetable with salad dressing on the side, raw vegetables, chef's salad with turkey or chicken (omit cold cuts)	Potato salad, macaroni salad, jello salad, coleslaw, taco salad with guacamole
MEATS	Baked, roasted or broiled: fish, poultry (chicken, turkey, Cornish hen) or lean meat cuts of beef, veal, lamb, pork, tenderloin steaks (filet, T-bone, top sirloin). Poached or boiled eggs; cottage cheese.	Fried, breaded, with gravy or sauce or combinations (stew, casseroles, hash, etc.) Fried or scrambled eggs; eggs benedict
SANDWICHES	Chicken, turkey, tuna fish, lean roast beef on wholewheat bread with lettuce and tomato, without mayonnaise	Luncheon meats (cold cuts), sausage, hot dogs, hamburgers, fried meat
POTATOES, STARCHES	Baked, boiled, mashed potatoes (with condiments on side); corn, rice, pasta with marinara or tomato sauce	Fried, au gratin, scalloped, hash browned, with meat or cream cheese sauces
VEGETABLES	Raw, boiled, steamed, baked; or vegetable plate as a meal	Fried, creamed, au gratin, with sauces or gravies
BREADS	All plain breads and rolls, plain muffins, breadsticks, crackers, graham crackers	Sweet rolls and muffins, coffee cake, Danish pastry, doughnuts, garlic bread
FATS	Margarine, salad dressing, mayonnaise (limited amounts)	Butter, cream, sour cream, gravy, sauces, olives, nuts, avocados, fried foods, bacon
DESSERTS	Fresh fruit, sherbet, angel food cake, nonfat frozen yogurt, sorbet, ice milk, fruit ice, popsicles	Pies, cakes, custards, puddings, cookies, sweetened fruits, ice cream
BEVERAGES	Coffee, tea, skim milk, buttermilk, diet drinks, water	Chocolate milk, regular soft drinks, milk shakes, lemonade, alcohol
MISCELLANEOUS	Chicken fajitas, soft chicken tacos, cheese pizza, bean soups	Sausage pizza, greasy or fried dishes

NOTE: Order all foods without butter or margarine, mayonnaise, gravy, sauces, salad dressing, etc. Add your own "on the side" topping to control portions.

MEALS OUT — COMPARISONS

(Select meals with 500-700 calories, ≤ 25 grams fat)

(See Legend Below)

APPETIZERS

	Amount	Cal.	Fat		Amount	Cal.	Fat
potato skins, loaded	3 pieces	125	6	chicken wings	2	150	8
chili con queso dip	1/2 cup	250	20	chicken fingers, fried	2	100	7
and chips	12 chips	300	18	vegetable soup	1 cup	100	5
fried zuccini	1/2 cup	200	12	gazpacho	1 cup	100	5
fried cheese	1 stick	200	20	cream soup	1 cup	200	10
nachos with cheese, sour	3 nachos	165	12	French onion soup	1 cup	250	12
cream, guacamole, refried				fruit cup	1 cup	100	0
beans				shrimp w/cocktail sauce	5 lg.	100	0

INSTEAD OF THIS . . .	TRY THIS . . .

STEAK HOUSE

	Cal.	Fat		Cal.	Fat
9-ounce prime rib	750	50	6-ounce filet steak (tenderloin)	360	19
1 medium baked potato, "loaded"	160	0	1 medium baked potato	160	0
w/ 1 Tbsp butter, 1 Tbsp sour	130	13	with 1 tsp margarine* and chives	35	4
cream, 1 Tbsp cheese, 1 tsp	40	4	tossed salad	25	0
bacon bits			with 1 Tbsp red.-cal. dressing**	20	2
1 dinner roll	80	1	water	0	0
with 1 tsp margarine	35	4			
tossed salad	25	0	*add salsa or soy sauce = 0 cal, 0 gm fat,		
with 4 Tbsp dressing	320	32	or add 1 Tbsp sour cream = 30 cal, 3 gm fat		
			**1 Tbsp regular dressing = avg. 80 cal.,		
TOTALS:	**1650**	**104**	8 gm fat	**600**	**25**

MEXICAN RESTAURANT

	Cal.	Fat		Cal.	Fat
20 large chips	500	30	3 soft corn tortillas; salsa	200	0
with salsa	0	0	Fajitas:		
2 large beef enchiladas	1000	70	2 flour tortillas	200	5
1/2 cup refried beans	250	8	with 4 oz. chicken (grilled with oil)	270	16
1 Margarita	300	0	and pico de gallo, lettuce, tomato, onion	0	0
			water or tea	0	0
TOTALS	**2050**	**108**		**670**	**21**

NOTE: Skip guacamole and sour cream.
Ask for "no oil" with chicken to save 70 cal, 6 gm fat.
Taco salad with picante sauce = 670 cal, 40 gm fat.

Cal = calories   Fat = fat in grams   gm = grams   oz = ounce   tsp = teaspoon   red cal = reduced calorie Tbsp = tablespoon

TEXAS STYLE

	Cal.	Fat		Cal.	Fat
Barbecue Beef Sandwich (4 oz. brisket)	600	40	Barbecue Chicken Breast (4-oz.)	210	5
1/2 cup fried okra	200	12	1 medium corn-on-the-cob*	100	2
1 fried pie	400	24	with 1 tsp margarine	35	4
12-oz. soft drink or beer	150	0	1/2 cup coleslaw	120	7
			1 dinner roll	80	1
			water	0	0
TOTALS	**1350**	**76**		**545**	**19**

*or 1 bun = 150 cal, 2 gm fat

SEAFOOD RESTAURANT

	Cal.	Fat		Cal.	Fat
6-oz. fried fish			6-oz. baked or broiled fish		
with batter (3 pieces)	400	23	with lemon, no butter*	240	3
3 hush puppies	150	7	1/2 cup broccoli w/ margarine	60	4
1/2 cup coleslaw	120	7	1/2 cup rice w/ margarine	135	4
1 large order French fries	375	20	1 wholewheat roll	80	1
12-oz. soft drink	150	0	water	0	0
TOTALS	**1195**	**57**		**515**	**12**

*add 100 cal, 10 gm fat if lemon-butter used

ITALIAN RESTAURANT

	Cal.	Fat		Cal.	Fat
4" square lasagna	700	36	1 cup spaghetti (no oil)	200	0
1 slice buttered garlic bread	200	12	with meat-free tomato sauce	150	10
tossed salad	25	0	2 slices Italian bread (no butter)	110	2
with 2 Tbsp Italian dressing	140	14	tossed salad	25	0
1 piece cheesecake	350	23	with 1 Tbsp Italian dressing	70	7
6 oz. red wine	150	0	1 serving cantaloupe or fruit	60	0
			water	0	0
TOTALS	**1565**	**85**		**615**	**19**

PIZZA

	Cal.	Fat		Cal.	Fat
4 pieces of 12-inch pepperoni pizza	900	32	2 pieces of 12-inch cheese pizza with		
2 beers (24 ounces)	300	0	mushrooms, green pepper, onion	340	10
			tossed salad	25	0
			with 1 Tbsp French dressing	55	6
			water or iced tea	0	0
TOTALS	**1200**	**32**		**420**	**16**

INSTEAD OF THIS . . .		**TRY THIS . . .**

CHINESE RESTAURANT

	Cal.	Fat		Cal.	Fat
1 egg roll	300	12	2 cups Chicken Lo-Mein*	300	10
6 oz. Sweet & Sour Pork w/vegetables	400	25	1 cup steamed rice	225	0
1 cup fried rice	270	5	1 fortune cookie	30	2
1 fortune cookie	30	2	Jasmine Tea	0	0
6 oz. sake (rice wine)	280	0			
TOTALS	**1280**	**44**		**555**	**12**

*any chicken, shrimp, or beef dish stir-fried with vegetables will be approx. 300 cal., 10 gm. fat

FAST FOOD RESTAURANT

	Cal.	Fat		Cal.	Fat
1 quarter pound cheeseburger	525	30	1 roast beef sandwich (medium)	350	15
1 order French fries	220	12	i.e. Arby's		
regular chocolate shake	350	8	1/2 order French fries	110	6
			tossed salad	25	0
			with 1 Tbsp reduced-cal. dressing**	20	2
			water	0	0
TOTALS	**1095**	**50**		**505**	**23**

**1 Tbsp regular dressing = avg. 80 cal., 8 gm. fat

FRENCH RESTAURANT

	Cal.	Fat		Cal.	Fat
6 oz. Chicken Kiev	500	33	6 oz. Chicken in Rosé Sauce	350	16
1 cup cream of celery soup	150	10	1/2 cup sautéed fresh vegetables	65	4
1/2 cup wild rice	150	5	watercress & romaine salad	15	0
1/2 cup sautéed mushrooms	45	4	w/ 1 Tbsp French or Ranch dressing	55	6
1 dinner roll	80	1	1 slice French bread	70	1
with 1 tsp margarine or butter	35	4	fresh seasonal fruit plate	100	0
watercress & romaine salad	15	0			
with 2 Tbsp French or Ranch dressing	110	12			
chocolate soufflé	300	22			
TOTALS	**1385**	**92**		**655**	**27**

| Cal = calories | Fat = fat in grams | gm = grams | oz = ounce | tsp = teaspoon | Tbsp = tablespoon |

TIPS: If you do eat more fat at a restaurant, eat lightly at the next meal. Let your week balance the fat. If you eat out frequently, ask for an all-vegetable meal 3-4 times a week. Ask to split an entre. Note that entrees contain the most calories and fat.

TYPICAL RESTAURANT CHOICES

MEXICAN	CALORIES	FAT (gms)
Chile con Carne	375	17
Quesadilla	475	33
Mexican chips (25)	625	36
Beef Fajitas	615	24
Tamale	415	25
Tacos, chicken (2)	420	30
Tacos, beef (2)	500	35
Tostada	650	37
Cheese Enchiladas (2)	830	60
Taco Salad in Taco Shell	1065	70
Arroz con pollo	1200	74

ITALIAN		
Caesar salad	300	25
Garlic bread (1/4 loaf)	515	25
Pasta e Fagioli	600	22
Tomato/Mozzarella Salad	275	23
Veal Picatta	300	21
Veal Parmigiana	500	30
Chicken Parmigiana	400	25
Chicken Cacciatore	600	42
Pasta Primavera	550	32
Manicotti with meat	560	32
Fettucini Alfredo	750	35
Lasagna (4" square)	700	36
Ravioli with meat	750	37
Calzone	850	38
Canelloni, beef	890	50

GREEK		
Greek Salad with feta	250	22
Humus, 1/2 cup	325	18
Gyro	520	17
Spinach Pie with feta	450	23
Moussaka	630	48

AMERICAN		
Broiled chicken (no skin) (1/2 chicken) (6 oz.)	240	7
Fried chicken (1 chicken breast)	325	18
Barbecued chicken (with skin)	350	20
Broiled fish filet (with butter)	250	7
Fried fish filet	400	16
Blackened Redfish (w/ 3 Tbsp butter)	700	45
Roast Beef (6 oz.)	320	14
T-bone, Porterhouse, Sirloin (6 oz.)	380	18
Prime Rib (6 oz.)	650	55
Turkey sandwich, deli	220	6
Ham & cheese croissant	850	40
Ham & cheese sandwich (no mayo), deli	600	23
Hamburger	500-700	30-50

SALAD BARS

SELECT SALADS SENSIBLY!

	AMOUNT	CAL.*	FAT*
0-10 calories			
Artichoke hearts	2	10	0
Bean sprouts	3 Tbsp	7	0
Beets	2 slices	8	0
Broccoli	1/4 cup	6	0
Celery (3-inch stick)	2	4	0
Cucumber	4 slices	2	0
Carrots	1/4	6	0
Cauliflower	1/4 cup	6	0
Green or red pepper	3 slices	6	0
Mushrooms	2 Tbsp	3	0
Lettuce, all types	1 cup	8	0
Olives	2 large	10	2
Onion	1 slice	2	0
Radishes	2 whole	5	0
Tomato	2 slices	5	0
15-25 calories			
Chick-peas	2 Tbsp	35	0
Garbanzo and Kidney beans	2 Tbsp	35	0
Raisins	1 Tbsp	25	0
30-50 calories			
Bacon bits, real or imitation	1 Tbsp	35	2
Cheese, all types grated	1 Tbsp	35	3
Coleslaw	1/4 cup	50	5
Fresh fruit	1/2 cup	50	0
60-80 calories			
Cottage cheese	1/4 cup	55	3
Egg	1	80	5
Sunflower seeds	1 Tbsp	50	5
3-bean salad	1/4 cup	50	3
100 calories			
Avocado	1/4	90	9
Canned fruit	1/2 cup	100	0
Chicken, crab and tuna salad	1/4 cup	100	5
Croutons	1/4 cup	100	6
Macaroni and Potato salad	1/4 cup	100	5
SALAD DRESSING			
Lemon juice, Vinegar, Picante sauce (salsa)	1 Tbsp	0	0
French, Ranch	1 Tbsp	55	6
Bleu Cheese, Thousand Island, Italian, Russian	1 Tbsp	80	8
Reduced-calorie and oil-free dressings	1 Tbsp	6-30	0-4
Cottage Cheese (as dressing)	1/4 cup	55	3

Be Aware: 1 ladle (4 Tbsp) = 250-300 calories! Use all dressings sparingly.

MISCELLANEOUS			
Breadsticks	2	45	5
Crackers	4	60	2
Cornbread	1 piece	180	6
Soup			
broth or tomato-based	1 cup	100-200	5-10
creamy or cheese-based	1 cup	200-350	7-20

IF YOU ARE SULFITE-SENSITIVE, ASK YOUR WAITER ABOUT THE SALADS BEFORE ORDERING!

* Cal. = calories, Fat = fat in grams

FAST FOODS

Of course you can eat fast foods! They are a part of the American lifestyle. We used to say "as American as Apple Pie". Today we hear "as American as a Big Mac and a Coke"!

To meet consumer demand for nutritional information about fast foods, many of the fast food chains have analyzed the nutrient content of their products. Consumers can choose fast foods wisely only when aware of this information. Ask for it. Be informed about your choices.

Limit fast foods. Studies show the average fast food meals costs you 1200 calories!! And they usually are high in fat, cholesterol and sodium (salt). You can change this. Here's how:

14 TIPS ON ORDERING AT A FAST FOODS RESTAURANT

1. Order grilled chicken sandwiches in place of fried chicken or fried fish sandwiches.
2. Order small burgers — not large ones.
3. Know the fat content of various food choices. Select a meal with less than 15-20 grams fat. For example, choose a grilled chicken sandwich without mayonnaise (for 8 grams of fat) and a regular order of fries (for 10 grams of fat); or a small burger or cheeseburger (for 15-20 grams fat) and skip the fries. See Appendix C for listings of Fast Foods and their fat content. Mark your best options. Be prepared before ordering!
4. Avoid desserts, sweets, milkshakes, pies, etc., unless 5 grams fat or less. Today you can find nonfat frozen yogurt and low-fat milkshakes.
5. To reduce fat calories, omit mayonnaise (1 tablespoon = 100 calories). Add mustard, tomatoes, lettuce, pickles, onions instead.
6. Avoid high-calorie beverages, such as regular soft drinks (150-250 calories) or milkshakes (400 calories).
7. Order 1% fat milk, low-calorie soft drinks, fruit juices, tea, water, etc.
8. Avoid fried foods — calories can more than double in foods that are deep-fried.
9. Cut down on fat in fried foods by removing the outer coating before eating (i.e. fried chicken). A fried chicken has 15 grams fat; remove the crust, and you'll eat 7 grams fat.
10. Order a small cheese pizza with low-calorie vegetables such as green pepper, onions or mushrooms. Eat 2 to 3 pieces. Have a salad to help satisfy your appetite and boost fiber, nutrition, and "fullness".
11. At salad bars, limit amounts of dressing, ham, croutons, pasta or potato salads, cheese, nuts and seeds. Eat lots of lettuce, tomato, mushrooms, green pepper, carrots, celery, and cucumber. Use a low-calorie dressing.
12. Carry a piece of fresh fruit to include with your meal or as dessert.
13. Select a baked potato. Top with cottage cheese, picante sauce, 2 tablespoons grated cheese and/or sour cream, or chili.
14. Order fat-free bakery products, i.e. fat-free apple muffins.

OTHER 500-CALORIE MEALS OUT
(and less than 25 grams fat!)

FAST FOOD MEALS

	Cal.	Fat		Cal.	Fat
McDonald's cheeseburger	305	13	Arby's Roast Beef (regular)	380	18
2 percent milk	120	5	Salad	25	0
Fresh fruit (from home)	60	0	1 Tbsp Italian Dressing	70	7
TOTALS	**485**	**18**	**TOTALS**	**475**	**25**
2 slices Pizza Hut Thin n Crispy			Wendy's chili	190	6
Standard cheese, 13-inch	400	17	6 crackers	70	2
Salad	25	0	2 percent milk	120	5
1 Tbsp Ranch Dressing	55	6	Salad	25	0
			1 Tbsp French or Ranch dressing	55	6
TOTALS	**480**	**23**	**TOTALS**	**460**	**19**
Deli Tuna, Turkey, Chicken Sandwich	300	5-10	Burger King's Grilled Chicken Sandwich	280	10
without mayonnaise added to bread			(BK Broiler)		
2 percent milk	120	5	Small French Fries	240	12
Fresh fruit	60	0			
TOTALS	**480**	**10-20**	**TOTALS**	**520**	**22**

STEAK DINNER

	Cal.	Fat		Cal.	Fat
6-oz. filet steak	360	19	*3-oz. filet steak	180	10
1 medium baked potato	160	0	*1/2 medium baked potato	80	0
with 2 pats margarine	70	8 ➔	with 1 pat margarine	35	4
and chives	0	0	and chives	0	0
tossed salad	25	0	tossed salad	25	0
with 1 Tbsp French or Ranch dressing	55	6	with 1 Tbsp reduced-calorie dressing	20	2
water	0	0	water	0	0
TOTALS	**740**	**33**	**TOTALS**	**340**	**16**

*split with a friend or take 1/2 home

APPETIZERS AS SUPPER

	Cal.	Fat
5 jumbo shrimp w/ 2 Tbsp cocktail sauce	100	0
salad w/ 1 Tbsp dressing	100	8
soup (1 cup vegetable)	100	5
large bread or roll without butter	100	1
TOTALS	**400**	**14**

Cal = calories	Fat = fat in grams	gm = grams	oz = ounce	tsp = teaspoon	Tbsp = tablespoon

TRAVELING AND VACATIONING

WHEN YOU TRAVEL, DO YOU QUIT YOUR EATING AND EXERCISE PROGRAMS? HERE'S HOW TO STAY "ON TRACK":

1. Choose a restaurant that allows more food choices than a fast food place with only fried foods, hot dogs, shakes.

2. Take an ice chest with you in your car for diet drinks, fruit, etc. or a picnic lunch. Avoid high-calorie foods like potato chips, nuts, cookies and candy.

3. When traveling in the car, stop for lunch — at a restaurant or picnic area. Don't eat in the car. You won't enjoy it as much.

4. When you stop for a meal, take a walk or stretch. Get some exercise.

5. Decide in advance to avoid peanuts on a plane; choose a diet drink, tomato or fruit juice, water or club soda. Take a snack with you (raisins, bagel, pretzels, fruit).

6. Order a "vegetarian" or "low-calorie" or "seafood" meal 24 hours prior to your flight.

7. "Balance" one rich meal with one all-vegetable meal daily such as a vegetable plate, soup and salad; or a baked potato and salad.

8. Don't center all your activities around eating as the main pleasure of the trip.

9. Take your exercise clothes and use them! You can jump rope in your hotel room, take brisk walks and stay at hotels with exercise facilities or club affiliations.

10. Your eating and exercise plans...Don't leave home without them!

11. Drink 8-10 cups of water. Air travel is dehydrating and fatiguing.

12. Avoid vending machine snacks. Carry a healthy alternative snack.

WEEKENDS

ARE WEEKENDS A CHALLENGE FOR YOU? HERE'S HOW TO HANDLE THEM:

1. Before the weekend arrives, plan fun activities that do not involve eating.

2. Break the habit of getting to Monday 5 pounds heavier and having to lose that "extra" weight before Friday. Adjust your eating and exercise on weekends to fit your schedule. Keep healthy foods on hand to help you eat well and not gain weight.

3. Do not use food as a form of relaxation or recreation. Plan special recreational activities, practice relaxation techniques, and relax!

4. Determine to not "let go" of your eating program. Practice your strategies!

5. Plan 2 meals per day on weekends if your time schedule is adjusted.

HOLIDAYS

WANT TO HANDLE THE HOLIDAYS WITHOUT GUILT?

1. Choose foods that, for you and your family, are an essential part of a particular holiday. Cut back on others.

2. Plan ahead — for food preparation, the holiday meal itself, and use of leftovers. Prepare in advance the least tempting foods (since exposure to these is longer) and save the preparation of the most tempting foods until last.

3. Holiday time is often an emotional time. Plan activities to avoid emotion-related eating (as from loneliness, loss, happiness, etc.). Feel involved with whatever the season and decorate. Attend special holiday events. Avoid eating alone.

4. Remove environmental food cues.

5. Plan fun activities not centered solely around food, such as picture albums, slides, card games, ping-pong, volleyball, basketball or a walk.

6. Don't assume you can make amends after the holidays. Those "extra" pounds can be very difficult to lose.

7. Plan relaxing times for yourself. Enjoy the time away from your regular routine to read, work on hobbies, etc.

8. Remember — giving your time and attention to someone says "I love you" much more effectively than giving or eating food.

9. If you get fatigued, nap instead of snack.

10. Continue with your exercise program throughout the holidays.

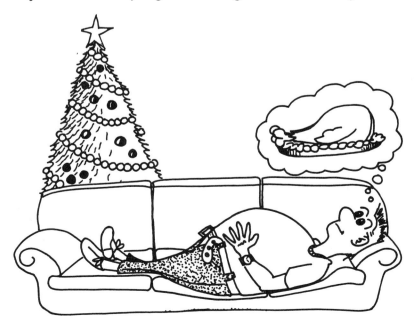

VIII
INNER PSYCHE AND
STRESS MANAGEMENT

INNER FOCUS

1. Think positive thoughts. Keep inner peace (187). Recognize weight loss as a source of strength, accomplishment, and stress reduction. It should RELIEVE — not create — stress!

2. Don't let bottled up feelings weight you down. Tune into you! Express your feelings in writing, to a friend, in prayer, or with exercise and physical activity.

HABIT FOCUS

1. Time Out! Identify stressors in your life and learn to relax without food (188-192).

2. Identify specific activities from your "Relaxation Check List" (193).

NUTRITION FOCUS

1. Make "Grocery Shopping" (194) less tempting by practicing positive shopping habits.

2. Read "Food Labels" (195-196).

GOALS

HABIT:	Identify stressors in your life and practice appropriate new responses to at least two stressors
FOOD:	Look for new food products as a result of reading food labels
EXERCISE:	Exercise when you feel stressed and experience your body tension dissipating
RECORDS:	Food, exercise, weight - reward yourself for handling stress without food

---

INNER PSYCHE

HOW WELL ARE YOU TAKING CARE OF YOUR INNER SELF?

Inner psyche refers to your spiritual, mental and emotional self. This "inner" health affects your **self-attitude** and **life-attitudes**. It motivates you to take care of yourself and promotes confidence to do so. Lack of inner contentment can disrupt any worthy goals and plans for weight control, healthy eating, and exercise ... because it zaps energy and enthusiasm.

Nourish and exercise your inner self with appropriate reading, family time and communication, fellowship with others (individually and in groups), challenges, and opportunities for growth. Self-reflect. Spend time with God. Take on a loving, giving attitude toward others. Try to "make it someone else's day." Your inner person will be enriched and you'll be able to meet your goals.

When you are content and fulfilled by your choices and activities, food becomes less of a focus in life.

> "It is the most beautiful of compensations of this life that no man can try to help another without helping himself."
> Ralph Waldo Emerson

NOURISH YOURSELF IN NUMEROUS WAYS

Develop your special gifts and talents. Wear flattering clothes. Enjoy varied activities and learning new skills. Seek personal growth. Expand your interests and friendships. Appreciate yourself and your own attractiveness. Remind yourself of qualities you like in yourself and in your appearance.

TUNE INTO YOURSELF

Do you eat for emotional reasons or for unmet needs? **Emotional eating** often results from unresolved conflict, anger, fatigue, boredom, stress, loneliness. Do you need more attention, more social activities, better relationships, more job fulfillment, more fun and recreation, more recognition, or a greater meaning in life? Food is a poor substitute.

The **counsel** of a professional, a trusted friend, a pastor, or religious leader, reading, or prayer may direct you to solutions.

To feel you are in **control of your weight** and your life, accept responsibility for your life and choices. Learn assertiveness skills, learn to express your feelings and needs, do things you enjoy, accept yourself, and pursue your own interests and enrichment times. You'll find new fulfillment and less hunger.

SEEK MODERATION

In place of an "all or none" attitude toward eating, and a chronic "losing weight" / "gaining weight" lifestyle, try a new approach of **moderation**. Set your own boundaries or "ground rules" for foods to limit, enjoy a freedom of **eating anything**, within your chosen guidelines.

STRESS AND RELAXATION

WHAT IS STRESS?

- Pressure from external circumstances that can cause internal tensions.
- A way of life. Man cannot live in complete freedom from stress.
- Stress can be a positive drive to stimulate your best efforts.
- Prolonged, unrelieved stress can lead to organic disease; too much stress may lead to excess eating, smoking, drinking, sleep difficulties, anxiety, depression, irritability and susceptibility to cancer, ulcers, headache, hypertension and heart problems.

HOW DO YOU HANDLE STRESS?

- Almost everyone encounters stressful periods — from some crisis (death, marriage, divorce, change in jobs, etc.) or from day to day hassles (traffic, losing keys, missing the bus, etc.).
- WHAT IS IMPORTANT IS HOW YOU HANDLE THE STRESS!
- Learn to cope with stress so it does not work against you.
- Learn how to change some stress into unstress (positive stress).
- Prevent excessive or chronic stress.
- IDENTIFY EVENTS THAT TRIGGER STRESS FOR YOU, (I.E., RUSH-HOUR TRAFFIC, TOO MANY PHONE CALLS IN THE DAY, FINANCES, LACK OF TIME).

  1.   5.
  2.   6.
  3.   7.
  4.   8.
- HOW DO YOU REACT TO STRESS?

  _____tension headache   _____back pain, neck/shoulder pain
  _____jaw tension   _____migraine headache
  _____high blood pressure   _____allergies
  _____constipation   _____diarrhea
  _____digestive disorders   _____fatigue
  _____overeating or bingeing   _____anxiety
  _____eating less/undereating   _____withdrawal, isolation
  _____depression   _____other:_____

"Learn to take care of your mind as well as your body ... the foundations of good health lie in love, laughter, and faith in oneself."

Dr. Don Dudley, SeattlePsychiatrist

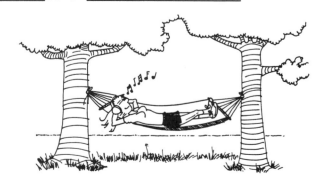

Tips To Relax & Handle Stress

1. Identify the causes of stress and work toward solutions.

2. Talk to someone you can trust.

3. Escape for awhile. Read a book, go to a movie, listen to music or take a walk. DO NOT escape to food, smoking, alcohol, etc.

4. Don't take on more than you can accomplish — set limits and say NO to excessive demands. BE ASSERTIVE.

5. Set priorities. List your necessary tasks in order of importance and tackle one at a time. Solve difficult tasks when you are energetic and simple tasks later in the day.

6. Organize your time. Pace yourself. Identify your most productive time and allow for rest periods. Avoid too many appointments and deadlines and unnecessary obligations.

7. Don't try to be perfect. Work to the best of your efforts and ability. Avoid criticism for not achieving an "impossible" task. Take deserved credit for a task well done.

8. Plan for change. Coping with the unexpected is a great stressor. Try to avoid too many big changes at the same time and try to accept and prepare for change.

9. Slow down. Practice walking slower, eating slower, driving slower, and talking slower. Really listen to someone talking with you. Look at others' faces.

10. Avoid situations and places that are noisy and crowded. Take the back streets, eat in quiet restaurants and shop in smaller stores.

11. Take time for yourself and have fun! Get involved in a hobby or something that helps you to forget stressors of the day. Learn to relax mentally and physically. Pamper your body — massage, facial or bath works wonders!

12. Make friends and work at keeping them. Help others. Practice complimenting others several times a day.

13. Build a positive self-image. Realistically accept your special gifts and limitations. Do a good job. Be dependable. Develop a life purpose. Stay close to your support system of friends.

14. Balance your life with work and play, seriousness and laughter, etc.

> *"Laughter is inner jogging."*
>
> - Norman Cousins

15. Take care of yourself — EAT RIGHT AND EXERCISE REGULARLY. A healthy well-nourished and well-exercised body handles stress better than a weak, poorly nourished one. Limit caffeine in coffee, tea, colas, and chocolate. Avoid salt and refined sugars. Eat breakfast and avoid late night snacks. Eat three meals daily at regular times. Eat slowly. This aids digestion and prevents overeating. Exercise relaxes your body.

16. Hug someone. Touching gives us a sense of well-being, comfort and security.

17. SMILE! It helps to relax you. Positive emotions help fight stress. Don't hold grudges — a mental drain. Learn to forgive.

18. Listen to quiet, soothing, relaxing music. Sounds of rain or waves at the seashore are relaxing. Wind chimes and a bird feeder in the backyard can be a source of relaxation. Enjoy beautiful pictures or photographs.

19. Avoid self-medication. Alcohol and drugs only reduce your resistance and cover up your problems.

20. Utilize the "Big 3" coping solutions:
    1. commitment — to self, work, family, friends, values
    2. control — sense personal control over your life
    3. challenge — see change as an opportunity

- **WHAT CAN YOU DO TO REMOVE OR REDUCE STRESS?** (for example, exercise daily, get enough rest, schedule 15 minutes quiet time daily, use a phone answering machine, eat nutritious, regular meals)
  1.
  2.
  3.
  4.
  5.

- **EXCESS CHANGE AT ONE TIME CAN PRODUCE STRESS.**
  LIST MAJOR CHANGES YOU ARE EXPERIENCING AND WAYS TO COPE:

CHANGE (i.e., new job)	COPING STRATEGIES (i.e., rest more, pace yourself)
1.	1.
2.	2.
3.	3.
4.	4.
5.	5.

RELAXATION TECHNIQUES

1. **LEARN TO BREATHE PROPERLY. THIS INCREASES OXYGEN IN YOUR BLOOD, STRENGTHENS ABDOMINAL AND INTESTINAL MUSCLES, AND RELEASES TENSION.**

　　a. Think of your lungs in 3 parts.
　　b. Breathe in and fill up the bottom part lifting your diaphragm and keep chest stiil.
　　c. Fill the middle area of your lungs and feel your chest expand.
　　d. Fill the upper portion and feel your shoulders rise slightly.
　　e. Set a regular time each day for deep, slow breathing and **not** rapid shallow breathing.
　　f. Do 10 breaths, 4 times a day.

2. **TRY THESE TECHNIQUES AND USE THE ONES THAT WORK BEST FOR YOU:**

　　a. Distract yourself. Keep a list of alternative activities you can enjoy — a hobby, music, reading a favorite magazine or book, talking, walking, etc. DO NOT use food to relax!
　　b. Talk to someone.
　　c. Take a nap, or just relax and close your eyes.
　　d. Practice muscle relaxing exercises.
　　e. Use your imagination and "GET AWAY" to relax — imagery techniques.
　　f. Meditate or pray.
　　g. Breathe deeply.

3. **PRACTICE THESE MUSCLE RELAXING EXERCISES — BREATHE DEEPLY THROUGHOUT THE EXERCISES AND FEEL THE TENSION LEAVE YOUR BODY:**

　　a. Clench each fist and hold 10 seconds. RELAX. Repeat 5 times.
　　b. Rigidly straighten both arms and hold for 10 seconds. RELAX. Repeat 2 times.
　　c. Shoulder rotation — stand with arms to side, rotate shoulders forward 10 times and then backward 10 times.
　　d. Neck rotation — take a full deep breath and exhale. Drop head to chest and rotate to right, then to left 8 times.
　　e. Shrug your shoulders, bringing them up to your ears. Hold 10 seconds and pull back down. Repeat 5 times.
　　f. Arm rotation — stand up and extend arms outward by your sides. Rotate arms, making 10 small circles in one direction. Increase the size of your circles and repeat 10 times. Repeat in opposite direction.
　　g. Overhead stretches — reach up with right arm 8 times and then with left arm 8 times.

> ## AT THE OFFICE OR AT HOME, TAKE A FEW MINUTES TO EXERCISE AND RELAX!

4. IMAGERY TECHNIQUES:

a. Be RELAXED. Find a quiet place to be alone, away from other persons, noise, activity, and the phone. Tensions block the success of visual suggestions.

b. Sit in a comfortable chair in comfortable clothing. Turn down the lights and close your eyes.

c. Take a deep, full breath and exhale fully and completely.

d. Keep your eyes shut and drift away to a time or special place that you found to be calm and relaxing and peaceful — the beach, a hike in a wooded area, a walk in the fields, vacation spot, etc.

e. Let your imagination go and put yourself completely into this environment — the smells, the cool or warm feeling, the sounds, the feelings that made it peaceful. Stay with this scene until you feel completely RELAXED — ENJOY for about 5 minutes.

f. When RELAXED, open your eyes and move your arms and legs. FEEL THE CALM.

g. Practice at least once a day and "get away from it all!"

RULE NO. 1: *Don't sweat the small stuff.*

RULE NO. 2: *It's all small stuff.*
— Robert Eliot, M.D.

If you can't fight and you can't flee, learn to flow.
- Robert Eliot, M.D.

Most folks are about as happy as they make up their minds to be.
- A. Lincoln

To err is human, to forgive divine.
- Alexander Pope

Other people are not in the world to live up to your expectations.
- Fritz Perls

I can't give you the formula for success, but I can sure give you the formula for failure ... try to please everybody.
- A. Lincoln

RELAXATION CHECK LIST

CHECK AND LIST SPECIFIC ACTIVITIES YOU CAN TURN TO FOR RELAXATION:

_____ Exercise — intense or recreational
_____ Movies, T.V.
_____ Concerts, plays
_____ Hobbies
_____ Music
_____ Rhythmic motion, such as dancing or rocking chair. Watch blowing trees, rain or swimming fish
_____ Sing
_____ Escape with your earphones
_____ Communicate — in person, phone, letter
_____ Use typewriter to transfer thoughts and frustration
_____ Talk to self
_____ Talk to significant other(s)
_____ Take a shower or long bath
_____ Meditate
_____ Think out and analyze problem
_____ Pray
_____ Read
_____ Sleep
_____ Daydream
_____ Socialize — attend meetings, programs with others
_____ Review picture albums of pleasant events and times
_____ Touch
_____ Laugh, cry — express feelings

USE YOUR HANDS:

_____ Carpentry
_____ Painting
_____ Sewing
_____ Gardening
_____ Needlepoint
_____ Gifts
_____ Ceramics
_____ Knitting
_____ Car Work
_____ Picture albums
_____ Artwork
_____ Musical instruments

GROCERY SHOPPING
Resist Grocery Store Temptations!

1. Make a **SHOPPING LIST** from your eating plan and stick to it! Avoid buying unnecessary and often high-calorie foods. Do not try to shop from memory on spur of the moment.

2. Shop **AFTER A MEAL** when you are not hungry, or at a time of the day when you are least susceptible to food cues. Hunger pangs often lead to overbuying and high-calorie foods.

3. Shop **ONCE WEEKLY** on a regular schedule. The less time spent in a grocery store, the better. Plus, you'll save money.

4. Avoid **TEMPTING** shopping AISLES.

5. Shop at "inviting" stores with beautiful, fresh produce. This makes the right food irresistible!

6. Buy **LOW-CALORIE SNACKS**. Avoid high-fat, sugary foods.

7. If you are tempted by a high-calorie "junk food," stop and think. Select a lower-calorie substitute.
   If you must have the "junk food" buy a very **small** quantity!

8. Put grocery bags in your trunk to avoid snacking on the way home.

9. When home, put foods away immediately — out of sight!

HONEY, I'M STARVING, LET'S GO GROCERY SHOPPING

Read the Food Labels!

1. Look for **SUGAR** as: ("ose" means sugar) sugar, corn syrup, maple syrup, molasses, honey, dextrin, sorghum, brown sugar, sorbitol, mannitol, sucrose, fructose, lactose, dextrose, galactose, glucose, maltose, mannose

2. Look for **SALT** as: salt, (sodium chloride), MSG (monosodium glutamate), sodium bicarbonate (baking soda), brine, sodium propionate, sodium alginate, sodium hydroxide, sodium sulfite, sodium saccharin, etc.

3. Look for **FATS** as: butter, oil, shortening, lard, hydrogenated fats, beef fat, cream, bacon, mayonnaise, dressing.
   Choose polyunsaturated oils (safflower, corn, sunflower, soybean, cottonseed).
   "vegetable oil" does not always mean polyunsaturated oil; coconut and palm oils are saturated fats and are added to many commercial products; hydrogenated or partially hydrogenated oil is saturated.

  © 1993, *The Balancing Act Nutrition and Weight Guide*, G. Kostas, M.P.H., R.D., Dallas, Texas

FOOD LABELS

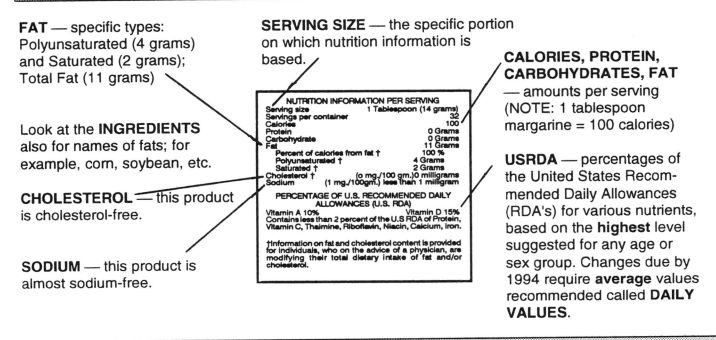

FAT — specific types: Polyunsaturated (4 grams) and Saturated (2 grams); Total Fat (11 grams)

Look at the **INGREDIENTS** also for names of fats; for example, corn, soybean, etc.

CHOLESTEROL — this product is cholesterol-free.

SODIUM — this product is almost sodium-free.

SERVING SIZE — the specific portion on which nutrition information is based.

CALORIES, PROTEIN, CARBOHYDRATES, FAT — amounts per serving (NOTE: 1 tablespoon margarine = 100 calories)

USRDA — percentages of the United States Recommended Daily Allowances (RDA's) for various nutrients, based on the **highest** level suggested for any age or sex group. Changes due by 1994 require **average** values recommended called **DAILY VALUES.**

The following nutrition information panel is from a package of potato chips:

CALORIES — 150 calories/ounce. This 1-5/8 ounce package = 245 calories.

FAT — 10 grams (90 calories). With 150 calories/ounce, this is 60% Fat.*

SODIUM — 200 milligrams per ounce. This 1-5/8 ounce package = 325 milligrams (1/4 teaspoon salt).

*HOW TO CALCULATE % FAT IN FOODS: Multiply grams of fat/serving × 9 cal/gm and divide by total number of calories in food. Example above: 10 gm fat × 9 cal/gm = 90 cal fat ÷ 150 cal/serving = 60% Fat by calories. This is not the same as 60% fat by weight (e.g., milk that is labeled 4% fat, contains 4% of its weight and 60% of its calories from fat.

HOW TO CONVERT GRAMS TO CALORIES: Example above:

Protein	: 4 cal/gm	× 2 gm	=	8 cal
Carbohydrate	: 4 cal/gm	× 14 gm	=	56 cal
Fat	: 9 cal/gm	× 10 gm	=	90 cal
	TOTAL CALORIES		=	154 (approx 150) per serving

CHOOSE FOODS WITH 3 OR LESS GRAMS FAT PER 100 CALORIES, AS OFTEN AS POSSIBLE.

UNDERSTANDING FOOD LABELS

List of Ingredients

Starting in 1993, all ingredients must be listed on the label. The ingredient present in the largest amount, by weight, must be listed first, followed in descending order of weight by the other ingredients. Specific names of additives, colors, flavors, preservatives, and seasonings, must be included on the new labels by 1994. It has been proposed that all sugars (honey, sugar, corn syrup solids, molasses, etc.) be collectively expressed by weight, and individually listed by name.

Nutrition Information on Food Labels

Nutrition information is given on a per serving basis. The label tells the **size** of a **serving** (for example: one cup, two ounces, one tablespoon), the **number** of **servings** in the container, the **number** of **calories** per serving, **fat calories** per serving, and the amounts (in grams) of **protein**, **carbohydrate** and **fat** per serving. New labels must also add the amounts of **cholesterol** (mg.), **fiber** (gm.), **saturated fat** (gm.), **sodium** (mg.), **sugar** or simple carbohydrate (gm.) and **total carbohydrates** (gm.) (meaning complex and simple carbohydrates). Only 2 vitamins and 2 minerals are required: Vitamins A and C, and minerals calcium and iron expressed as percentages of the **Daily Value** recommended. All other nutrients will be compared to **Daily Values Recommended**, listed by percentage and grams.

How to Interpret Nutrition Information
(U.S. RDA's, RDI's, RDV's, Daily Values)

Based on the highest level of nutrients recommended for any age group, the U.S. Recommended Daily Allowances **(U.S. RDA's)** are the amounts of protein, vitamins, and minerals that an adult should eat every day to keep healthy. Up to 1993, these values are listed on foods by percentage. For example, a label may state that one serving of the food contains 35 percent of the U.S. RDA for Vitamin A and 25 percent of the U.S. RDA for iron. The new labeling laws (effective 1993-1994) will compare nutrients with the **Daily Values** (average values) recommended, based on eating 2,000 calories daily. Daily Values are comprised of **Recommended Daily Intakes** (RDI's) for vitamins and minerals, and **Daily Reference Values** (DRV's) for fat, saturated fat, cholesterol, carbohydrates, fiber, and sodium. Proposed DRV's are 65 grams fat and 20 grams of saturated fat, based on eating 2,000 calories a day. For individuals consuming 1500 calories daily, DRV's would be 50 grams fat and 15 grams saturated fat. You must adjust these recommended values to your own calorie intake.

New Definitions

All terms on labels (i.e., "light", "low-fat", etc.) will be carefully defined and consistently used. For example, **"light"** can be used only if the product serving contains 1/3rd less calories and 1/2 the fat of the original product equivalent. **"Low-fat"** means the product contains less than 3 grams of fat per serving.

Nutrition Facts
Serving Size ½ cup (114g)
Servings Per Container 4

Amount Per Serving
Calories 260   Calories from Fat 12

	% of Daily Value
Total Fat 13g	**20%**
Saturated Fat 5g	**25%**
Cholesterol 30mg	**10%**
Sodium 660 mg	**28%**
Total Carbohydrate 31g	**11%**
Dietary Fiber 0g	**0%**
Sugars 5g	
Protein 5g	

Vitamin A 4% • Vitamin C 2%
Calcium 15% • Iron 4%

* Percents (%) of a Daily Value are based on a 2,000 calorie diet. Your Daily Values may vary higher or lower depending on your calorie needs:

Nutrient		2,000 Calories	2,500 Calories
Total Fat	Less than	65g	80g
Sat. Fat	Less than	20g	25g
Cholesterol	Less than	300mg	300mg
Sodium	Less than	2,400mg	2,400mg
Total Carbohydrate		300g	375g
Fiber		25g	30g

1g Fat= 9 calories
1g Carbohydrates= 4 calories
1g Protein= 4 calories

Sample New Label

IX
BUILDING SUPPORT &
MORE FOOD FACTS

HABIT FOCUS

1. Develop "Your Support Team" (199) to keep you moving forward! Learn to handle non-support.

2. List "My Support Team" (204). Take the lead and encourage teamwork.

NUTRITION FOCUS

1. "Bone Up On Calcium!" (205)

2. Get the "Fiber Facts" (207)

3. Limit "Caffeine" (208)

4. Water Unlimited! (212)

5. Additives — To Eat or Not to Eat (213)

GOALS

HABIT:	take control - work with your support team
FOOD:	increase calcium, fiber foods - drink more water
EXERCISE:	continue your aerobics program
RECORDS:	food, exercise, weight - identify calcium sources, fiber foods and water intake

---

YOUR SUPPORT TEAM

WHEN TRYING TO LOSE WEIGHT, HAVE YOU EVER FELT THAT...

- No one cares or is interested?
- You are teased about your weight and made to feel different even though you are changing and losing weight?
- Your friends and/or family are pessimistic or non-supportive?
- You are being sabotaged — given high-calorie foods? Have only food-related social activities? Given food as a sign of affection? Told that you are becoming too skinny?
- People insist that you eat dessert, seconds, etc.?

THE PEOPLE IN YOUR ENVIRONMENT PLAY A VERY IMPORTANT AND INFLUENTIAL ROLE IN YOUR PROGRAM AND IN YOUR LIFE! People can be a source of reinforcement and rewards — noticing changes, complimenting you, giving you feedback and encouragement.

!!TAKE CONTROL!!

BE VOCAL! No one can read your mind. Be explicit about what you need and want.

1. Ask for **daily** support and encouragement. Be specific. Tell others **how** to support you.

2. Ask for feedback. Be specific. What type of feedback do you desire? When?

3. Ask for praise.

4. Ask for cooperation and assistance. Tell others **how** to assist.

5. Ask for participation — in exercise, shopping, cooking, counseling, education , pre-planning, cue elimination, etc.

6. Entertain with low-calorie, attractive, fun foods.

7. Do not use food for sharing and affection. Request that love be expressed in other ways. Ask for flowers, books, music, etc.

8. Ask for food. Let others know that you do not want it offered to you.

9. Minimize conversations about food.

10. Exercise with your family and friends or with a class.

11. Ask that people not continue to eat tempting foods around you.

12. Get involved in activities that take you outside of yourself — ceramics, sewing, gift-making, bowling, team sports, painting, carpentry, yard work, church groups, charities, etc.

13. Plan family gatherings to include **activities** — not just food.

14. Thank others for their support and encouragement.

HOW DO YOU HANDLE NON-SUPPORT?

- People have different ways of reacting to someone losing weight.

- Be sensitive to the factors that may cause **negative responses**, conscious or unconscious, from others:

    1. Others may feel threatened by your self-discipline and self-control and not want to have to match your accomplishments!

    2. Your improved appearance may create new, uncertain feelings within others. With a "new look," will you want a "new type relationship"?

- Do not let others control you. You must control your own life.

- Learn to cope with non-supportive behaviors:

    1. Are your expectations of others unrealistic?

    2. How do you reinforce others' supportive behaviors?

    3. How can you positively cope? Respond?

    4. How can you let others get involved?

    5. Ask for support you want. Others may not know how to help you.

- **Remember:** Your program and the education you give others may benefit them!!!

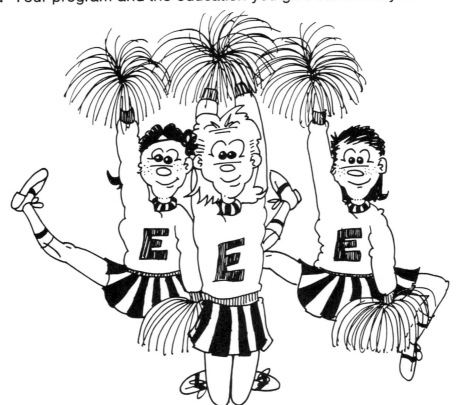

Social and Community Support

HERE'S HOW TO SURROUND YOURSELF WITH ON-GOING SUPPORT:

1. **Associate and socialize** with others of similar values, motives, goals and "coping skills" to acquire stronger behavioral skills and easier social adjustment skills.

2. Join **clubs or groups** that reinforce your interests — spas, gyms, low-fat cooking classes, bike club, dance group, etc.

3. Join **self-help groups** — their benefits:

   (a) social outlet/peer support

   (b) role models (participants) representing obtainable goals

   (c) motivation and self-confidence

   (d) problem-solving practice

   (e) self-responsibility

4. Participate in **self-help activities**:

   (a) lead the class

   (b) check buddy's food records or exercise log

   (c) write newsletter

   (d) contribute recipes

   (e) develop phone check system

5. Take **classes** that motivate your desired behaviors and knowledge:

   (a) swimming, tennis, aerobics classes, etc. — the discipline of regular meetings will reinforce and commit your behaviors

   (b) enriched skills make tasks easier and more desirable

   (c) a camaraderie of class friends provide support and encouragement

6. Find a **"partner"** with whom you can communicate and work. Commit to a common goal and action plan.

7. Develop **communication skills** and **interpersonal relation skills**.

Environmental Support

HERE'S HOW TO MOTIVATE YOURSELF TO STAY FIT AND EAT WELL:

1. **PARTICIPATE IN ACTIVE EVENTS:**

   (a) walks, races, swim meets, tennis tournaments, etc.

   (b) hiking trips, ski trips, bike trips

   (c) intramural sports

   (d) treadmill tests

   (e) vacations

   (f) children's activities

   (g) charity bike-a-thons, etc.

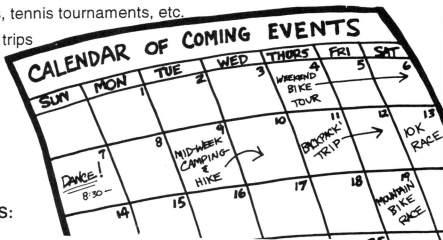

2. **GO TO THE RIGHT PLACES:**

   (a) gyms and exercise facilities — a healthier after-work activity than bars

   (b) non-food environments — socialize with a friend outdoors, not in front of the television or at a food counter

   (c) church, charity groups — activities that put others first

   (d) home and work — keep your surroundings free of "food cues"

3. **MANAGE YOUR TIME WELL:** don't use food as a . . .

   (a) procrastinator

   (b) transition

   (c) time-filler, such as when waiting for a bus

   (d) coffee break

   (e) leisure or recreational activity or pastime

4. **KNOW YOUR REACTION TO MEDIA:**

   (a) enjoy health, fitness, weight control magazines and tapes instead of high-fat cooking magazines and food catalogs

   (b) distinguish healthy versus unhealthy food ads on T.V. and radio, in newspapers and magazines

Self-Support

YOU CAN TALK AND THINK YOURSELF INTO HEALTHIER BEHAVIORS:

1. Practice positive **self-talk** when excuses and discouragement seep in. Write down your positive responses.

Negative Thoughts	Positive Thoughts
(a) I over-ate and feel guilty. I might as well keep eating and forget this program.	It's O.K. I enjoyed it. Now it is time to get back on track and start again.
(b) I shouldn't have had that candy. That blows the whole day. I'll start over tomorrow.	I won't procrastinate; I'll start back right now. A small mistake won't hurt. I'll exercise more this afternoon and eat less tonight.
(c) When I eat out, I have to eat everything on my plate. After all, I paid for it.	I'm eating out because of the company or the convenience. That's what I'm paying for. I don't want to pay the waistline price tomorrow.
(d) I always blow it on weekends or at parties or after dinner.	I'll plan ahead to avoid undesirable situations.
(e) If I don't eat this now, I might never have another chance.	Ridiculous! There are always fun foods to enjoy. I'll enjoy it more when I've lost some weight.

2. Be your **own best friend**. Treat yourself to activities that please you as you make progress. Refer to your Pleasure Activities list on page 30.

3. **Compliment** yourself daily for reorienting your lifestyle and practicing new behaviors, attitudes, self-confidence, etc. (The scales are not the only sign of progress!)

4. Monitor your progress with **records** — food, exercise, weight, inches, clothing sizes. View any progress as a step in the right direction.

5. Manage your **thinking**.

   (a) Improve your **self-attitude**:
   - be ASSERTIVE — you must help yourself.
   - be REALISTIC — allow room for imperfection. Take small steps of change.
   - be OPTIMISTIC — feel positive about yourself, your successes and your ability to reach and maintain health goals.
   - be PROUD — you are living a healthier lifestyle.

   (b) Practice **self-imagery**:
   - envision yourself being more slender, confident and content
   - picture yourself living an active lifestyle
   - see yourself managing eating occasions in a positive way

6. List your priorities in life. Arrange your commitments to give your health and weight the attention they deserve.

© 1993, *The Balancing Act Nutrition and Weight Guide*, G. Kostas, M.P.H., R.D., Dallas, Texas

203

My Support Team

WHO DO YOU TURN TO FOR SUPPORT OF YOUR NEW LIFESTYLE? IDENTIFY PEOPLE AND FACTORS THAT ENCOURAGE YOU. SURROUND YOURSELF WITH THESE.

SOCIAL (individuals, groups)
- best friend Mary
- weight control class
1.
2.
3.

ENVIRONMENTAL
- join YMCA
- charity walk/run
1.
2.
3.

SELF-SUPPORT
- positive self-attitude

- encourage self daily
- be realistic

- be alert
1.
2.
3.

NON-SUPPORTIVE BEHAVIORS
- family snacking at night
1.
2.
3.

PSYCHE
- positive self-image
- appearance, fitness

- confidence boosters
1.
2.
3.

HOW:
- exercise partner; emotional support
- team motivation
1.
2.
3.

HOW:
- exercise class and participants
- motivational goal
1.
2.
3.

HOW:
- keep thinking of positive steps and ability to reach goals
- take 1 day at a time
- lose 1 pound a week; don't expect to be perfect
- keep food + exercise records; weigh weekly
1.
2.
3.

HOW I COPE:
- drink low-calorie beverages; enjoy family
1.
2.
3.

HOW:
- focus on positive qualities — fitness
- smaller clothing size, feeling good, compliments
- focus on challenges achieved
1.
2.
3.

BONE UP ON CALCIUM!

At all ages, men and women need calcium for strong bones, teeth, and exercising muscles. In particular, women need extra calcium after age 30 to prevent osteoporosis, "softening of the bones" which occurs in women after age 50. Do you eat enough calcium?

ADULTS (ages)		CALCIUM (mg) NEEDED DAILY	DAILY NUMBER OF 300 mg CALCIUM EQUIVALENT FOODS*
Men	(20 +)	800	2-3 servings
Women	(20-30)	1000	3-4 servings
Women	(30-50)	1200	3-4 servings
Women	(50 +)	1500	3-4 servings + supplement

CALCIUM-RICH FOODS

Item	Serving Size	Calcium (mg)
Yogurt	1 cup	400
Ricotta cheese, part-skim	1/2 cup	340
Milk, all types	1 cup	300
Orange juice w/ calcium	1 cup	300
Swiss cheese	1 ounce	260
Cheddar cheese	1 ounce	200
American cheese	1 ounce	175
Total cereals, wheat or corn	1 ounce	200
Oysters	3/4 cup	170
Salmon, canned with bones	3 ounces	170
Collard greens; most greens	1/2 cup	145
Spinach, cooked	1/2 cup	100
Ice cream or ice milk	1/2 cup	100
Mustard greens, cooked	1/2 cup	100
Beans, cooked	1 cup	90
Cottage cheese, 2% low-fat	1/2 cup	80
Kale, cooked	1/2 cup	75
Broccoli, cooked	1/2 cup	70
Orange	1 medium	55

*CALCIUM EQUIVALENTS
(300 mg/serving)

Item	Serving Size
Milk, all types	1 cup
Nonfat dry milk	5 tablespoons
Alba hot cocoa mix	1 cup
Alba High Calcium Shake	1 cup
Yogurt	1 cup
Cheddar cheese	1-1/2 ounces
Processed cheese	1-1/2 ounces
Mozzarella cheese	2 ounces
Cottage cheese	2 cups
Ice cream or ice milk	1-1/2 cups
Tofu	8 ounces
Broccoli	2 cups
Collards; turnip greens	1 cup
Kale; mustard greens	1-1/2 cups
Oysters	1-1/2 cup
Salmon, canned with bones	4 ounces
Sardines w/ bones	2-1/2 ounces
Orange juice w/ calcium	1 cup
Supplement, i.e., Citracal	1 tablet

SAMPLE HIGH-CALCIUM, LOW-CALORIE MENU

Daily Food	Calcium (mg)	Calories	Fat (gms)
2 cups skim milk	600	180	trace
2 ounces mozzarella cheese	300	160	10
1/2 cup spinach, cooked	100	25	0
1 orange, medium	50	50	0
1 apple, large	10	80	0
3 slices bread	75	210	3
3 ounces chicken, baked	12	150	6
Tossed salad	30	25	0
1 baked potato, medium	15	140	0
1 carrot	25	25	0
TOTALS:	1217 mg	1045 calories	19 gms

TIPS TO INCREASE CALCIUM:

- Add nonfat dry powdered milk to:

oatmeal	macaroni and cheese
cooked cereals	mashed potatoes
soup	cornbread or muffins
casseroles	liquid milk
spaghetti sauce	high-calcium Alba cocoa
pizza sauce	homemade yogurt make from skim milk
pancakes	homemade milk-fruit shakes

- Add grated cheese to salads, baked potatoes, casseroles.
- Eat low-fat diet cheese (same calcium, less fat).

> 1 Tablespoon dry powdered milk = 60 milligrams calcium

FACTORS TO PROMOTE STRONG BONES:

- Eat adequate calcium.
- Eat a balanced, healthy diet.
- Lose weight to avoid stress on bones.
- Do regular weight-bearing exercise such as walking (not biking or swimming), at least five times a week.
- Get sunlight exposure at least 15 minutes a day. Sunlight stimulates vitamin D production in skin. Vitamin D aids calcium absorption.
- Do not smoke.
- Avoid "mega-doses" of vitamins A and D which accelerate bone resorption.
- Use estrogen replacement as directed by your physician.
- Avoid soft drinks and caffeine.

CALCIUM SUPPLEMENTS — WHICH ARE BEST?

Various forms of calcium are available:
- calcium citrate (in Citracal) or calcium citrate maleonate (in orange juice w/ calcium); these forms of calcium are the best absorbed and are recommended at the Cooper Clinic
- calcium carbonate (also in Tums and other antacid tablets)
- calcium phosphate
- calcium lactate
- calcium gluconate

Avoid bone meal and dolomite due to potential lead contamination. Take calcium as your physician directs.

WAYS TO BOOST CALCIUM SUPPLEMENT ABSORPTION:

- take supplement on an empty stomach, or
- take calcium with a dairy product, such as milk (lactose and vitamin D aid absorption), or
- take calcium with orange juice or tomato juice (vitamin C boosts calcium absorption)
- never take supplements with caffeine-containing beverages such as tea, coffee and cola drinks or high-fiber foods (caffeine and fiber impair calcium absorption)
- take supplements with vitamin D only if you are shut-in and without daily sunlight exposure
- take supplements at different times of day, if you take more than one calcium supplement daily. Smaller amounts, consumed at regular intervals, are absorbed better.

FIBER FACTS

FIBER IS CRITICAL TO OPTIMAL HEALTH AND EASE WITH WEIGHT CONTROL.

WHAT IS FIBER?

- Plant "roughage" — peels, seeds, kernels, wholegrains, bran, "strings" in foods (bananas, pears, melons, oranges) — and plant carbohydrate content
- "Bulk" in the diet which "pushes" food through the digestive tract more smoothly, aiding digestion and elimination
- Two types of fiber — insoluble and soluble
- Insoluble fiber — is in plant coatings, peels, seeds, kernels, strings (Sources: apple peels, nuts, beans, seeds, bran kernels, popcorn, orange or pear or celery strings)
- Soluble fiber — is in water-soluble complex carbohydrate content of food and characterized by "stickiness" after cooking (apples, oats, beans, vegetables, peas, barley, psyllium); also in gums (guar, locust beans) used to thicken foods (fat-free salad dressings, fat-free frozen desserts, etc.)

8 REASONS TO EAT MORE FIBER — IT:

1. Promotes weight control — fiber-rich foods take longer to eat and create a feeling of fullness and satiety.
2. Enhances good digestion.
3. Acts as a "natural laxative" to reduce constipation and promote regular elimination.
4. Decreases the risk of colon cancer.
5. Helps prevent and treat diverticulosis.
6. Prevents and treats spastic colon, hemorrhoids and other digestive problems.
7. Insoluble fiber reduces cholesterol levels.
8. Insoluble fiber stabilizes blood sugar levels, which helps control appetite and lowers insulin requirements in persons with diabetes.

WHERE IS FIBER?

KEY SOURCES: wholegrain breads and cereals, wheat bran, fresh fruits and vegetables, peas, beans, nuts, seeds, oats, psyllium, popcorn, barley, and brown rice.

EXTRA SOURCES: unprocessed bran flakes (such as Millers Bran), Fibermed crackers, Metamucil, etc.

EAT FOODS WITH BRAN FOR MAXIMUM FIBER!

HOW MUCH FIBER SHOULD YOU EAT?

Eat at least 20-35 grams (gm) per day.
TIP: Eat at least 8-9 high-fiber foods daily. Refer to the list on the next page.

FIBER CONTENT OF FOODS *

A simple way to make sure you consume enough fiber is to eat daily at least 3 fruits (6 gms fiber), 3 vegetables (6 gms fiber), 3 starches (6 gms fiber) and one serving bran cereal or beans (5-10 gms fiber). You want to eat 20-35 grams of fiber daily.

GRAINS (1 oz unless otherwise indicated)	Dietary Fiber (gm)	VEGETABLES (1/2 cup)	Dietary Fiber (gm)
All-Bran w/ Extra Fiber (Kellogg)	13.0	Sweet potato (1 large)	4.2
Fiber One (General Mills)	12.0	Peas	4.1
100% Bran (Nabisco)	9.1	Brussels sprouts	3.9
All-Bran (Kellogg)	8.6	Corn	3.9
Bran Buds (Kellogg)	7.7	Potato, baked (1 medium)	3.8
Wheat bran (1/3 c. dry)	6.4	Carrots (1 raw or 1/2 c. cooked)	2.3
Corn Bran (Quaker)	5.9	Collards	2.2
Wheat germ (1/4 c.)	5.5	Asparagus	2.1
Bran Chex (Post)	5.0	Green beans	2.1
Natural Bran Flakes (Post)	5.0	Broccoli	2.0
40% Bran Flakes (all brands)	4.3	Spinach	2.0
Oat bran (1/3 c. dry)	4.2	Turnips	1.7
Cracklin Oat Bran (Kellogg)	4.1	Mushrooms, raw	0.9
Fruit 'n Fiber (Post)	4.0	Summer squash	0.7
Fruitful Bran (Kellogg)	4.0	Lettuce, raw	0.3
Shredded Wheat n Bran (Nabisco)	4.0		
Wheatena (Uhlmann)	4.0	**FRUITS** (raw)	
Ralston Instant (Ralston)	3.3	Blackberries (1/2 c.)	4.5
Shredded Wheat (Nabisco)	3.3	Prunes, dried (3)	3.7
Popcorn, air-popped (2 c.)	3.2	Apple w/ skin (1)	2.6
Frosted Mini-Wheats (Kellogg)	3.0	Banana (1 medium)	2.0
Raisin Bran (Kellogg, Post)	2.9	Strawberries (3/4 c.)	2.0
Graham crackers (2 squares)	2.8	Grapefruit (1/2 medium)	1.7
Total (General Mills)	2.5	Peach (1 medium)	1.6
Wheat Chex (Ralston)	2.5	Cantaloupe (1/4 small)	1.4
Wheaties (General Mills)	2.5	Raisins (2 T)	1.3
Brown rice, cooked (1/2 c.)	2.4	Orange (1 small)	1.2
Grapenuts (Post)	2.2	Grapes (12)	0.5
Nutri-Grain (Kellogg)	2.1		
Millet, cooked (1/2 c.)	1.8	**LEGUMES** (1/2 cup cooked)	
Whole wheat bread (1 slice)	1.6	Kidney beans	5.8
Rye bread (1 slice)	1.0	Pinto beans	5.3
Spaghetti, cooked (1/2 c.)	0.8	Split peas	5.1
White bread (1 slice)	0.6	White beans	5.0
White rice, cooked (1/2 c.)	0.1	Lima beans	4.9
		Nuts/Seeds (1/4 cup)	3.0

EXTRA SOURCES

1. Unprocessed bran flakes (such as Millers Bran) may be added to foods, such as: soups, beverages, cooked or dry cereals, spaghetti sauce, stews, casseroles, meat loaf, muffins, bread, rolls, pancakes, vegetable salads, fruit salads, yogurt and fruit, etc. (2 tablespoons = 5.4 grams fiber; 70 calories).
2. One Fibermed cracker contains 5 grams of dietary fiber; 70 calories as supplied by corn, wheat and oats.

NOTE: There is **NO FIBER** in: milk, cheese, yogurt, poultry, fish, meat, margarine, oils, dressings.

* Sources: Anderson, J. *Plant Fiber in Foods*. (HCF Diabetes Research Foundation, Inc., P.O. Box 22124, Lexington, KY 40522) 1986 and USDA Handbook #8-8.

WAYS TO EAT MORE FIBER:

1. Eat a variety of fiber-rich foods, since different foods contain varied types of fiber with different benefits.

2. Eat foods with bran or beans every day. By eating 1/2 cup to 1 cup bran cereal (i.e., Fiber One) or beans daily, you consume 50% of the fiber you need. Add bran or bran cereal to other cereals, muffins, cookies, pancakes, bread recipes, meat loaf, or add as a topping on tossed or fruit salads, or on yogurt.

3. If you use unprocessed bran, gradually add increasing amounts, up to 3 tablespoons a day. Excessive amounts may lead to impaired absorption of some nutrients.

4. Eat vegetables raw or slightly cooked. Do not overcook!

5. Eat fresh fruit instead of canned, peeled, or pureed fruit or juices.

6. Choose breads and cereals labeled "wholewheat" or "wholegrained" as the first ingredient. Avoid brown-colored breads labeled "wheat flour" with "caramel" coloring; look for "wholewheat flour".

7. Eat hot oat bran, oatmeal, wholegrained cereal rather than cream of wheat and cream of rice, etc.

HOW TO IMPROVE DIGESTION:

1. Drink at least 10-12 glasses of fluids per day, at least half of which is water. Fiber absorbs liquid to form larger and softer stools that are easier to pass. Too little fluid may cause dehydration and constipation.

2. Eat slowly in a relaxed environment and chew food well.

3. Eat regular meals and adequate fluids, exercise daily, and get adequate rest to help promote good digestion and elimination and good health.

CAFFEINE

Caffeine (in coffee) is a drug belonging to a family of chemical compounds called *xanthines*. Other substances in this group are *theophylline* (in tea), and *theobromine* (in chocolate and cocoa).

- More than 200 milligrams of caffeine a day (2 cups brewed coffee) has been associated with the development of unpleasant symptoms — nervousness, anxiety, irritability, insomnia, gastrointestinal problems, irregular heart beat.
- Drink up to 2 cups or 1 mug coffee daily to not exceed 200 mg caffeine per day.

HOW CAFFEINE AFFECTS YOUR BODY

- Is absorbed immediately into your bloodstream!
- Stimulates the release of insulin which lowers blood sugar and produces hunger!
- May lead to a rise in blood pressure and body temperature.
- May cause rapid heart beats or skipped heart beats.
- Promotes acid secretion in the stomach (not advisable for persons with ulcers or gastric irritation; avoid decaffeinated coffee also since it has the same effect).
- Relaxes muscles or respiratory system, digestive tract, and kidneys causing increased urinary output — a dehydrating effect.
- Can cause diarrhea.
- Can cause central nervous system disturbances including nervousness, insomnia, irritability, anxiety, headaches, twitching muscles, difficulty sleeping, etc.
- In pregnant women, it may interfere with normal fetal development because it readily crosses the placenta.
- May lead to the development of fibrocystic breast disease in some women.
- Interferes with calcium and iron absorption.

HOW MUCH IS SAFE

Caffeine is a drug; 3 to 4 cups of caffeine-containing beverages (300-400 mg of caffeine) per day may make you psychologically and physically dependent. Be healthy — stay within 200 mg of caffeine (or 2 cups of coffee) per day. **GRADUALLY BREAK THE CAFFEINE HABIT COMPLETELY!** (Especially if you have heart disease, gastrointestinal problems, hypertension, emotional problems, ulcers, gastritis, diverticulosis, spastic colon, indigestion, hypoglycemia, diabetes.) Caffeine withdrawal may result in undesirable symptoms, i.e., headaches, nervousness, depression, drowsiness, irritability.

ALTERNATIVES

- Decaffeinated coffee, tea, and colas contain only a minute amount of caffeine. However, they may still stimulate stomach acid which may produce heartburn.
- Choose steam-decaffeinated coffee to avoid chemical solvents.
- Drink water, juice, herb teas — all naturally caffeine-free.
- Read labels for caffeine.
- Try grain based beverages as alternatives to caffeine — Postum, Cafix, Pero. Postum is made from bran, wheat and molasses.

Sources of Caffeine

FOOD	Mg PER SERVING
Coffee — 6-ounce serving	
brewed, ground	85
percolated	110
dripolated	150-180
instant	60
flavored — Cafe Francias, Vienna, etc.	30
grain blends — Mellow Roast, Sunrise, Luzianne-chicory	15-40
decaffeinated	3
Tea — 6-ounce serving	
regular, bagged	45
regular, loose	40
instant	30
decaffeinated	0
Cocoa, Hot chocolate beverages — 6-ounce serving	15
Cola beverages — 12-ounce serving	
Coca-Cola	65
Dr. Pepper — regular and diet	55
Pepsi Cola — regular and diet	40
Tab	45
RC Cola — regular and diet	30
RC 100	0
Non-Cola beverages — 12-ounce serving	
Mountain Dew	55
Sunkist	40
Diet Sunkist, Fanta drinks, Shasta drinks, Sprite — regular and diet, A&W Root Beer, Hires Root Beer, Diet Barq's Root Beer, 7-Up, Team, Nehi — orange, strawberry, peach	0
Barq's Root Beer	20
Nehi Red	5
Chocolate — 1 ounce	20
Drugs — per pill	
Aspirin, Cope, Midol, etc.	30
Excedrin, Anacin	60
No Doz, Vivarin	100-200
Dristan, Sinarest	30

WATER

MAKE WATER AN IMPORTANT PART OF YOUR DAILY EATING FOR OPTIMAL HEALTH AND MAXIMUM ENERGY!!!

WHY WATER IS SO IMPORTANT — IT:

1. Regulates every living cell's processes and chemical reactions.
2. Aids digestion and absorption of foods and nutrients.
3. Transports nutrients and oxygen.
4. Excretes waste products.
5. Helps to maintain normal bowel habits and prevent constipation.
6. Assists new tissue development.
7. Lubricates joints in your body, providing a protective cushion for tissues.
8. Maintains normal body temperature. Loss of water through perspiration cools the body and prevents it from building up internal heat (dehydration).
9. Contributes to the proper functioning of enzymes.
10. Contributes to the proper concentrations of blood electrolytes.

DRINK AT LEAST 6 - 8 GLASSES OF WATER PER DAY (2 QUARTS)

- The average adult human body is approximately 60 percent water, found in muscle, blood, brain, bone, etc.
- You can live for weeks without food. Without WATER you could only survive 3 days.
- A 5 percent loss of body water causes you to become weak; 15 to 20 percent lost is fatal. That means a loss of 7 pounds for a 150 pound person = 5 percent loss.
- You lose body water through: perspiration (skin), lungs, body functions, urine, stool, air travel.
- Water loss, not salt or sodium loss, impairs an athlete's performance.
- In the heat of the summer, increase your fluids!
- For every 1 hour of air travel, you lose 1 pint of water. Drink ample water to prevent fatigue.
- With increased fiber intake, increase fluids to prevent constipation.
- Caffeine in coffee, tea, etc. and alcohol have a dehydrating effect. They decrease body fluids.

TIPS TO INCREASE WATER INTAKE DAILY:

- Add lemon, lime, or orange slices to a glass of water
- Keep a clear pitcher of water (2 qt.) on your desk or work area
- Carry a squeeze bottle filled with water — in your car, at meetings, etc.

ADDITIVES

"TO EAT OR NOT TO EAT"

Food additives serve a multitude of purposes. They are used as stabilizers, thickening agents, flavor enhancers (i.e., sugar and salt), emulsifiers, acidic or alkaline or neutralizing agents, preservatives, anti-oxidants (to protect fats from becoming rancid during storage), nutritional supplements and food colors.

There are **benefits** and **risks** involved with their use.

- **Benefits**: prolonged shelf-life, spoilage prevention, enhanced food appearance of flavor or texture, and added nutrients.

- **Risks**: related to the quantity and choice of additives used and their known and unknown potential dangers. It is important to realize that all foods, as well as additives, are essentially chemical compounds. Therefore, additives are not "un-natural" nor automatically harmful.

The Food and Drug Administration has compiled a Generally Recognized as Safe, GRAS, list of 415 additives tested and approved as safe at specified levels. This list, first started in 1958, is updated on a regular basis. According to the last assessment, the vast majority of additives are considered safe at levels currently used. Their benefits of longer food shelf-life, convenience, a greater food supply and variety, added nutrients and food appeal seem to outweigh their risks. Furthermore, the human body is able to handle minute levels of almost any substance without serious health consequences. Some believe the decline in stomach cancer in America, since the 1930s, is related to the use of additives during this time span. On the other hand, most authorities agree that excessive amounts of any substance can be potentially dangerous. The less used, the better.

How then can we eat nutritiously and avoid excessive levels of additives in our diets?

The most sensible suggestion is grandmother's long-standing advice: eat a well-balanced diet, with a variety of foods, in moderation. The more varied our diets, the more healthful nutrients we are likely to consume and the less likely we are to eat excessive levels of potentially dangerous substances. Eat fresh foods to maximize nutrients and minimize additives.

The following page lists common additives.

Some Common Additives

CLASSIFICATION	TYPES	PURPOSE	USED IN
ANTITOXIDANTS	BHT, BHA, Vitamin E, ascorbic acid (Vitamin C), citric acid, EDTA	prevent oxidation that leads to rancidity of fats and discoloration of fruits; extend shelf-life	breakfast cereals, baker products, margarine, sauces, salad dressings, processed fruit, snack foods, fats, oil, shortening
PRESERVATIVES	benzoic acid, sodium benzoate, calcium propianate, citric acid, lactic acid, propionic acid, potassium sorbate, sulfur dioxide, sodium nitrate, salt, sugar, paraben	inhibit growth of bacteria, yeast and mold; extend shelf-life	pastries, baked goods, dried fruit, canned fruit, and vegetables and meat and soup, acidic foods, cured meat, bacon, olives, cheese, salad dressing
EMULSIFIERS	monoglycerides, diglycerides, lecithin, propylene glycol mono sterate, polysorbate, carrageenan	blend liquids together for more uniform consistency, texture and stability	mayonnaise, salad dressings, margarine, chocolate, whipped toppings, gelatin, pudding, ice cream
STABILIZERS AND THICKENERS	agar, cellulose, guar gum, gelatin, pectin, dextrin, alginate compounds, propylene glycol	maintain uniform color, flavor and smooth texture	mayonnaise, salad dressings, ice cream, dessert dairy products, jam, jelly
COLORING AGENTS	Natural or Synthetic: Natural: chlorophyll (green), beet or tomato powder (red), caramelized sugar (brown), carotene (yellow). Synthetic: Red No. 3 and No. 40, yellow No. 5	enhance color	canned fruit and vegetables, bakery products desserts
FLAVORING AGENTS	Natural or Synthetic: Natural: vanilla, cocoa, lemon, orange, spices, sweeteners. Synthetic: fruit flavors, monosodium glutamate (MSG), saccharin	enhance flavor or modify original taste and/or aromas	beverages, baked goods, cereals, dessert mixes, candy, sauces, many canned foods, soup, oriental foods, dietary products

 © 1993, *The Balancing Act Nutrition and Weight Guide*, G. Kostas, M.P.H., R.D., Dallas, Texas

X
TIPS TO CONTINUE ONWARD

HABIT FOCUS

Congratulations for your accomplishments thus far!

How far have you climbed the "Ladder to Success"?

How will you maintain your new lifestyle and success?

1. Reassess your progress. (217)
2. Have you thought about trying these eating goals? (219)
3. Practice and record your "Positive Eating Strategies". (220-222)
4. Continue your successful weight loss and/or maintenance with the tips outlined. (223)

GOALS

HABIT: practice, practice, practice!

FOOD: keep healthy food choices at home

EXERCISE: continue exercising 3-5 times a week; make exercise part of your lifestyle

RECORDS: food, exercise, weight - continue records daily until you reach your target weight; then keep records off and on for lifetime lifestyle modification

Complete "End of Month Progress Check (Appendix A)

NUTRITION AND EXERCISE FOCUS

Keep your new habits a part of your lifestyle for a lifetime!

FUTURE DIRECTIONS

Repeat a section of this manual weekly until you reach your target weight. Keep going! Small changes add up. Keep focusing on your newly forming lifestyle and the benefits and rewards you are enjoying.

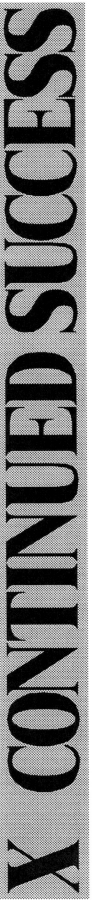

X CONTINUED SUCCESS

216   © 1993, *The Balancing Act Nutrition and Weight Guide,* G. Kostas, M.P.H., R.D., Dallas, Texas

MAINTAIN YOUR NEW LIFESTYLE

Congratulations!

- By now, you have made progress in modifying your eating habits and managing your weight.

- You have made personal decisions regarding appropriate goals and strategies, have taken appropriate actions, and have enjoyed success and beneficial effects of weight management.

- The purpose of this manual has been to teach you skills and techniques with which to manage your social, physical and private environments...**THE SKILLS TO TAKE CHARGE OF YOUR EATING BEHAVIOR AND WEIGHT.**

- Continue your efforts to make necessary habit changes and to strengthen changes you have already made.

- **REMEMBER -** It takes time and repeated practice to establish permanent new eating patterns. **BE PATIENT AND OPTIMISTIC!**

- You must **RE-ASSESS YOUR PROGRESS** and problem areas on a regular basis, set small goals, reach these and continue moving forward.

1. **TAKE THE FOLLOWING SELF-ASSESSMENT QUIZ:**

   A. Turn to your **Assessment of Eating Habits** form (page 33). What eating behaviors did you improve on?

1.	4.
2.	5.
3.	6.

   B. Which eating habits do you need to concentrate on improving now?

1.	4.
2.	5.
3.	6.

   C. **"My Plan"** - What goals did you achieve? (page 35)

1.	4.
2.	5.
3.	6.

   What areas need work?

   1.
   2.
   3.

D.   What new **PLEASURES** are you enjoying, other than food?
        1.   4.
        2.   5.
        3.   6.

     List others you will enjoy:
        1.   4.
        2.   5.
        3.   6.

E.   List your priorities in life. Arrange your commitments to give your health and weight
     the attention they deserve.
        1.   4.
        2.   5.
        3.   6.

F.   Identify your greatest challenge in your weight reduction efforts:

G.   List and test potential solutions:

H.   My most successful solution(s) are:

I.   Where are you in your positive progress toward health and fitness? List areas you
     need to focus on and refer to appropriate sections to reinforce your good habits.

2.   SET WEEKLY EATING GOALS: (see page 217)

- Meatless week
- Fish or poultry all lunches
- Meat - 3 times a week
- Vegetarian week
- 2 fruit a day week
- No ice cream week
- No nachos week
- No alcohol week
- No soft drinks week
- "3 pre-planned meals a day" week
- Slower eating week
- Smart snacks week
- Breakfast daily
- "Brown bag lunch" week
- "5 fish meals" week
- "Remove food cues" week
- "All homemade meals" week
- "3 vegetables a day" week
- "Sugar-free" week
- "Measure portions" week
- Treat self without food
- Relax without food
- Choose a non-food entertainment
- Exercise if angry
- Eat sitting down only
- Low-fat week
- 2 crunchy foods per meal

> **EAT TO LIVE, DO NOT LIVE TO EAT.**

POSITIVE EATING STRATEGIES

WHAT NEW HABITS DO YOU NEED TO PRACTICE?

MARK YOUR "SUCCESS" DAYS

PLANNING AHEAD

	S	M	T	W	TH	F	S
____Start each day with breakfast	___	___	___	___	___	___	___
____Eat three regular, planned meals	___	___	___	___	___	___	___
____Choose small, planned snacks	___	___	___	___	___	___	___
____Eat lunch daily	___	___	___	___	___	___	___
____Eat meals at scheduled times	___	___	___	___	___	___	___
____Use a Meal-Menu Planner daily	___	___	___	___	___	___	___
____Think before you eat. Predict/plan eating out choices	___	___	___	___	___	___	___

PROBLEM FOODS

	S	M	T	W	TH	F	S
____Don't buy my problem food: i.e., _____	___	___	___	___	___	___	___
____Choose low-cal alternatives, i.e., _____	___	___	___	___	___	___	___
____Eat a low-cal instead of a high- cal snack, i.e., _____	___	___	___	___	___	___	___
____Chew sugarless gum while cooking	___	___	___	___	___	___	___
____Don't sample food during meal preparation	___	___	___	___	___	___	___
____Drink sugar-free drinks	___	___	___	___	___	___	___

FOOD QUANTITY

	S	M	T	W	TH	F	S
____Measure portions	___	___	___	___	___	___	___
____Leave some food on your plate	___	___	___	___	___	___	___
____Take 20 minutes to eat a meal	___	___	___	___	___	___	___
____Enjoy one portion; skip seconds	___	___	___	___	___	___	___
____Use smaller dishes — portions look larger	___	___	___	___	___	___	___
____Sit down while eating	___	___	___	___	___	___	___
____Put utensils down between bites	___	___	___	___	___	___	___
____Let someone else scrape dishes	___	___	___	___	___	___	___
____Put left-overs away immediately	___	___	___	___	___	___	___
____Share a single serving — particularly an entree, dessert, appetizer, or richer food — with someone.							

ENVIRONMENTAL CONTROL	S	M	T	W	TH	F	S
_____Keep tempting foods out of sight	___	___	___	___	___	___	___
_____Take healthy, low-cal snacks to parties	___	___	___	___	___	___	___
_____Tell fellow peers not to offer me food	___	___	___	___	___	___	___
_____Avoid places that give me trouble	___	___	___	___	___	___	___
_____Eat a low-cal snack before eating out to reduce appetite	___	___	___	___	___	___	___
_____Make special requests in restaurants — be assertive	___	___	___	___	___	___	___

COOKING AND ENTERTAINING	S	M	T	W	TH	F	S
_____Fix lower-calorie foods for company	___	___	___	___	___	___	___
_____Substitute lower-calorie ingredients	___	___	___	___	___	___	___
_____Try new, low-cal recipes	___	___	___	___	___	___	___
_____Broil or bake instead of frying	___	___	___	___	___	___	___

YOUR INDIVIDUAL STRATEGIES	S	M	T	W	TH	F	S
(Write in)_____	___	___	___	___	___	___	___
_____	___	___	___	___	___	___	___
_____	___	___	___	___	___	___	___

FEELINGS/SELF-IMAGE	S	M	T	W	TH	F	S
_____I see myself as slender	___	___	___	___	___	___	___
_____I see my clothes fitting better	___	___	___	___	___	___	___
_____I enjoy healthy, balanced meals	___	___	___	___	___	___	___
_____I feel terrific without food	___	___	___	___	___	___	___
_____I find comfort in the outdoors, in peace and quiet, with family and friends	___	___	___	___	___	___	___
_____Activities and exercise make me feel good — food doesn't	___	___	___	___	___	___	___
_____I have more confidence in me	___	___	___	___	___	___	___
_____I enjoy life and people a lot more	___	___	___	___	___	___	___

EMOTIONS AND THOUGHTS	S	M	T	W	TH	F	S
_____Avoid persons or situations that upset me	___	___	___	___	___	___	___
_____Interpret events objectively	___	___	___	___	___	___	___
_____Express feelings objectively	___	___	___	___	___	___	___
_____Counter excuses and negative thoughts with positive self-talk	___	___	___	___	___	___	___
_____Use relaxation techniques	___	___	___	___	___	___	___
_____Go for a walk or talk to someone instead of eating	___	___	___	___	___	___	___

EATING SITUATIONS

	S	M	T	W	TH	F	S
____Don't eat in the car	__	__	__	__	__	__	__
____Let others get their own snacks	__	__	__	__	__	__	__
____Do nothing else while eating	__	__	__	__	__	__	__
____Remove food cues	__	__	__	__	__	__	__
____Eat only at my designated eating place	__	__	__	__	__	__	__
____Eat only while sitting down	__	__	__	__	__	__	__
____Eat healthy foods, even "on the run"	__	__	__	__	__	__	__

BUYING AND STORING FOODS

	S	M	T	W	TH	F	S
____Shop when not hungry	__	__	__	__	__	__	__
____Shop from a list	__	__	__	__	__	__	__
____Don't buy "problem foods"	__	__	__	__	__	__	__
____Avoid tempting aisles	__	__	__	__	__	__	__
____Put groceries in trunk on way home	__	__	__	__	__	__	__
____Do not open package until ready to use	__	__	__	__	__	__	__
____Use opaque instead of clear wrap when storing foods							

EATING OUT

	S	M	T	W	TH	F	S
____Choose restaurants with varied food selections	__	__	__	__	__	__	__
____Order skim milk or low-cal drink	__	__	__	__	__	__	__
____Eat a low-cal snack before eating out	__	__	__	__	__	__	__
____Take own low-cal salad dressing, food, or drink	__	__	__	__	__	__	__
____Share entreés, desserts, and sauces	__	__	__	__	__	__	__
____Ask for salad dressing "on the side"	__	__	__	__	__	__	__
____Order menu items "grilled", "steamed", "without butter", etc."	__	__	__	__	__	__	__
____Avoid reading dessert list	__	__	__	__	__	__	__
____Call hostess about her menu beforehand; plan strategies	__	__	__	__	__	__	__
____Make special requests in restaurants	__	__	__	__	__	__	__

© 1993, *The Balancing Act Nutrition and Weight Guide,* G. Kostas, M.P.H., R.D., Dallas, Texas

FINAL TIPS

FOR CONTINUED SUCCESS:

1. **RE-ASSESS** your problem areas from time to time.

2. Continue **RECORD-KEEPING.**

3. Re-read this **MANUAL** and concentrate on lessons that deal specifically with your eating concerns.

4. Practice **STRATEGIES** suggested and devise new ones.

5. Maintain a **SUPPORTIVE** environment.

6. Be prepared for weight **PLATEAUS. These are normal.** Continue your program and the weight will **inevitably** disappear.

7. Expect problems from time to time. Anticipate ways to **COPE.**

8. When you reach your desired weight, gradually add 200 calories per week, until you reach your weight maintenance calorie level.

MAINTENANCE:

1. Know your weight! **WEIGH** frequently (at least once weekly) and record.

2. Keep food **RECORDS** periodically.

3. **ENJOY** your new weight and rewards associated with it.

4. Maintain your good eating **HABITS.** Do not eat like a fat person. You know how to eat for your well-being.

5. Get rid of, or alter, old **CLOTHES.** Buy new, flattering clothes. Do not allow yourself an easy road back to your old sizes.

6. Set a three pound weight gain **LIMIT** for yourself. As soon as you are over this limit, start immediately to re-establish sound eating habits.

7. If you need a break, decide to **MAINTAIN** your weight for a week, rather than to **LOSE** that week.

8. Remind yourself of all the work it took to reach your ideal weight. Do not let it be wasted effort.

9. Stay **ACTIVE.** Continue to increase daily activity.

10. **CARE ABOUT YOURSELF.**

Our Best Wishes For Your Success!

© 1993, *The Balancing Act Nutrition and Weight Guide*, G. Kostas, M.P.H., R.D., Dallas, Texas   223

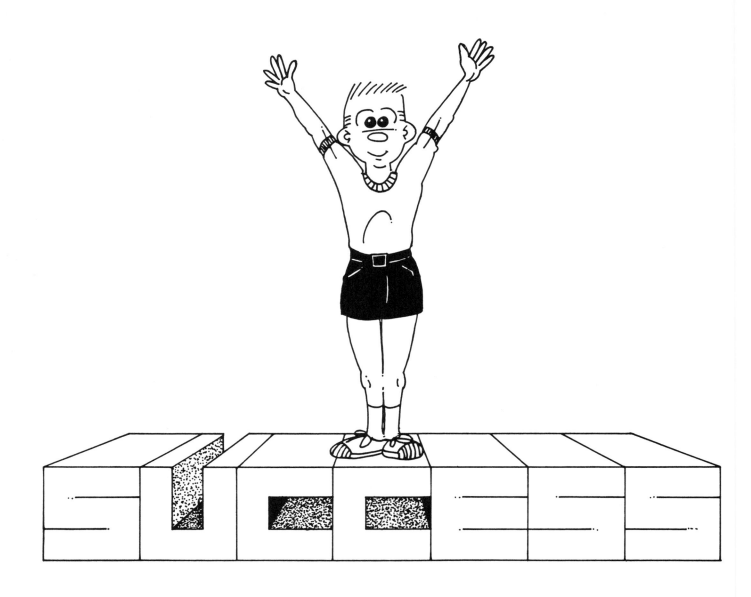

APPENDIX A

Progress Records

- Food Records
- Exercise Logs
- Weight Graphs
- Ladder to Success Weekly Achievement List
- End-of-Month Progress Check

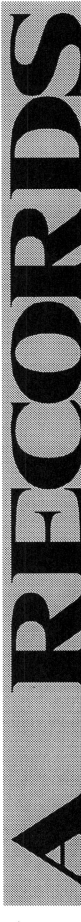

FOOD RECORDS

FOOD RECORD

NAME _____

DATE _____

Write ONE food on each line.
May record thoughts, etc.

	Plan		Actual		Actual
	_____	milk	_____		_____
	_____	meat	_____		_____
	_____	starch	_____		_____
	_____	fruit	_____		_____
	_____	veg.	_____		_____
	_____	fat	_____		_____

Time/Min. Eating and Place/Who With	Mood or Circum-stances	Amt.	Food – How Prepared	Food Groups or Calories	Fat grams

EXERCISE:

FOOD RECORDS

FOOD RECORD

NAME _____

DATE _____

Write ONE food on each line.
May record thoughts, etc.

	Plan		Actual		Actual
	_____	milk	_____		_____
	_____	meat	_____		_____
	_____	starch	_____		_____
	_____	fruit	_____		_____
	_____	veg.	_____		_____
	_____	fat	_____		_____

Time/Min. Eating and Place/Who With	Mood or Circum-stances	Amt.	Food – How Prepared	Food Groups or Calories	Fat grams

EXERCISE:

© 1993, *The Balancing Act Nutrition and Weight Guide*, G. Kostas, M.P.H., R.D., Dallas, Texas

FOOD RECORDS

FOOD RECORD

NAME _____

DATE _____

Write ONE food on each line.
May record thoughts, etc.

	Plan	Actual	Actual
	_____ milk _____	_____	
	_____ meat _____	_____	
	_____ starch _____	_____	
	_____ fruit _____	_____	
	_____ veg. _____	_____	
	_____ fat _____	_____	

Time/Min. Eating and Place/Who With	Mood or Circum- stances	Amt.	Food – How Prepared	Food Groups or Calories	Fat grams

EXERCISE:

FOOD RECORDS

FOOD RECORD

NAME _____

DATE _____

Write ONE food on each line.
May record thoughts, etc.

	Plan	Actual	Actual
	_____	milk _____	_____
	_____	meat _____	_____
	_____	starch _____	_____
	_____	fruit _____	_____
	_____	veg. _____	_____
	_____	fat _____	_____

Time/Min. Eating and Place/Who With	Mood or Circum-stances	Amt.	Food – How Prepared	Food Groups or Calories	Fat grams

EXERCISE:

FOOD RECORDS

FOOD RECORD

NAME _____

DATE _____

Write ONE food on each line.
May record thoughts, etc.

	Plan	Actual	Actual
milk	_____	_____	_____
meat	_____	_____	_____
starch	_____	_____	_____
fruit	_____	_____	_____
veg.	_____	_____	_____
fat	_____	_____	_____

Time/Min. Eating and Place/Who With	Mood or Circum- stances	Amt.	Food – How Prepared	Food Groups or Calories	Fat grams

EXERCISE:

FOOD RECORDS

FOOD RECORD

NAME _____

DATE _____

Write ONE food on each line.
May record thoughts, etc.

	Plan	Actual	Actual
milk	_____	_____	_____
meat	_____	_____	_____
starch	_____	_____	_____
fruit	_____	_____	_____
veg.	_____	_____	_____
fat	_____	_____	_____

Time/Min. Eating and Place/Who With	Mood or Circum-stances	Amt.	Food – How Prepared	Food Groups or Calories	Fat grams

EXERCISE:

FOOD RECORDS

FOOD RECORD

NAME _____

DATE _____

Write ONE food on each line.
May record thoughts, etc.

	Plan	Actual	Actual
milk	_____	_____	_____
meat	_____	_____	_____
starch	_____	_____	_____
fruit	_____	_____	_____
veg.	_____	_____	_____
fat	_____	_____	_____

Time/Min. Eating and Place/Who With	Mood or Circum-stances	Amt.	Food – How Prepared	Food Groups or Calories	Fat grams

EXERCISE:

FOOD RECORDS

FOOD RECORD

NAME _____

DATE _____

Write ONE food on each line.
May record thoughts, etc.

	Plan	Actual	Actual
milk	_____	_____	_____
meat	_____	_____	_____
starch	_____	_____	_____
fruit	_____	_____	_____
veg.	_____	_____	_____
fat	_____	_____	_____

Time/Min. Eating and Place/Who With	Mood or Circum-stances	Amt.	Food – How Prepared	Food Groups or Calories	Fat grams

EXERCISE:

EXERCISE LOGS

			EXERCISE LOG				
Sunday	Monday	Tuesday	Wednesday	Thursday	Friday	Saturday	**Weekly Totals**

EXERCISE LOGS

EXERCISE LOG							
Sunday	Monday	Tuesday	Wednesday	Thursday	Friday	Saturday	**Weekly Totals**

EXERCISE LOGS

			EXERCISE LOG				
Sunday	Monday	Tuesday	Wednesday	Thursday	Friday	Saturday	**Weekly Totals**

EXERCISE LOGS

			EXERCISE LOG				
Sunday	Monday	Tuesday	Wednesday	Thursday	Friday	Saturday	**Weekly Totals**

WEEKLY WEIGHT GRAPHS

NAME: _Mary Jones_

STARTING WEIGHT: _172_   DATE: _Sept 1_

DESIRED WEIGHT: _130_   DATE: _June 23_

WEEK NO.	DATE	WEIGHT	WEIGHT CHANGE	TOTAL WEIGHT CHANGE
0	Sept 1	172		
1	Sept 8	171	−1	−1
2	Sept 15	170 ½	−½	−1½
3	Sept 22	169	−1½	−3
4	Sept 29	168	−1	−4
5	Oct. 6	167	−1	−5
6	Oct. 13	168	+1	−4
7	Oct. 20	166	−2	−6
8	Oct. 27	166	0	−6
9	Nov. 3	164	−2	−8
10	Nov. 10	162	−2	−10
11	Nov. 17	161 ½	−½	−10½
12	Nov. 24	160	−1½	−12
13				
14				
15				
16				
17				
18				
19				
20				
21				
22				
23				
24				
25				
26				

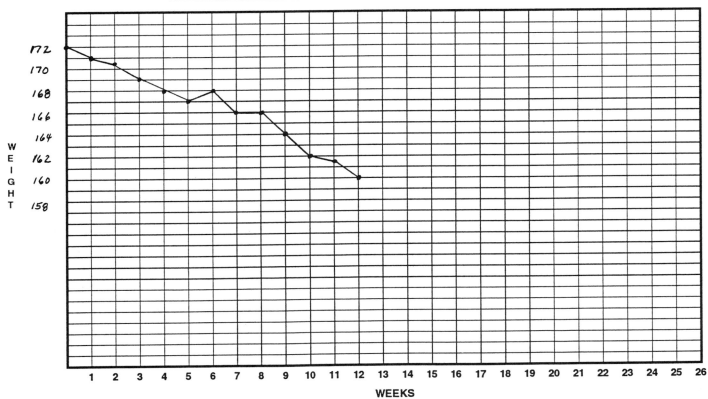

WEEKS

WEEKLY WEIGHT GRAPHS

NAME: _____

STARTING WEIGHT: _____ DATE: _____

DESIRED WEIGHT: _____ DATE: _____

WEEK NO.	DATE	WEIGHT	WEIGHT CHANGE	TOTAL WEIGHT CHANGE
0				
1				
2				
3				
4				
5				
6				
7				
8				
9				
10				
11				
12				
13				
14				
15				
16				
17				
18				
19				
20				
21				
22				
23				
24				
25				
26				

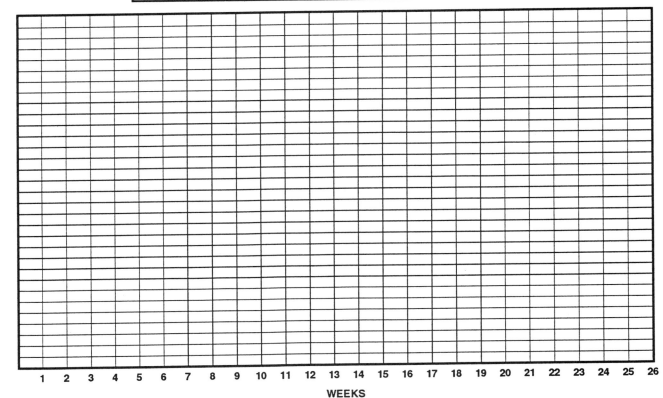

WEIGHT

WEEKS

1 2 3 4 5 6 7 8 9 10 11 12 13 14 15 16 17 18 19 20 21 22 23 24 25 26

© 1993, *The Balancing Act Nutrition and Weight Guide*, G. Kostas, M.P.H., R.D., Dallas, Texas

LADDER TO SUCCESS CHARTS

WEEKLY ACHIEVEMENTS

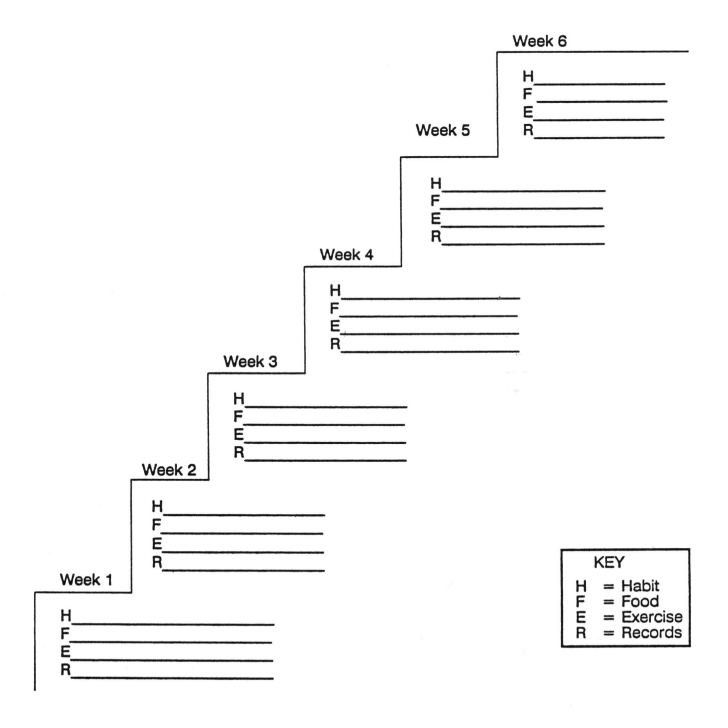

KEY

H	=	Habit
F	=	Food
E	=	Exercise
R	=	Records

END-OF-MONTH PROGRESS CHECK

MONTH: _____

1. Identify your greatest challenge in your weight reduction efforts:

2. List and test potential solutions:

3. My most successful solutions are:

4. Where are you in your positive progress toward health and fitness? List areas you need to focus on and refer to appropriate sections to reinforce your good habits.

MONTH: _____

1. Identify your greatest challenge in your weight reduction efforts:

2. List and test potential solutions:

3. My most successful solutions are:

4. Where are you in your positive progress toward health and fitness? List areas you need to focus on and refer to appropriate sections to reinforce your good habits.

END-OF-MONTH PROGRESS CHECK

MONTH: _____

1. Identify your greatest challenge in your weight reduction efforts:

2. List and test potential solutions:

3. My most successful solutions are:

4. Where are you in your positive progress toward health and fitness? List areas you need to focus on and refer to appropriate sections to reinforce your good habits.

MONTH: _____

1. Identify your greatest challenge in your weight reduction efforts:

2. List and test potential solutions:

3. My most successful solutions are:

4. Where are you in your positive progress toward health and fitness? List areas you need to focus on and refer to appropriate sections to reinforce your good habits.

END-OF-MONTH PROGRESS CHECK

MONTH: _____

1. Identify your greatest challenge in your weight reduction efforts:

2. List and test potential solutions:

3. My most successful solutions are:

4. Where are you in your positive progress toward health and fitness? List areas you need to focus on and refer to appropriate sections to reinforce your good habits.

_____

MONTH: _____

1. Identify your greatest challenge in your weight reduction efforts:

2. List and test potential solutions:

3. My most successful solutions are:

4. Where are you in your positive progress toward health and fitness? List areas you need to focus on and refer to appropriate sections to reinforce your good habits.

APPENDIX B

Recommended Reading and Resources

- Nutrition
- Weight Control
- Sports Nutrition
- Cookbooks
- Calorie and Nutrient Counters
- Newsletter / Magazines

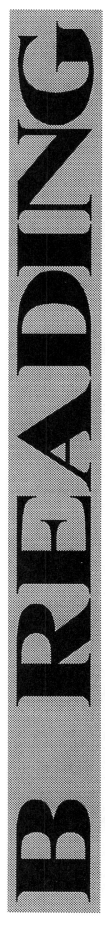

RECOMMENDED READING

With the abundance of nutrition and diet books available, be selective in choosing a nutrition resource that is reliable and factual. Some nutrition materials are based on fads which give erroneous information.

Be sure to scrutinize the author and content before buying the book. It should:
1. Describe a credible author including —
   - degrees
   - work experience
   - distinguish between "nutritionist" and R.D. (registered dietitian); "doctor" or M.D.
2. Describe a credible diet including —
   - emphasis on a variety of foods and not just a single food and/or beverage
   - a realistic, livable approach
   - a healthy balance of protein, carbohydrate and fat intake
3. At the Cooper Clinic, we recommend these books:

NUTRITION

Brody, J. *Jane Brody's Nutrition Book - A Lifetime Guide to Good Eating For Better Health and Weight Control.* Bantam, 1988.

Cooper, K. *The Aerobics Program for Total Well-Being.* M. Evans and Co., 1983.

Deutsch, R.M. and Morrill, J.S. *Realities of Nutrition,* 1993.

Gershoff, S. *The Tufts University Guide to Total Nutrition.* Harper Perrineal: 1990.

Herbert, V. and Gubak-Sharp, G. *Vitamins and "Healthy Foods": The Great American Hustle.* St. Martin's Press, 1990.

Herbert, V. *The Mt. Sinai School of Medicine Complete book of Nutrition.* St. Martin's Press, 1990.

Mayer, J. and Goldberg, J. *Dr. Jean Mayer's Diet and Nutrition Guide.* Pharos Books, 1990.

Stare, F. et al. *Your Guide to Good Nutrition.* Prometheus Books, 1991.

Tribole, E. *Eating on the Run.* Leisure Press, 1992.

Wotcki, C. and Thomas, P. *Eat for Life.* Washington D.C. National Academy Press, 1992.

WEIGHT CONTROL

American Dietetic Association's The Healthy Weigh: A Practical Food Guide. ADA, 1991.

Bailey, C. *The New Fit or Fat.* Houghton Mifflin Co., 1991.

Cooper, K. *The Aerobics Program for Total Well-Being.* M. Evans and Co., 1983.

Brownell, K. *The Learn Program.* American Health Publishing Co., 1994.

Ferguson, J. *Habits, not Diets.* Bull Publishing Co., 1990.

Ferguson, J. *Learning to Eat.* Bull Publishing Co., 1993.

Katahn, M. *The T-Factor Diet.* W.W. Norton and Co., 1993.

Kostas, G. *The Balancing Act Nutrition & Weight Guide.* Balancing Act Nutrition Books, 1995.

Nash and Long, R.D. *Managing Your Weight and Well-Being.* Bull Publishing Co., 1978.

Nash, J. *Maximize Your Body Potential.* Bull Publishing Co., 1991.

Tribole, E. and Resch, E. *Intuitive Eating: A Recovery Book for the Chronic Dieter.* St. Martin's Press, 1995.

SPORTS NUTRITION

Berning, J. and Seen, S. *Sports Nutrition for the '90's*. Aspen Publications, 1992.
Clark, N. *Nancy Clark's Sports Nutrition Guidebook*. Leisure Press, 1990.
Coleman, E. *Eating for Endurance*. Bull Printing Co., 1992.
Elserman, P. and Johnson, D. *Coaches Guide to Nutrition and Weight Control*. Human Kinetics
    Publishers, Inc., 1982.
Katch, F., and McCardle, W. *Nutrition Weight Control and Exercise*. Houghton Mifflin Co., 1983.
Neiman, D. *The Fitness Handbook*. Bull Publishing Co., 1986.
Nutrition and Athletic Performance edited by W. Haskell, J. Scala and J. Whittam. Bull Publishing Co.,
    1991.
Peterson, M. and Peterson, K. *Eat to Compete*: A Guide to Sports Nutrition. YearBook Medical
    Publishers, 1988.
Smith, N. *Food for Sport*. Bull Publishing Co., 1989.
Williams, M. *Nutritional Aspects of Human Physical and Athletic Performance*. Charles C. Thomas, 1991.

COOKBOOKS

ADA Family Cookbook. The American Dietetic Association and American Diabetic Association.
    Englewood Cliffs, NJ: Prentice-Hall, 1991.
The American Heart Association Low-Fat, Low Cholesterol Cookbook.Times Books, 1991.
Brody, J. *Jane Brody's Good Food Book*. Bantam, 1987.
Brody, J. *Jane Brody's Good Food Gourmet*. Bantam, 1992.
Cookery Classics. Cooper Wellness Programs. 12300 Preston Rd., Dallas, TX 75230.
Cooking Light. Southern Living. Susan M. McIntosh. Oxmoor House, Birmingham, 1991.
Cooper Clinic. *What's Cooking at the Cooper Clinic*. 12200 Preston Rd., Dallas, TX 75230.
DeBakey, M., et.al. *The Living Heart Diet*. Raven Press/Simon & Schuster, 1984.
Hachfeld, L. and Eykyn, B. *Cooking a la Heart*. Appletree Press, 1991.
Jones, J. *Cook It Light Classics*. MacMilliam, 1992.
Kostas, G. *The Guilt-free Comfort Food Cookbook*. Thomas Nelson. 1995.
Lowry, E. *Living Lean and Loving It*. St. Louis, MO: Mosby Co., 1988.
McDonald, H.B. *Eat Well, Live Well*. Canada: Macmillan, 1990.
Piscatella, J. *Don't Eat Your Heart Out Cookbook*. Workman Publishing, 1987.
Piscatella, J. *Controlling Your Fat Tooth*. Workman Publishing, 1991.
Ponichtera, B. *Quick and Healthy Recipes and Ideas*. 1519 Hermits Way The Dalles, OR 97058. 1991.
Robertson, L. and Flinder C. *Laurel's Kitchen - A Handbook for Vegetarian Cookery and Nutrition*. CA:
    B. Ruppenthal's, 1987.
Weight Watcher's Cookbook. Weight Watcher's International, 1995.

CALORIE AND NUTRIENT COUNTERS

Bellerson, Karen. *The Complete and Up-to-Date Fat Book*. Avery Publishing Group, 1993.
Carper, J. *Total Nutrition Guide*. Bantam Books, 1987.
Health Counts: A Fat and Calorie Guide. Kaiser Permanente: Wiley, 1991.
Netzer, Corinne. *The Complete Book of Food Counts*. Dell Publishing, 1994.
Nutritive Value of foods, Agricultural Handbook No. 456. U.S. Department of Agriculture. Superintendent
    of Documents, U.S. government Printing Office. Washington, D.C., 20402, 1981.
Pennington, J. and Church, H. *Bowles and Church's Food Values of Portions Commonly Used. 16th Ed.*,
    Perennial Library, 1994.
Pope-Cordle, J. and Katahn, M. *The T-Factor Fat Gram Counter*. W.W. Norton, 1994.
Roth, Harriet. *Fat Counter*. Signet Publishing Co., 1992.

NEWSLETTERS AND MAGAZINES

Supermarket Scoop Newsletter
(New Products)
Supermarket Savvy
P.O. Box 7069
Reston, VA 22091

Brand-New / Brand-Name Shopping List
(Comprehensive Healthy Product List - 2x/yr)
Supermarket Savvy
P.O. Box 7069
Reston, VA 22091

Environmental Nutrition
2112 Broadway, Suite 200
New York, NY 10023

Tufts University Diet & Nutrition Letter
53 Park Place
New York, NY 10007

University of California, Berkeley Wellness Newsletter
Health Letter Associates
P.O. Box 420148
Palm coast, FL 32142

Nutrition Action Healthletter
Center for Science in the Public Interest
1875 Connecticut Ave., NW, Suite 300
Washington, DC 20009-5728

Consumer Reports on Health
Box 56356
Boulder, CO 80322-6356

Vitality Magazine
Vitality Inc.
8080 N. Central, LB 78
Dallas, TX 75206

HOTLINES

Toll-free American Dietetic Association National Referral Service
Call for Registered Dietitions in your area.
1-800-877-1600 ext. 4853

Toll-Free Department of Agriculture, Meat, and Poultry Hotline
Call for safe preparation and storage of meat and poultry.
1-800-535-4555

American Anorexia & Bulemia Association
1-212-891-8656

National Association of Anorexia Nervosa & Associated Disorders
1-708-831-3138

Toll-Free Consumer Nutrition Hotline
Call for educational materials or questions regarding nutrition.
1-800-366-1655

Toll-Free National Osteoporosis Foundation
Call for educational material.
1-800-223-9994

APPENDIX C

Calorie Information

- Recommended Daily Calorie Needs & Weights
- Food Calories
- Fast Foods
- Exercise Calories
- Nutrient Sources

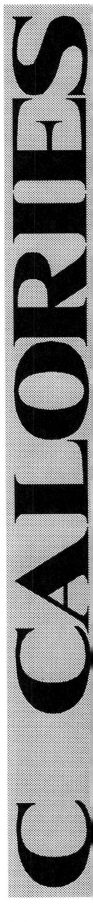

RECOMMENDED DAILY CALORIE NEEDS

ADULT DAILY CALORIE NEEDS	WOMEN	MEN
Baseline Needs	1200-1700	1800-3000
With Aerobic Exercise	1400-2000	2000-4000
With Competitive Athletics	2000-4000	3000-6000
For Weight Loss	1000-1500	1500-2000

See pages 27-29 to calculate your calorie needs more specifically.

RECOMMENDED WEIGHTS

		WOMEN					MEN		
Height Feet	Inches	Small Frame	Medium Frame	Large Frame	Height Feet	Inches	Small Frame	Medium Frame	Large Frame
5	0	100	109	118	5	3	118	129	141
5	1	104	112	121	5	4	122	133	145
5	2	107	115	125	5	5	126	137	149
5	3	110	118	128	5	6	130	142	155
5	4	113	122	132	5	7	134	147	161
5	5	116	125	135	5	8	139	151	166
5	6	120	129	139	5	9	143	155	170
5	7	123	132	142	5	10	147	159	174
5	8	126	136	146	5	11	150	163	178
5	9	130	140	151	6	0	154	167	183
5	10	133	144	156	6	1	158	171	188
5	11	137	148	161	6	2	162	175	192
6	0	141	152	166	6	3	165	178	195
					6	4	168	181	198

Source: Hathaway, M.L., and Foard, E.D.: Heights and Weight of Adults in the United States. Home Economics Research Report No. 10, U.S. Department of Agriculture, Washington, D.C., Table 80 p.111.

FOOD CALORIES

Food	Amount	Calories	Fat (gm)	Cholesterol (mg)	Sodium (mg)
Apple, fresh	1 medium	80	0	0	1
juice	1/2 cup	60	0	0	1
Applesauce, canned, sweetened	1/2 cup	105	0		3
unsweetened	1/2 cup	50	0	0	2
Apricots, fresh	3 small	50	0	0	1
canned, sweetened	1/2 cup(4 halves)	100	0	0	1
dried	1/4 cup(4 halves)	80	0	0	9
nectar	1/2 cup	70	0	0	0
Asparagus, fresh	1/2 cup	20	0	0	1
canned	1/2 cup	20	0	0	235
Avocado, fresh	1/2 medium	190	18	0	5
dip(guacamole)	1/2 cup	140	13	0	165
Banana, fresh	1 6-inch long	100	0	0	1
Bacon, cooked	2 slices	109	10	16	303
bits	1 tablespoon	36	2	0	432
Canadian	1 slice	65	4	10	442
Baking powder	1 teaspoon	4	0	0	405
Baking soda	1 teaspoon	0	0	0	821
Bean dip	1 tablespoon	20	1	2	177
Bean sprouts	1 cup	35	0	0	5
Beans	1/2 cup	118	0	0	7
baked	1/2 cup	190	6	0	485
garbanzo, cooked	1/2 cup	134	2	0	6
green, cooked	1/2 cup	15	0	0	2
kidney, canned	1/2 cup	112	0	0	4
navy, cooked	1/2 cup	88	0	0	0
pinto, cooked	1/2 cup	92	0	0	0
pork and beans, cooked	1/2 cup	160	4	1	59
refried beans	1/2 cup	230	12	0	340
Beef, barbecued sandwich w/bun	1 sandwich	509	37	81	506
brisket, baked	3 ounces	367	33	80	46
barbecued	3 ounces	382	34	80	176
chicken fried steak	4 ounces	370	22	130	350
chop suey	1 cup	300	17	64	1052
chuck roast, baked	3 ounces	240	17	60	40
corned beef	3 ounces	372	30	83	1740
flank steak	3 ounces	158	5	50	47
hamburger patty, broiled	3 ounces	190	10	50	60
jerky	1 piece	38	2	10	418
liver, fried	3 ounces	200	9	255	155
meatloaf	3 ounces	171	11	50	555
pateé	1 tablespoon	41	14	40	91
pot pie	1 piece	443	24	41	1008
prime rib, baked	3 ounces	380	33	80	40
round steak	3 ounces	220	13	60	60
short ribs	1 rib	290	24	24	39
sirloin steak, broiled	3 ounces	330	27	80	50
stew	1 cup	220	11	63	90
stroganoff	1 cup	470	33	130	860
sweetbreads	3 ounces	143	3	466	0
tenderloin (fillet)	3 ounces	174	8	72	54
Beet greens, cooked	1/2 cup	15	0	0	55
Beets, canned	1/2 cup	30	0	0	200
Beverages, beer	12 ounces	150	0	0	25
beer, non-alcoholic	12 ounces	65	0	0	0
club soda	6 ounces	0	0	0	30
coffee	1 cup	3	0	0	2
Gatorade	1 cup	39	0	0	123
ginger ale	12 ounces	105	0	0	4

	Amount	Calories	Fat (gm)	Cholesterol (mg)	Sodium (mg)
Beverages, beer (cont'd)					
Kool Aid	1 cup	100	0	0	1
lemonade	1 cup	110	0	0	1
mineral water	1 cup	0	0	0	5
quinine water	1 cup	74	0	0	16
soft drinks, all canned	12 ounces	150	0	0	10-30
Tang	1 cup	135	0	0	17
tea	1 cup	3	0	0	0
tonic water	12 ounces	132	0	0	0
V-8 juice	6 ounces	31	0	0	364
whiskey	1 1/2 ounces	107	0	0	0
wine	4 ounces	85	0	0	5
Blackberries, fresh	1 cup	80	0	0	2
Blackeyed peas, canned	3/4 cup	81	0	0	602
dried, cooked	1 cup	72	1	0	2
Blueberries, fresh	1 cup	90	0	0	2
Bouillon cube	1 cube	18	1	0	960
low-sodium	1 cube	18	1	0	10
Bread, bagel	1 piece	180	2	0	260
biscuit	1 piece	90	3	2	270
diet	1 slice	40	0	0	115
breadstick	1 piece	23	0	0	100
cornbread	1 piece	180	6	3	265
cornbread muffin	1 2-inch muffin	130	4	2	190
croissant	1 piece	180	11	48	270
croutons	2 cups	359	1	0	1360
English muffin	1 muffin	138	1	0	203
French bread	1 slice	70	0	0	145
mixed grain bread	1 slice	64	1	0	103
pita pocket	1 pita	170	2	0	53
popover	1 medium	112	5	74	110
raisin bread	1 slice	65	0	1	90
roll, dinner	1 small	85	2	1	140
hard	1 small	160	2	0	315
wholewheat	1 small	90	1	0	197
rye bread	1 slice	65	0	1	140
sweet roll	1 medium	270	16	46	240
white bread	1 slice	70	0	1	130
wholewheat bread	1 slice	65	0	1	130
Broccoli, cooked	1/2 cup	20	0	0	8
raw	1 cup	24	0	0	24
Brussel sprouts	1/2 cup	30	0	0	8
Butter, regular	1 teaspoon	35	4	13	40
unsalted	1 teaspoon	36	4	11	0
Cabbage, cooked	1/2 cup	15	0	0	10
Cake(1 piece), angel food	1/12 cake	135	0	0	60
brownie without icing	2 inch x 2 inch	146	10	25	75
cheese cake, plain	1/12 cake	255	13	60	170
chocolate cake with icing	1/12 cake	379	16	62	322
cupcake with icing	1 cupcake	190	6	54	160
fruitcake	1/30 cake	55	2	0	21
gingerbread	2 inch x 2 inch	170	5	0	190
pound cake	1/17 cake	140	9	48	35
Candy, caramels	3 pieces	120	3	2	65
chocolate chips	2 tablespoons	148	8	2	64
fudge	1 ounce	120	5	5	50
gum	1 piece	9	0	0	0
gum drop, small	2 tablespoons	100	0	25	10
hard candy	1 ounce	110	0	0	10
jelly beans	1/4 cup	66	0	0	0
milk chocolate	1.65 ounces	140	9	4	25
peanut brittle	1 ounce	120	3	2	10
peanut butter cup	1 piece	130	8	1	75
Cantaloupe	1/4 melon	50	0	0	20
Carrots, cooked	1/2 cup	20	0	0	25
Cauliflower, cooked	1/2 cup	15	0	0	10

	Amount	Calories	Fat (gm)	Cholesterol (mg)	Sodium (mg)
Celery, raw	1 stalk	15	0	0	100
Cereals, All-Bran	1 cup	210	2	0	960
Alpha Bits	1 cup	119	0	0	227
bran	1 cup	120	2	0	60
Bran Buds	1 cup	210	2	0	516
bran flakes	1 cup	127	0	0	363
Cheerios	1 cup	89	1	0	297
corn flakes	1 cup	95	0	0	325
Cream of Wheat, cooked	1/2 cup	50	0	0	175
granola	1 cup	503	20	0	232
Grape Nuts	1 cup	402	0	0	299
Malt-O-Meal, cooked	1/2 cup	61	0	0	1
oat bran, dry	1/3 cup	110	2	0	0
oatmeal, cooked	1/2 cup	69	1	0	218
Product 19	1 cup	126	0	0	386
Puffed Rice	1 cup	54	0	0	1
Puffed Wheat	1 cup	50	0	0	1
Raisin Bran	1 cup	155	1	0	293
Ralston, cooked	1/2 cup	67	0	0	2
Rice Chex	1 cup	110	0	0	240
Rice Krispies	1 cup	112	0	0	340
Shredded Wheat	1 cup	180	1	0	2
Special K	1 cup	76	0	0	154
Sugar Crisp	1 cup	121	0	0	29
Sugar Pops	1 cup	109	0	0	103
Team flakes	1 cup	109	1	0	175
Total	1 cup	109	1	0	352
wheat flakes	1 cup	100	0	0	310
wheat germ	1/3 cup	120	4	0	0
Cheese, American	1 ounce	110	9	50	405
bleu cheese	1 ounce	100	8	21	395
brie	1 ounce	95	8	28	178
camembert	1 ounce	85	7	20	239
cheddar	1 ounce	115	10	28	175
colby	1 ounce	112	9	27	171
cottage cheese, regular	1/2 cup	120	5	24	455
low-fat	1/2 cup	81	1	12	459
cream cheese	2 tablespoon	100	10	32	85
edam	1 ounce	101	7	25	274
feta	1 ounce	75	6	25	316
gouda	1 ounce	101	8	32	232
gruyere	1 ounce	117	9	31	95
low-calorie cheese	1 ounce	52	2	5	606
low-cholesterol cheese	1 ounce	110	9	5	150
monterey jack	1 ounce	106	9	26	152
mozzarella, part-skim	1 ounce	72	5	16	132
muenster	1 ounce	104	9	27	178
neufchatel	1 ounce	74	6	22	113
parmesan	1/3 cup	130	9	28	247
pimiento	1/4 cup	106	9	27	405
provolone	1 ounce	100	8	20	248
ricotta cheese, regular	1/2 cup	216	16	63	104
part-skim	1/2 cup	170	10	38	153
roquefort	1 ounce	100	8	45	395
Swiss	1 ounce	110	8	35	75
Cherries, fresh	1/2 cup	45		0	1
Chicken, breast, baked w/o skin	3 ounces	190	7	89	86
breast, fried	3 ounces	327	23	89	498
canned	1/2 cup	200	12	91	42
chow mein	1 cup	95		15	725
pot pie	1 piece	503	25	13	863
salad	1/2 cup	127	8	28	345
Chili, beef and bean	1 cup	340	15	34	1355
Chow mein noodles	1/2 cup	200	8	0	320
Cocoa powder	1 tablespoon	18	0	0	25
Coconut	4 tablespoons	180	12	0	7

	Amount	Calories	Fat (gm)	Cholesterol (mg)	Sodium (mg)
Coffee creamer, non-dairy					
liquid	1 tablespoon	20	2	0	12
powder	1 teaspoon	11	1	0	4
Coleslaw	1 cup	118	8	7	149
Cookies, animal crackers	5	43	1	4	30
chocolate chip	1	57	8	2	64
Fig Newton	1	50	1	17	35
ginger snaps	3	50	1	0	69
graham cracker	1	55	1	8	95
molasses cookie	1	71	3	7	58
oatmeal cookie	1	80	3	7	69
Oreo cookie	1	49	2	0	63
peanut butter cookie	1	232	10	0	85
Rice Krispie bar	2 inch x 2 inch	225	10	0	80
shortbread cookie	1	42	2	0	36
sugar cookie	1	98	3	9	109
vanilla wafers	3	51	2	9	28
Cool Whip	1 tablespoon	14	1	0	1
Corn, on-the-cob	1 ear	169	1	0	0
canned	1/2 cup	70	1	0	195
creamed, canned	1/2 cup	110	1	0	300
frozen	1/2 cup	70	0	0	0
Crackers (see Snack foods)					
Cranberry, fresh	1 cup	46	0	0	0
juice	3/4 cup	106	0	0	0
Cream, half and half	1 tablespoon	20	2	6	6
heavy	1 tablespoon	52	6	24	6
sour	1 tablespoon	26	3	5	6
whipped	1/2 cup	210	22	80	20
whipping cream, heavy	1 tablespoon	52	6	21	6
light	1 tablespoon	44	5	17	5
Cucumber	1/2 cup	10	0	0	4
Custard	1/2 cup	150	8	139	105
Dates	1/2 cup	220	0	0	1
Donuts, cake	1	160	8	33	210
glazed	1	180	11	16	100
Egg	1	80	6	252	60
Egg substitute	1/4 cup	25	0	0	80
Egg noodles, cooked	1 cup	220	3	55	15
Figs, fresh	1 piece	80	0	0	2
dried	2 pieces	274	1	0	34
Fish, bass, baked	3 ounces	82	2	68	59
caviar	1 tablespoon	42	2	94	352
cod, baked	3 ounces	180	6	56	115
crab	3 ounces	100	2	100	850
fish sticks	4	200	10	70	115
flounder, baked	3 ounces	200	8	51	235
haddock, baked	3 ounces	180	7	66	195
halibut, baked	3 ounces	175	4	51	86
herring, canned	1/2 cup	208	11	85	74
lobster	3 ounces	90	2	85	205
mackerel, baked	3 ounces	250	17	95	35
mussels	1/4 cup	48	1	16	104
oysters, fresh	6	80	2	60	90
fried	6	138	8	131	116
perch	3 ounces	227	13	55	153
pike	3 ounces	116	2	55	64
red snapper	3 ounces	93	1	55	67
salmon, baked with butter	3 ounces	189	12	58	116
canned in water	1/2 cup	160	6	75	425
patty, fried	3 ounces	239	12	64	96
smoked	3 ounces	150	8	85	425
sardines	1/4 cup	58	3	28	184
scallops	3 ounces	105	2	53	250
shrimp, boiled	1 cup	100	1	119	250
fried	1 cup	380	19	240	320

	Amount	Calories	Fat (gm)	Cholesterol (mg)	Sodium (mg)
Fish (cont'd)					
sole, baked	3 ounces	141	1	51	235
sushi (raw fish)	3 ounces	93	1	50	67
swordfish, baked	3 ounces	174	6	43	98
trout	3 ounces	196	5	55	61
tuna, canned in oil	3 ounces	176	9	19	535
canned in water	3 ounces	109	2	30	399
canned in water, low-sodium	3 ounces	106	2	30	33
steak	3 ounces	145	4	60	0
Frankfurter	1	261	17	45	776
Fruit cocktail, canned, sweetened	1/2 cup	95	0	0	5
Grapefruit, fresh	1/2 medium	40	0	0	1
juice, unsweetened	1 cup	93	0	0	3
Grapes, fresh	1 cup	70	0	0	4
juice	3/4 cup	120	0	0	4
Green chilies, canned	1 tablespoon	14	0	0	0
Green pepper, raw	1/2 cup	15	0	0	10
Greens, collard, cooked	1/3 cup	20	0	0	35
kale, cooked	1 cup	41	0	0	30
spinach, cooked	1/2 cup	20	0	0	50
spinach, raw	1/2 cup	7	0	0	19
Swiss chard, cooked	1/2 cup	15	0	0	60
turnip, cooked	1/2 cup	15	0	0	19
Grits, cooked	1/2 cup	73	0	0	0
Ham, baked, lean	3 ounces	203	8	74	1684
Honey	1 tablespoon	65	0	0	1
Honeydew	1/4 melon	55	0	0	20
Ice cream, regular (10 percent fat)	1/2 cup	135	7	36	60
rich (16 percent fat)	1/2 cup	266	14	72	120
soft serve	1/2 cup	165	10	0	51
Ice milk	1/2 cup	90	3	13	50
Instant breakfast	1 cup	280	8	28	242
Jalapeno pepper, canned	1/4 cup	132	0	0	497
Jam or jelly	1 tablespoon	55	0	0	2
Jello	1/2 cup	70	0	0	0
Kiwi	1 piece	46	0	0	4
Knockwurst	3 ounces	278	23	65	483
Lamb chop, baked	3 ounces	340	28	85	50
roast, baked	3 ounces	160	6	59	60
Lasagna	1 cup	380	12	67	43
Lemon, fresh	1/4 lemon	22	0	0	3
juice	1 tablespoon	5	0	0	0
Lentils	2/3 cup	110	0	0	10
Lettuce	1 cup	6	0	0	6
Lima beans	1/2 cup	95	0	0	2
Lime, fresh	1/4 lime	20	0	0	1
juice	1 tablespoon	3	0	0	2
Luncheon meats, bologna	1 ounce	85	8	28	370
pepperoni	1 ounce	139	13	70	492
pimento loaf	1 ounce	74	6	10	394
salami	1 ounce	130	11	15	350
Macaroni and cheese	1 cup	430	22	42	1085
Macaroni, cooked	1 cup	210	1	0	0
Mandarin oranges, canned	1/2 cup	76	0	0	8
Mango	1 cup	110	0	0	10
Margarine, low-calorie	1 teaspoon	16	2	0	49
regular	1 teaspoon	35	4	0	50
unsalted	1 teaspoon	35	4	0	0
Marshmallows	1/2 cup	90	0	0	10
Milk, buttermilk, skim	1 cup	90	0	5	318
chocolate, low-fat	1 cup	180	5	5	150
evaporated milk, regular	1 cup	340	20	77	265
evaporated milk, skimmed	1 cup	199	0	10	293
hot chocolate	1 cup	110	3	35	154
low-fat (1 percent fat)	1 cup	102	3	3	122

	Amount	Calories	Fat (gm)	Cholesterol (mg)	Sodium (mg)
Milk (cont'd)					
low-fat (2 percent fat)	1 cup	140	5	5	145
nonfat (dry)	1/4 cup	109	0	6	161
skim	1 cup	90	0	5	125
whole (4 percent fat)	1 cup	155	9	34	120
Mixed vegetables, canned	1/2 cup	38	0	0	121
frozen	1/2 cup	54	0	0	45
stir-fried	1/2 cup	59	5	0	17
Mushrooms, canned	1/3 cup	17	0	0	400
fresh	1/2 cup	10	0	0	5
Nectarine, fresh	1	64	0	0	6
Nuts and seeds, almonds, unsalted	1/4 cup	180	16	0	56
brazil nuts, unsalted	1/4 cup	180	19	0	0
cashews, unsalted	1/4 cup	320	26	0	120
macadamia nuts, unsalted	1/4 cup	109	12	0	60
mixed nuts, unsalted	1/4 cup	214	20	0	4
peanuts, salted	1/4 cup	330	28	0	157
peanuts, unsalted	1/4 cup	330	28	0	1
pecans, unsalted	1/4 cup	200	20	0	0
pistachio nuts, salted	1/4 cup	88	8	0	60
sunflower seeds, unsalted	1/4 cup	200	17	0	10
walnuts, unsalted	1/4 cup	200	20	0	0
Okra, cooked	1/2 cup	30	0	0	2
Olives, black	5	35	4	0	150
green	5	20	3	0	465
Onion, green	1 tablespoon	1	0	0	0
Orange, fresh	1 medium	80	0	0	1
juice	3/4 cup	85	0	0	2
Pancakes (4-inch diameter)	3 medium	210	2	63	600
Papaya	1/2 medium	60	0	0	4
Parsnips	1/2 cup	66	0	0	8
Peach, fresh	1 medium	40	0	0	1
canned, sweetened	2/3 cup	120	0	0	4
canned, unsweetened	2/3 cup	43	0	0	9
Peanut butter, regular	1 tablespoon	95	8	0	95
unsalted	1 tablespoon	95	9	0	5
Pear, fresh	1 medium	100	0	0	3
canned, sweetened	1/2 cup	65	0	0	2
canned, unsweetened	1/2 cup	35	0	0	3
Peas, canned	1/2 cup	75	0	0	200
frozen	1/2 cup	55	0	0	90
split	1/2 cup	115	0	0	15
Pickles, dill	1 large	15	0	0	1930
sweet	1 small	50	0	0	200
relish	1 tablespoon	20	0	0	105
Pie (1 slice), banana cream	1/8 pie	285	12	40	252
chocolate cream	1/8 pie	264	15	0	273
lemon meringue	1/8 pie	257	14	130	395
mincemeat	1/8 pie	365	16	0	604
pecan	1/8 pie	334	18	92	177
pumpkin	1/8 pie	320	17	150	325
rhubarb	1/8 pie	190	17	10	432
strawberry	1/8 pie	228	9	10	227
Pimientos, canned	1/4 cup	11	0	0	0
Pineapple, fresh	1 cup	80	0	0	2
canned, sweetened	1 cup	190	0	0	4
canned, unsweetened	1 cup	150	0	0	4
Pizza, cheese (13-inch diameter)	2 slices	340	11	2	900
combination (13-inch diameter)	2 slices	400	17	13	1200
pepperoni (13-inch diameter)	2 slices	370	15	27	1000
Plum, fresh	1 large	30	0	0	1
canned, sweetened	1/2 cup	110	0	0	1
canned, unsweetened	1/2 cup	51	0	0	1
Pork chop, broiled	3 1/2 ounces	357	26	77	60
roast, baked	3 ounces	310	24	59	50
Potatoes, au gratin	1/2 cup	95	3	6	529

	Amount	Calories	Fat (gm)	Cholesterol (mg)	Sodium (mg)
Potatoes (cont'd)					
baked	1 medium	140	0	0	5
French fries	1/2 cup (10 pieces)	220	10	13	120
mashed	1/2 cup	100	5	15	350
tater tots	1/2 cup	200	12	20	545
Prunes, canned	1 cup	245	0	0	6
dried (5 pieces)	1/4 cup	130	0	0	4
Pudding, banana	1/2 cup	241	6	25	11
chocolate	1/2 cup	167	5	65	160
low-calorie	1/2 cup	76	0	0	146
tapioca	1/2 cup	110	4	9	130
vanilla	1/2 cup	140	5	16	85
Quiche (1 slice), cheese	1/8 pie	448	39	305	869
cheese and bacon	1/8 pie	520	42	310	970
Radishes	1/2 cup	7	0	0	10
Raisins	1/4 cup	100		0	10
Raspberries, fresh	1/2 cup	40	0	0	1
frozen	1/2 cup	128	0	0	0
Rhubarb, cooked, sweetened	1/2 cup	190	0	0	2
Rice, brown	2/3 cup	160	1	0	370
white	2/3 cup	150	0	0	2
wild	1 tablespoon	33	0	0	1
Rice-a-Roni	2/3 cup	165	5	13	820
Rice cake	1 cake	31	0	0	8
Salad dressings					
blue cheese	1 tablespoon	75	8	4	165
blue cheese, low-calorie	1 tablespoon	10	1	4	177
French	1 tablespoon	65	6	1	220
French, low-calorie	1 tablespoon	22	0	1	128
green goddess	1 tablespoon	68	7	1	150
Italian	1 tablespoon	85	9	1	315
Italian, low-calorie	1 tablespoon	15	2	1	118
mayonnaise	1 tablespoon	100	11	8	85
mayonnaise, low-calorie	1 tablespoon	50	5	1	100
oil and vinegar	1 tablespoon	71	8	0	0
Ranch or buttermilk	1 tablespoon	53	5	4	185
Russian	1 tablespoon	76	8	0	133
thousand island	1 tablespoon	80	8	8	110
thousand island, low-calorie	1 tablespoon	24	2	2	153
Sauces and Condiments					
barbecue	1 tablespoon	15	1	0	130
bearnaise	1 cup	701	68	189	1265
catsup	1 tablespoon	15	0	0	155
chili	1 tablespoon	17	0	0	228
chocolate	2 tablespoons	100	0	2	36
gravy	1/4 cup	164	14	7	720
hollandaise	1/4 cup	361	39	382	400
mustard	1 teaspoon	4		0	65
picante or salsa	1 1/2 tablespoons	10	0	0	111
soy	2 tablespoons	25	0	0	2665
soy, low-sodium	2 tablespoons	25	0	0	1200
steak	1 tablespoon	18	0	0	149
tartar	2 tablespoons	75	8	10	100
terriyaki	1 tablespoon	15	0	0	690
white	1/2 cup	200	16	16	475
worcestershire	1 teaspoon	4	0	0	49
Sauerkraut	1/2 cup	20	0	0	880
Sausage, link	1	134	12	0	175
patty	1	122	8	34	418
Polish	3 ounces	276	24	60	744
Scallions	1/4 cup	10	0	0	1
Shallots	1/3 cup	36	0	0	6
Sherbet	1/2 cup	134	1	0	10
Snack foods and crackers					
Cheetos	1 cup	153	10	9	329
corn chips	1 cup	155	10	0	183

	Amount	Calories	Fat (gm)	Cholesterol (mg)	Sodium (mg)
Snack food and crackers (cont'd)					
peanut butter cracker sandwich	1 sandwich	61	4	3	103
popcorn, air-popped	2 cups	80	1	0	0
popcorn, caramel	2 cups	270	2	0	0
popcorn, cheese	2 cups	130	8	5	280
popcorn, cooked with oil	2 cups	106	5	13	466
potato chips	1 cup	115	8	0	200
pretzels, sticks	50 sticks	109	1	0	875
pretzels, 3-ring	10 rings	120	2	0	500
rice cake	1 cake	31	0	0	8
Ritz crackers	5 crackers	76	3	8	180
Rykrisp crackers	2 crackers	40	0	0	110
saltines	4 squares	50	2	8	125
saltines, unsalted tops	4 squares	50	2	8	83
shoestring potato sticks	1 cup	152	10	3	280
tortilla chips	1 cup	135	6	0	99
trail mix	1/3 cup	189	10	0	236
Triscuit crackers	2 crackers	60	2	0	90
Wheat Thin crackers	4 crackers	70	3	0	120
Soups, bean	1 cup	170	6	10	1010
beef noodle	1 cup	84	3	5	952
black bean	1 cup	116	2	0	110
broth, beef	1 cup	16	0	0	782
broth, beef, low-sodium	1 cup	16	0	0	12
broth, chicken	1 cup	16	0	0	782
broth, chicken, low-sodium	1 cup	16	0	0	7
chicken noodle	1 cup	75	2	7	1107
cream of mushroom	1 cup	203	14	20	1076
gazpacho	1 cup	57	2	0	1183
gumbo, chicken	1 cup	200	4	22	970
lentil	1 cup	108	0	0	1038
minestrone	1 cup	83	3	2	911
onion	1 cup	65	2	5	1051
onion, dehydrated	2 tablespoons	21	0	0	636
pea	1 cup	140	3	4	940
potato	1 cup	148	7	22	1060
tomato	1 cup	90	3	4	970
turkey	1 cup	136	4	9	923
vegetable	1 cup	78	4	0	1010
vegetable beef	1 cup	80	2	4	1050
vegetable, chunky	1 cup	122	4	0	1010
won ton	1 cup	92	2	1	2027
Spaghetti, cooked	1 cup	210	1	0	5
Spam	1 ounce	87	7	15	336
Squash (winter), baked	1/2 cup	65	0	0	1
Strawberries, fresh	2/3 cup	35	0	0	1
frozen, sweetened	2/3 cup	160	0	0	2
frozen, unsweetened	2/3 cup	119	0	0	2
Succotash	1 cup	222	2	0	32
Sweet potato or yam, baked	3/4 cup	160		0	15
canned	3/4 cup	216	5	10	67
Syrup, corn	1 tablespoon	58	0	0	14
maple	1 tablespoon	50	0	0	2
Taco shell	1 piece	135	6	0	99
Tangerine, fresh	1 medium	46	0	0	2
Tofu	1/2 cup	85	5	0	10
Tofutti	1/2 cup	230	14	0	95
Tomato, fresh	1/2 cup	25	0	0	4
canned, regular	1/2 cup	25	0	0	155
canned, no-salt added	1/2 cup	25	0	0	20
juice	3/4 cup	35	0	0	365
juice, low-sodium	3/4 cup	31	0	0	18
paste	1/2 cup	110	1	0	50
sauce, canned	1/2 cup	43	0	0	656
sauce, canned, no salt added	1/2 cup	43	0	0	25

	Amount	Calories	Fat (gm)	Cholesterol (mg)	Sodium (mg)
Tortilla, corn (6-inch diameter)	1	65	1	0	1
flour (8-inch diameter)	1	105	3	0	134
Turkey, dark meat, baked w/o skin	3 ounces	170	7	64	85
light meat, baked w/o skin	3 ounces	150	4	64	70
roll, light and dark meat	3 ounces	126	6	48	498
turkey ham	3 ounces	73	3	0	563
Turnips	1/2 cup	20	0	0	25
Veal cutlet	3 ounces	231	13	76	55
patty	3 ounces	298	19	90	51
Waffle	4-inch square	124	5	32	340
Water chestnuts, canned	1/4 cup	20	0	0	5
Watercress	1 cup	5	0	0	20
Watermelon	2 3/4 cup	110	0	0	5
Yogurt, plain, non-fat	1 cup	127	0	4	174
frozen	1/2 cup	108	0	0	0
Zucchini, cooked	1 cup	22	0	0	2
raw	1 cup	38	0	0	3

FAST FOODS

(Goal: Meals with 10-25 gm fat per meal)

N.A. = Data Not Available

	Calories	Fat (gm)	Cholesterol (mg)	Sodium (mg)
ARBY'S				
Junior Roast Beef	233	11	22	519
Regular Roast Beef	383	18	43	936
Arby Q	389	15	29	1268
Philly Beef'N Swiss	467	25	53	1144
Super Roast Beef	552	28	43	1174
Beef'N Cheddar	508	27	52	1166
Bac'N Cheddar Deluxe	512	32	38	1094
Chicken Breast Filet	445	23	45	958
Turkey Sub	486	19	51	2033
Roast Beef Sub	623	32	73	1817
Roast Chicken Club	503	27	46	1143
Grilled Chicken Deluxe	430	20	44	901
Grilled Chicken BBQ	386	13	43	1002
Tuna Sub	663	37	43	1342
French Dip	368	15	43	1018
Roast Chicken Salad	204	7	43	508
Light Roast Chicken Deluxe	276	7	33	777
Light Roast Turkey Deluxe	260	6	33	1262
Light Roast Beef Deluxe	294	10	42	826
Hot Ham'N Cheese	355	14	55	1400
Fish Fillet Sandwich	526	27	44	872
Potato Cakes	204	12	0	397
Plain Baked Potato	240	2	0	58
Side Salad	25	3	0	30
Chef Salad	205	10	126	796
Lumberjack Mixed Vegetable Soup	89	4	4	1075
Peanut Butter Cup Polar Swirl	517	24	34	385
BURGER KING				
Whopper Sandwich	570	31	80	870
w/cheese	660	38	105	1190
Bacon Double Cheeseburger	470	28	100	800
Whopper, Jr.	300	15	35	500
w/cheese	350	19	45	650
Hamburger	260	10	30	500
Cheeseburger	300	14	45	660
BK Broiler	280	10	50	770
Chicken Sandwich (Fried)	620	32	45	1430
Chicken Tenders (6 pcs.)	236	13	38	541
Ocean Catfish Filet Sandwich	450	28	30	760
Garden Salad	95	5	15	125
Side Salad	25	0	0	27
Chef Salad	178	9	103	568
Chunky Chicken Salad	142	4	49	443
Breakfast Croissan'wich	315	20	222	607
w/ bacon	353	23	230	780
w/ sausage	534	40	258	985
w/ ham	351	22	236	1373
Breakfast Buddy w/ Sausage, Egg, Cheese	255	16	127	492
Blueberry Mini Muffins	292	14	72	244
French Toast Sticks	440	27	0	490
Snickers Ice Cream Bar	220	14	15	65
Lemon Pie	290	8	35	105

	Calories	Fat	Cholesterol	Sodium
		(gm)	(mg)	(mg)
DAIRY QUEEN				
Single Hamburger	310	13	45	580
w/ cheese	365	18	60	800
Double Hamburger	530	28	85	660
w/cheese	650	37	95	980
Breaded Chicken Sandwich	430	20	55	760
Fish Sandwich	370	16	45	630
w/cheese	440	21	60	1035
Hot Dog	280	16	25	700
w/ chili	320	19	30	720
w/ cheese	330	21	35	920
Super Hot Dog	590	38	60	1360
Regular DQ Dip Cone	330	16	20	100
Banana Split	510	11	30	250
Hot Fudge Brownie Delight	710	29	35	340
Heath Blizzard, regular	820	36	60	410
Vanilla Cone, small	140	4	15	60
regular	230	7	20	95
large	340	10	30	140
JACK IN THE BOX				
Hamburger	267	11	26	556
Cheeseburger	315	14	41	746
Double Cheeseburger	467	27	72	842
Jumbo Jack	584	34	73	733
Jumbo Jack w/cheese	677	40	102	1090
Bacon Cheeseburger	705	45	113	1240
Bacon Old Fashioned Patty Melt	713	46	92	1360
Ultimate Cheeseburger	942	69	127	1176
Chicken Supreme	641	39	85	1470
Grilled Chicken Fillet	431	19	65	1070
Chicken Strips (6 pcs.)	451	20	82	1100
Fish Supreme	510	27	55	1040
Chicken & Mushroom Sandwich	438	18	61	1340
Chicken Fajita Pita	292	8	34	703
Taco	187	11	18	414
Super Taco	281	17	29	718
Guacamole	55	5	0	130
Egg Rolls (3 pcs.)	437	24	29	957
Chef Salad	325	18	142	900
Taco Salad	503	31	92	1600
Side Salad	51	3	0	84
Supreme Crescent	547	40	178	1053
Sausage Crescent	584	43	187	1012
Sourdough Breakfast Sandwich	381	20	236	1120
Breakfast Jack	307	13	203	871
Scrambled Egg Platter	559	32	378	1060
Hash Browns	156	11	0	312
Pancake Platter	612	22	99	888
Cheesecake	309	18	63	208
Tortilla Chips	140	6	0	134
Sesame Bread Stick (1)	70	2	0	110
Taquitos (5 pcs.)	362	15	24	462

N.A. = Data Not Available

	Calories	Fat (gm)	Cholesterol (mg)	Sodium (mg)
KENTUCKY FRIED CHICKEN				
ORIGINAL RECIPE CHICKEN				
Wing	172	11	59	383
Side Breast	245	15	78	604
Center Breast	260	14	92	609
Drumstick	152	9	75	269
Thigh	287	21	112	591
EXTRA CRISPY CHICKEN				
Wing	231	17	63	319
Side Breast	379	27	77	646
Center Breast	344	21	80	636
Drumstick	205	14	72	292
Thigh	414	31	112	580
HOT & SPICY CHICKEN				
Wing	244	18	65	460
Side Breast	400	27	83	922
Center Breast	382	25	84	905
Drumstick	207	14	75	406
Thigh	412	30	105	750
SKINFREE CRISPY				
Side Breast	293	17	63	410
Center Breast	296	16	59	435
Drumstick	166	9	42	256
Thigh	256	17	68	394
Kentucky Nuggets (6 pcs.)	284	18	66	865
Chicken Little Sandwich	169	10	18	331
Colonel's Chicken Chicken	482	27	47	1060
Hot Wings	471	33	150	1230
Mashed Potatoes w/ Gravy	71	2	0	339
Corn-on-the-Cob	90	2	0	11
Cole slaw	114	6	4	177
Potato Salad	177	12	14	500
Baked Beans	133	2	1	500
Buttermilk Biscuit	235	12	1	655
LONG JOHN SILVER'S				
Crispy Fish (1 pc.)	150	8	20	240
Batter-Dipped Fish Sandwich (No Sauce)	340	13	30	890
Batter-Dipped Chicken Sandwich (No Sauce)	280	8	15	790
Batter-Dipped Fish (1 pc.)	180	11	30	490
Batter-Dipped Shrimp (1 pc.)	30	2	10	80
Ala Carte (Baked)				
3 pc. Fish-Lemon Crumb	150	1	110	370
Chicken Light Herb	120	4	60	570
Seafood Chowder w/cod (7oz.)	140	6	20	590
Seafood Gumbo (7 oz.)	120	8	25	740
Seafood Salad (No Drsg)	380	31	55	980
Ocean Chef Salad (No Drsg)	110	1	40	730
Chicken Planks (2 pcs.)	240	12	30	790
Cole Slaw	140	6	15	260
Corn Cobette (1 pc.)	140	8	0	0
Hushpuppies (1 pc.)	70	2	<5	25
Green Beans	20	0	0	320
Small Salad	25	0	0	20
Lemon Pie (1 slice)	340	9	45	130

	Calories	Fat	Cholesterol	Sodium
McDONALD'S		(gm)	(mg)	(mg)
Hamburger	255	9	37	490
Cheeseburger	305	13	50	725
Quarter Pounder	410	20	85	645
Quarter Pounder w/ Cheese	510	28	115	1110
Big Mac	500	26	100	930
McLean Deluxe	320	10	60	670
McLean Deluxe w/ Cheese	370	14	75	890
Chicken McNuggets (6 pcs.)	270	15	55	580
McChicken	415	19	50	830
Filet-O-Fish	370	18	50	730
Chicken Fajita	190	8	35	310
Chef Salad	170	9	111	400
Garden Salad	50	2	65	70
Chunky Chicken Salad	150	4	78	230
Side Salad	30	1	33	35
Egg McMuffin	280	11	235	710
Sausage McMuffin	345	20	57	770
Sausage McMuffin w/ Egg	430	25	270	920
Biscuit, Plain	260	13	1	730
Biscuit w/ Sausage	420	28	44	1040
Biscuit w/ Sausage & Egg	505	33	260	1210
Biscuit w/ Bacon, Egg, & Cheese	440	26	240	1215
Scrambled Eggs (2)	140	10	425	290
Hot Cakes w/ Butter & Syrup	440	12	8	685
Sausage	160	15	43	310
Hash Brown Potatoes	130	7	0	330
English Muffin w/ Spread	170	4	0	285
Breakfast Burrito	280	17	135	580
Apple Bran Muffin (Fat Free)	180	0	0	200
Breakfast Apple Danish	390	17	25	370
Wheaties Cereal (1/2 Cup)	90	1	0	220
Cheerios Cereal (3/4 Cup)	80	1	0	210
Soft Serve Cone	105	0	3	80
Sundae, all flavors	280	6	6	175
McDonaldland Cookies	290	9	0	300
Chocolate Chip Cookies	300	15	4	280
Low-Fat Milkshake	320	1	10	170

PIZZA HUT

(Serving Size - 2 slcs of med 13 inch pizza; 4 per pizza)

	Calories	Fat	Cholesterol	Sodium
THIN'N CRISPY				
Standard Cheese	398	17	33	867
Standard Pepperoni	413	20	46	986
Supreme	459	22	42	1328
Super Supreme	463	21	56	1336
PAN PIZZA				
Cheese	492	18	34	940
Pepperoni	540	22	42	1127
Supreme	589	30	48	1363
Super Supreme	563	26	55	1447
HAND-TOSSED				
Cheese	518	20	55	1276
Pepperoni	500	23	50	1267
Supreme	540	26	55	1470
Super Supreme	556	25	54	1648
PERSONAL PAN PIZZA (1)				
Pepperoni	675	29	53	1335

	Calories	Fat	Cholesterol	Sodium
		(gm)	(mg)	(mg)
TACO BELL				
Bean Burrito	381	14	9	1148
Beef Burrito	431	21	57	1311
Burrito Supreme	440	22	33	1181
Chicken Burrito	334	12	52	880
Combo Burrito	407	16	33	1136
Totasda	243	11	16	596
Nachos Supreme	367	27	18	471
Mexican Pizza	575	37	52	1031
Pintos & Cheese	190	9	16	642
Nachos	346	18	9	399
Nachos Bellgrande	649	35	36	997
Taco	184	11	32	246
Soft Taco Supreme	272	16	32	554
Chicken Soft Taco	213	10	52	615
Soft Taco	225	12	32	554
Taco Supreme	230	15	32	276
Taco Salad	905	61	80	910
Taco Salad w/o Shell	434	31	80	680
Chicken Mexi Melt	257	15	48	779
Beef Mexi Melt	266	15	38	689
Cinnamon Twists	171	8	0	234
Guacamole	34	2	0	113
Nacho Cheese Sauce	103	8	9	393
WENDY'S				
Hamburger, Jr. *	270	9	35	590
Cheeseburger, Jr. *	320	13	45	760
Single Hamburger *	350	15	70	510
Single w/ Everything	440	23	75	850
Jr. Cheeseburger Deluxe	390	20	50	800
Hamburger, Kid's Meal *	270	9	35	590
Bacon Cheeseburger, Jr.	440	25	65	870
Wendy's Big Classic	480	23	75	850
Chicken Club Sandwich	520	25	75	980
Grilled Chicken Sandwich w/ Honey Mustard	290	7	60	670
Breaded Chicken Sandwich	450	20	60	740
Fish Sandwich w/ Tartar Sauce	460	25	55	780
Crispy Chicken Nuggets (6 pcs,)	280	20	50	600
Chili, small (8 oz.)	190	6	40	670
Hot Stuffed Baked Potatoes				
Plain (10 oz.)	300	0	0	20
Sour Cream w/ Chives	370	6	15	35
Cheese	550	24	30	640
Chili & Cheese	600	25	45	740
Bacon & Cheese	510	17	15	1170
Broccoli & Cheese	450	14	0	450
Deluxe Garden Salad (take out)	110	5	0	380
Side Salad	60	3	0	200
Caesar Side Salad	160	6	10	700
Grilled Chicken Salad	200	8	55	690
Taco Salad	640	30	80	960
Three Bean Salad (1/4 Cup)	60	1	N.A.	20
Potato Salad (1/4 Cup)	140	10	N.A.	340
Pasta Salad (1/4 Cup)	160	8	10	230
California Cole Slaw (1/4 Cup)	90	6	10	120
Turkey Ham (1/4 Cup)	60	2	30	420
Taco Shell (1)	50	3	N.A.	45

(* No Mayonnaise)

 © 1993, *The Balancing Act Nutrition and Weight Guide*, G. Kostas, M.P.H., R.D., Dallas, Texas

	Calories	Fat	Cholesterol	Sodium
WENDY'S *(CONT'D)*		(gm)	(mg)	(mg)
Flour Tortilla	100	3	N.A.	210
Taco Chips (8)	160	6	N.A.	15
Fettucini (1/2 Cup)	120	4	10	0
Rotini (1/2 Cup)	90	2	0	0
Pasta Medley (1/2 Cup)	60	2	0	0
Alfredo Sauce (1/4 Cup)	30	1	N.A.	260
Spaghetti Sauce (1/4 Cup)	30	0	0	340
Cheese Sauce (1/4 Cup)	40	2	N.A.	310
Cheese, Shredded Imitation (2 Tbsp.)	50	4	0	280
Cottage Cheese (2 Tbsp.)	30	1	5	125
Chicken Salad (1/4 Cup)	140	10	0	270
Tuna Salad (1/4 Cup)	200	12	0	540
Seafood Salad (1/4 Cup)	70	4	0	300
Breadstick (1)	130	3	5	250
Frosty, small (12 oz.)	340	10	40	200
Pudding, all flavors (1/4 Cup)	80	3	0	60

MISCELLANEOUS

BEVERAGES

	Calories	Fat	Cholesterol	Sodium
Coffee	3	0	0	2
Tea	3	0	0	0
Orange Juice (6 oz.)	80	0	0	2
Chocolate Milk	160	5	15	135
1% Milk	110	2	10	130
2% Milk	120	5	18	122
Whole Milk	155	9	34	120
Soft Drink (12 oz.)	167	0	0	30
Diet Soft Drink (12 oz.)	1	0	0	58
Milkshake, Vanilla (10 oz.)	314	8	32	232
Milkshake, Chocolate (10 oz.)	360	11	37	273

EXTRAS

	Calories	Fat	Cholesterol	Sodium
Ketchup (2 Tbsp.)	150	0	0	155
Jelly (1 Tbsp.)	55	0	0	2
Table Syrup (1 Tbsp.)	50	0	0	2
Coffeemate (1 pkt.)	17	1	0	6
Dressings (1 Tbsp.) *				
Lemon Juice or Vinegar	0	0	0	0
Bleu Cheese	75	8	4	165
French	65	6	1	214
Italian	69	7	0	116
Thousand Island	60	6	2	110
Ranch	53	6	10	276
Oil & Vinegar	72	8	0	0
Low-Calorie Dressings (Avg.)	35	3	0	173
French Fries, small order	240	12	0	150
French Fries, medium order	360	17	0	220
French Fries, large order	450	22	0	280
Onion Rings	360	21	0	540
Fried Pie	260	15	6	240
Tartar Sauce (1 Tbsp.)	130	14	15	115
Sweet & Sour Sauce (1 pkt.)	45	0	0	55
BBQ Sauce (1 pkt.)	50	N.A.	N.A.	100
Cocktail Sauce (1 pkt.)	32	0	0	206
Picante Sauce (1 Tbsp.)	5	0	0	0

(* 2 Tbsp. = 1 oz.)

EXERCISE CALORIES
(calories expended per hour)

To calculate the exercise calories you expend per hour, find your "exercise" in the left column and your "weight" in the right column. In the place where they intersect is the figure indicating the calories burned **per hour**. For example, if you aerobic dance for 1 hour and weigh 125 pounds, you will expend 285 calories.

Exercise	Weight (in pounds)				
	110	125	150	175	200
	Calories expended per hour				
Aerobic dancing	250	285	340	395	450
Archery	225	255	305	360	410
Baseball	225	255	305	360	410
Basketball	415	470	565	660	750
Bowling	180	205	245	285	325
Calisthenics (vigorous)	225	255	305	360	410
Cross country skiing					
- moderately hilly	595	675	810	945	1080
- indoor machine (11 mph)	330	375	450	525	600
Cycling					
- outdoor (5.5 mph)	195	220	260	305	350
- outdoor (9.4 mph)	300	340	410	475	545
- outdoor racing (19 mph)	505	575	690	805	920
- Schwinn Aerodyne	510	580	695	810	925
- stationary (mod tension)	330	375	450	525	600
Golf					
- w/ Cart (90-120 minutes)	145	165	200	230	265
- no Cart (90-120 minutes)	185	210	255	295	340
Handball/Squash	635	725	870	1015	1155
Hiking - 4 mph, 20 lb pack	355	405	490	570	650
Horseback Riding	225	255	305	360	410
Ice Skating	275	300	350	390	425
Nordic Ski Machine					
Heavy (18 mph)	1100	1250	1500	1750	2000
Medium (11 mph)	330	375	450	525	600
Light (6 mph)	225	255	305	360	410
Racquetball	550	625	750	875	1000
Roller Skating/Blading	275	300	350	390	425
Rope Skipping (100 skips/min)	560	640	765	895	1020
Rowing (sculling or machine)	620	705	845	990	1130

Exercise	Weight (in pounds)				
	110	125	150	175	200
	Calories expended per hour				
Running (Jogging)					
5:30 min/mile (11 mph)	870	985	1185	1380	1575
6:00 min/mile (10 mph)	755	860	1030	1200	1375
7:00 min/mile (8.5 mph)	685	780	935	1090	1245
7:30 min/mile (8 mph)	655	745	890	1040	1190
8:00 min/mile (7.5 mph)	625	710	850	990	1135
8:30 min/mile (7 mph)	603	685	825	960	1100
9:00 min/mile (6.5 mph)	580	660	790	920	1050
10:00 min/mile (6 mph)	535	605	730	850	970
11:00 min/mile (5.5 mph)	470	530	640	745	850
11:30 min/mile (5.25 mph)	405	460	550	645	735
12:00 min/mile (5 mph)	375	425	510	600	680
Scuba Diving	355	405	490	570	650
Snow Skiing - Downhill	300	340	410	480	545
Softball	225	255	305	360	410
Stair Climbing (moderate)	515	600	750	850	960
Stairmaster (machine)	595	675	810	945	1080
Step Aerobics - 120 steps/min	550	625	750	875	1000
Swimming - 45 min/mile	385	435	525	610	700
- 60 min/mile	300	335	405	475	540
Table Tennis (moderate)	200	225	270	315	360
Tennis - Doubles	225	255	305	360	410
- Singles	325	370	445	520	600
Treadmill - 12 min/mile	375	425	510	600	680
- 13.5 min/mile	330	375	450	525	600
Volleyball - Competitive	435	495	595	700	800
- Recreational	165	185	225	260	300
Walking/Race Walking					
12 min/mile (5 mph)	435	495	595	700	800
Walk/Jog Combination					
13:30 min/mile (4.5 mph)	330	375	450	525	600
Walking					
15:00 min/mile (4 mph)	300	345	415	480	550
17:00 min/mile (3.5 mph)	250	285	345	400	450
20:00 min/mile (3 mph)	225	255	310	360	410
30:00 min/mile (2 mph)	145	165	200	230	265
Weight Training/Lifting (Light)	270	310	370	430	500

NUTRIENT SOURCES

NUTRIENT	WHY NEEDED	FOOD SOURCES
CALORIES	Energy from food. Adequate calories are necessary to sustain life processes and provide energy; excesses stored as fat.	All foods, beverages, alcohol.
PROTEIN	Incorporated in all body tissues and organs, bones, muscle, hormones, enzymes. Regulates acid-base balance. Helps disease resistance.	Dried beans and peas, fish, poultry, veal (10 meals per week); lean meat (4 meals per week); low-fat dairy products; eggs (3 per week).
COMPLEX CARBOHYDRATE	Chief most efficient energy source. Supplies essential fiber. Spares protein as an energy source. Rich in vitamins and minerals.	Fresh fruits; vegetables; whole-grain bread; cereals with bran, oats, wheat, corn, rye, barley; oatmeal; legumes: pinto beans, lentils; starches: potatoes, rice, pasta; unsalted popcorn; pretzels.
FAT	Long-term energy source. Contains essential fatty acids for skin and health. Carries fat-soluble vitamins.	Eat unsaturated (vegetable) fats: safflower, corn, sunflower, olive oils; tub margarine; mayonnaise; salad dressing (Italian, French). Avoid animal fats.
CHOLESTEROL	Precursor of Vitamin D and many vital body compounds; component of hormones and cell walls. Excesses deposited in artery walls may lead to atherosclerosis.	Eggs, organ meats, shellfish, beef, lamb, pork, butter, whole mild dairy products (cheese, ice cream, sweet and sour cream, dips, creamy dressings, etc.).
SUGAR (Simple Carbohydrate)	High-calorie source, but devoid of vitamins and minerals.	Sugar, brown sugar, honey, jam, jellies, soft drinks, candy, cookies, pastries, cake, sugar-coated cereals, other sources.
ALCOHOL	A drug and high-calorie source; devoid of vitamins and minerals.	Beer, wine, liquor.
CAFFEINE	Stimulant — may cause insomnia, irregular heart beat, nervousness. Irritant — may increase stomach acidity. Diuretic; muscle relaxant. May aggravate fibrocystic breast disease.	Coffee, tea, cola drinks, chocolate. Over 200 milligrams per day (2 cups coffee) may have adverse effects.
WATER	Vital to normal body processes, hydration, temperature control; waste excretion; digestion and absorption of nutrients	At least 4 (8-ounce) glasses daily; and at least 4 of other beverages.
FIBER	Aids and promotes good digestion; reduces constipation; prevents and treats diverticulosis; decreases risk of colon cancer.	Wheat, bran, wholegrain bread and cereals, fresh fruits and vegetables, beans, nuts, seeds, popcorn, peels, potatoes - 8 per day minimum.

MINERAL	WHY NEEDED	FOOD SOURCES
CALCIUM	Promotes strong bones, teeth, nails. Aids muscle tone, blood clotting, nerve function, heart beat. Prevents osteoporosis and cramping.	Low-fat dairy products: mile, yogurt, cheese, etc. Dark green leafy vegetables: broccoli, spinach, etc. Eat at least 3 dairy products daily.
PHOSPHORUS	Promotes strong bones and teeth. Produces energy. Regulates blood chemistry and internal processes.	Lean meat, fish, poultry; low-fat dairy products
MAGNESIUM	Promotes energy production. Normalizes heart rhythm and muscle/nerve function. Prevents muscle cramps.	Wholegrain cereals, nuts, legumes, seafood, dark green leafy vegetables.
SODIUM	Regulates normal water balance inside and outside cells and blood pressure. Maintains electrolyte and chemical balance.	In processed foods: ham, bacon, crackers, pickles, sauces, soups, fast foods, pizza.
POTASSIUM	Regulates balance and volume of body fluids. Prevents muscle cramping, weakness. Normalizes heart rhythm and electrolyte balance in blood.	In all protein foods: meat, cheese; citrus fruits, leafy green vegetables, potatoes, tomatoes, wholegrains and bran.
ZINC	Aids appetite; taste acquity. Promotes growth; healthy skin; wound healing. Structural part of cells in body.	Lean meat, liver, milk, fish, poultry, shellfish, wholegrain cereals.
IRON	Aids formation of red blood cells and oxygen transport to cells. Prevents nutritional anemia.	Liver, lean meats, dried beans, peas, eggs, dark leafy vegetables, wholegrain cereals, dried fruit.

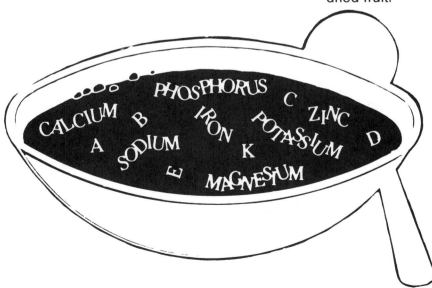

VITAMIN	WHY NEEDED	FOOD SOURCES
VITAMIN A	Normal vision, healthy eyes. Prevents night "blindness." Healthy skin, mucous membrane. Boosts resistance to infection. Aids tissue growth and repair.	Liver, dark green leafy vegetables; spinach, carrots, broccoli, cantaloupe, apricots, plums, tomato.
VITAMIN D	Promotes calcium and phosphorus absorption. Normal growth; healthy bones, teeth, nails.	Sunshine and fortified milk. Vitamin D is formed by action of sunlight on skin.
VITAMIN E	Prevents spoilage of fats; preserves foods. Protects cell membranes.	Vegetable oils, margarine. You need 3 teaspoons daily!
THIAMIN (B1)	Energy production. Normal appetite; digestion. Functioning of nerves, heart, muscle. Growth; fertility.	Pork, liver, lean meat, enriched and fortified wholegrains, legumes, nuts.
RIBOFLAVIN (B2)	Energy production. Good vision. Healthy skin and mouth tissue.	Low-fat dairy products, lean meat, liver, eggs, enriched and fortified wholegrains, green leafy vegetables.
NIACIN (B3)	Energy production. Healthy skin, tongue, digestive and nervous system. Normal appetite, digestion.	Liver, lean meats, port, poultry, fish, nuts, legumes. Enriched and fortified wholegrains.
PYRODOXINE (B6)	Energy production. Red blood cell formation; growth.	Liver, pork, lean meats, fish, legumes. Enriched and fortified wholegrains, green leafy vegetables.
PANTOTHENIC ACID	Energy production. Growth and maintenance of body tissues.	Liver, eggs, lean meats, low-fat milk, wholegrains, legumes, potatoes.
FOLIC ACID	Energy production. Red blood cell formation; growth.	Liver, lean meat, fish, legumes, nuts. Green leafy vegetables, wholegrains.
VITAMIN B12	Energy production. Healthy nerve tissue. Normal red blood cell formation. Utilization of folic acid.	Liver, lean meat, poultry, fish, eggs, low-fat dairy products.
VITAMIN C	Promotes growth, wound healing. Aids disease and infection resistance. Bone, teeth formation; increases iron absorption.	Citrus fruits, cantaloupe, strawberries, potatoes, tomatoes, green vegetables: greens, broccoli, cabbage, kale, collards, liver.

NOTE: Limit liver (rich in cholesterol), nuts and seeds (rich in fat), even though they are listed as nutrient-dense foods.

APPENDIX D

Recipes

- Fishy Ideas
- Chicken Ideas
- Meat-Free Dishes
- High-Calcium Recipes
- Soups
- Low-Calorie Dressings
- High-Fiber Recipes
- Low-Sodium Recipes
- Low-Sugar Desserts

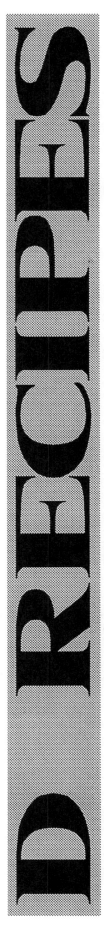

Fishy Ideas

BUYING FISH:

Fish marked "fresh" means that it has never been frozen.
For good-quality frozen fish:

- Buy solidly frozen packages. (Wrapping should be moisture and vapor proof.)
- Little or no odor present.
- Avoid fish with excessive ice build-up, torn packages, or discoloration.
- Avoid fish with freezer burn. the longer a fish is frozen, the more it deteriorates.

SECRETS TO PREPARING FISH:

- Do not overcook
- Bake at 350-400 degrees for 8-10 minutes only
- Season with lemon, onion
- It's "done" if flaky
- Allow 1/3 pound of fish per person

TO AVOID "FISH" SMELL:

- Bake fish — do not fry it
- Burn vanilla candle
- Use exhaust vent

EASY FISH DISHES:

- Poached fish
- Stir-fried vegetables with fish
- Mixed fish dishes: crab or tuna salad, cold shrimp, salmon or tuna patties, tuna casserole, etc.

FUSS-FREE BASICS:

- **Baked Fish** — Make tray with foil. Bake onion slices (uncovered) in tray. Place fish on top cooked onion. Add lemon juice, dill, oregano, salt, pepper, etc.

  Variation: Line pan with onion slices; top with lemon slices. Add fish. On top fish layer lemon, then onion slices. Bake at 375 degrees for 10 minutes.

  Variation: Bake fish with topping of low-calorie zesty Italian dressing.

- **Broiled Fish** — Preheat oven on "broil" for 10 minutes. Place fish fillet on rack. (May add seasonings and lemon or low-calorie Italian dressing.) Broil fish 3-4 inches from heat source on one side only. Done in 5-10 minutes.

  Variation: Add chopped green onions to fish...and a little white wine for flavor.

  Variation: Mix low-calorie mayonnaise and parmesan cheese. Spread thin layer over fish.

- **Salmon or Tuna Patty** — Mix together 1 small can pink salmon or tuna, 1 chopped onion and 1 egg. Form patties. Roll in cracker crumbs. Bake at 375 degrees for 45 minutes.

- **Tuna Salad** — Add to water-packed tuna: low-calorie Italian dressing or fat-free mayonnaise or non-fat yogurt (to replace mayonnaise). Add fruit (apple, pineapple, grapes) or vegetables (celery, pickle, onion).

- **Poached Fish** — Barely cover fish with a liquid (milk or water seasoned with wine, vinegar, lemon juice, onion and spices). Bring liquid to boil, reduce heat and simmer until fish flakes easily with a fork.

- **Steamed Fish** — Place fish on a rack above simmering liquid such as broth (onion, celery, carrot, water), wine or water, or combination. Cover container. Steam for 10-12 minutes.

- **Fish Shish-a-Bob** — Put fish chunks on skewers with vegetables (onion, tomato, mushroom, pepper, etc.). Broil 3-4 inches from heat source. To prevent drying out, lightly brush with oil or place a container of boiling water in perforated rack to allow seam to moisten fish.

Italian Fish Fillets

2 pounds sole, cod or walleye fillets
2 tablespoons oil
2 cups sliced onion
6 cups sliced zucchini
2 cups green pepper slices
1 1/2 cups chopped tomatoes
1/3 cup dry sherry

2 tablespoons lemon juice
1 teaspoon salt
1 teaspoon basil
1/4 teaspoon pepper
4 drops Tabasco sauce
1/2 cup shredded Parmesan cheese

1. Place fillets, single layer, in an oiled 9 x 13 inch baking pan.
2. Sauté sliced vegetables in oil until crisp-tender; spoon over fillets.
3. Top with chopped tomatoes.
4. Combine sherry, lemon juice, salt, basil, pepper and Tabasco; pour over fillets.
5. Bake until fish flakes easily with fork (25-30 minutes).
6. Remove fish and vegetables to a heated platter; sprinkle with Parmesan cheese.

Yield: 8 servings

One serving = 210 calories, 7 grams fat
= 3 meat + 1 vegetable + 1 fat

Shrimp Creole

1/2 cup chopped onion
1/2 cup chopped celery
1/2 cup diced bell pepper
1/2 teaspoon minced garlic
2 tablespoons diet margarine
2 (8oz.) cans tomato sauce

1/8 teaspoon black pepper
1/4 teaspoon chili powder
1 pound cooked, small shrimp (as frozen or
     canned) or fresh, peeled
4 cups cooked rice

1. Melt margarine in skillet. Sauté garlic and vegetables in melted margarine.
2. Add tomato sauce and seasonings. Simmer 15 minutes.
3. Add shrimp. Cook 10 minutes more.
4. Serve over rice.

Yield: 6 servings

One serving = 230 calories, 2 grams fat, 55 mg cholesterol
= 2 bread + 1 1/2 meat

Chicken Ideas

Marinated Chicken Breasts

Chicken Breasts, any number
  (approx. 6 oz. each, if with bone and skin; or 3-4 oz. each if without bone and skin)
Low-calorie Italian dressing
Paprika (Optional)

1. Remove skin from chicken pieces. Wash. Drain.
2. Pierce chicken with fork prongs to allow marinade to soak in. Place in glass Pyrex pan.
3. Cover chicken with low-calorie or oil-free Italian salad dressing.
4. Marinate overnight in refrigerator, covered, or for at least 20 minutes before cooking.
5. Pour off marinade. Sprinkle with paprika for color, if needed.
6. Bake (covered) at 350 degrees for 45 minutes. Or, grill outdoors over hot coals, cooking each side for 5-7 minutes.

One chicken breast (3 oz.) = 125 calories, 3 grams fat
                          = 3 meat

Poultry Hawaiian

1 large onion, chopped
3 garlic cloves, minced
4 carrots, julienne strips
1 green pepper, julienne strips
1 cup celery, sliced
1 tablespoon vegetable oil
6 ounce chicken broth or 2 bouillon
  cubes + 3/4 cup water

2 tablespoons cornstarch
1/3 cup soy sauce
1/3 cup pineapple liquid
1/4 can pineapple tidbits, drained
4 ounce can mushroom bits, drained
5 ounce can water chestnuts, sliced and drained
3 cups turkey or chicken , julienne strips

1. Sauté onion and garlic in vegetable oil.
2. Stir in carrots, green pepper, celery.
3. Add chicken broth.
4. Cover and simmer 5 minutes.
5. Blend soy sauce and cornstarch until smooth in separate container. Add pineapple liquid. Blend.
6. Add liquid mixture to vegetable mixture.
7. Cook, stirring often, until sauce thickens. Boil 5 minutes.
8. Stir in pineapple, mushrooms, water chestnuts and poultry.
9. Cover and heat slowly until hot. May serve hot over rice.

Yield: 6 servings

One serving = 270 calories, 6 grams fat
            = 3 meat + 1 vegetable + 1 fruit

Fried Chicken

6 (4 oz.) chicken breasts (no skin, no bone)　　Herb blend seasoning
1 cup bread crumbs　　Skim milk

1. Pre-heat oven to 350 degrees.
2. Coat each piece with skim milk and roll in 3 tablespoons bread crumbs and herb blend. Place in shallow baking pan.
3. Bake at 350 degrees for 40 minutes or until tender.

Yield: 6 servings

One serving =　200 calories, 3 grams fat
　　　　　　 =　3 meat + 1/2 bread

Lemon-Baked Chicken

One chicken (2 1/2-3 pound),　　　　1 teaspoon mined garlic
　　cut into serving pieces　　　　2 teaspoon oregano
1 tablespoon lemon juice　　　　　 1 teaspoon pepper
1 tablespoon olive oil

1. Remove skin from pieces; wash; pat dry. Place in shallow baking pan.
2. In a bowl, blend oil, lemon juice, seasonings. Pour mixture over chicken pieces.
3. Cover and bake in pre-heated 350 degree oven about 40 minutes, basting occasionally.
4. Uncover and bake 10 minutes longer for browning.

Yield: 4 servings

One serving =　200 calories, 9 grams fat
　　　　　　 =　3 meat, 1 fat

Quick Italian Chicken

3 (4 oz.) chicken breasts (no skin, no bone)
8 oz. jar spaghetti sauce

1. Wash chicken pieces; pat dry. Place in covered saucepan or crockpot.
2. Add spaghetti sauce and simmer 1 hour in saucepan or 2-3 hours in crockpot.

Yield: 3 servings

One serving =　170 calories, 5 grams fat
　　　　　　 =　3 meat

Meat-Free Dishes

Spinach Lasagna

10 ounce (1 pkg) frozen chopped spinach,
    thawed *
1 onion, chopped
2 garlic cloves, minced
1/2 cup chicken broth
3 cups tomato sauce
1 tablespoon chopped fresh basil, or
    1/3 teaspoon dried basil

1 tablespoon marjoram
1 tablespoon oregano
1 tablespoon parsley
1 bay leaf
1 teaspoon black pepper
8 ounces lasagna noodles
1 1/2 cups nonfat or low-fat cottage cheese
4 ounces part-skim mozzarella cheese, shredded

* Can substitute other vegetables, i.e., broccoli, zucchini, yellow squash, etc.

1. Squeeze thawed spinach dry, or use a salad spinner to spin dry.
2. Sauté onions and garlic in broth.
3. Add tomato sauce and seasonings. Simmer 20-30 minutes.
4. Cook lasagna noodles in a separate pot; drain well.
5. Spread half of sauce in a shallow 9-inch baking pan.
6. Layer half the: noodles, spinach, cottage cheese mixture, and mozzarella.
7. Add remaining tomato sauce and repeat layers, ending with mozzarella.
8. Baked (covered) at 350 degrees for 45 minutes.

Yield: 8 servings

One serving =   220 calories, 5 grams fat
           =   2 bread + 1 meat + 1 vegetable

Pasta Salad Meal

8 ounces pasta of choice
    (curls, shells, noodles, etc.)
4 cups vegetables, chopped in bite-size
    pieces (broccoli, red pepper, zucchini,
    peas, mushrooms, cauliflower, etc.)

2 tablespoons grated Parmesan cheese
1/8 teaspoon black pepper
1/2 teaspoon oregano leaves, crushed
1 cup low-fat (or oil-free) Italian salad dressing

1. Cook pasta and drain.
2. Meanwhile, blanch vegetables in boiling water until just crisp - 2-3 minutes. Drain.
3. Toss together gently, pasta, vegetables, seasonings, cheese, and salad dressing.
4. Chill, if desired, before serving.

Yield: 4 servings (Approx. 2 cups per serving.)

			If no-oil dressing is used:
One serving =	350 calories, 10 grams fat	=	250 calories, 0 fat
	3 bread + 1 vegetable + 2 fat	=	3 bread + 1 vegetable

     © 1993, *The Balancing Act Nutrition and Weight Guide*, G. Kostas, M.P.H., R.D., Dallas, Texas

Vegetable Chili

1 onion, chopped
1 garlic clove, minced
2 cans (15 oz. each) whole tomatoes
3 cups fresh mushrooms, chopped
2 green peppers, chopped
2 carrots, grated

2 zucchini, chopped
1/8 teaspoon black pepper
1 teaspoon dried oregano, crushed
3 teaspoons chili powder
1/1/2 tablespoon flour
1 can (16 oz.) kidney beans, drained

1. In a large skillet, steam onion and garlic in a little water until tender.
2. Add all vegetables and seasonings (all ingredients except flour and beans).
3. Cover and simmer until all vegetables are tender, about 15 minutes.
4. Combine flour with 3 tablespoons water. Add to saucepan with beans.
5. Cook, stirring often, until thickened, about 5 minutes.

Yield: 8 servings   *Yield: 6 servings*

                                     OR

One serving =   100 calories, 1 gram fat   =   140 calories, 1 gram fat
             =   1 starch + 1 vegetable   =   1 1/2 starch + 1 1/2 vegetable

Mexican Bean Bake

6 tortillas
2 cups cooked kidney beans
1 onion, chopped
1 garlic clove, minced
1/8 teaspoon black pepper
1 tablespoon dried basil
1 tablespoon dried oregano

1 tablespoon parsley flakes
1 bouillon cube
15 ounce can tomato sauce
8 ounce can tomato paste
1/2 cup skim ricotta cheese
4 ounces shredded part-skim mozzarella cheese

1. Stir and heat in a saucepan the beans, onion, garlic, seasonings, bouillon cube.
2. Add tomato sauce and paste. Cook 20 minutes, stirring occasionally.
3. Add ricotta cheese. Stir and heat.
4. Line bottom of a 11 x 7 x 1 1/2 inch shallow glass baking pan with 6 tortillas.
5. Layer with bean mixture and then mozzarella cheese.
6. Bake uncovered in a pre-heated 400 degree oven for 30 minutes.

Yield: 4 servings

One serving =   300 calories, 7 grams fat
             =   3 bread + 2 meat

High-Calcium Recipes

Herb Spinach-Cheese Pie

1 wholewheat loaf frozen bread dough, thawed
3 eggs or 3/4 cup egg substitute equivalent
1 1/2 cups skim milk
1/2 tablespoon Italian seasoning
  or low-sodium herb blend
1 small tomato, sliced

1/4 teaspoon garlic powder
1/4 teaspoon black pepper
10 ounce (1 pkg) frozen chopped spinach
8 ounces (2 cups) shredded part-skim
    mozzarella cheese

1. Pre-heat oven to 450 degrees.
2. Spread thawed bread dough into greased shallow cooking pan.
3. Bake about 10 minutes, until just browning. Remove and let cool.
4. Reduce oven to 350 degrees.
5. Combine eggs, milk, seasonings. Blend well.
6. Squeeze spinach dry, then add to egg mixture.
7. Add 1 cup of cheese.
8. Pour mixture over crust. Top with tomato slices and remaining cheese.
9. Bake until done - knife inserted comes out clean...about 50 minutes.

Yield: 6 servings

One serving =   350 calories, 9 grams fat, 510 milligrams calcium
            =   3 bread + 2 meat + 1 vegetable

Cheese Enchiladas

2 cans (15 oz. each) tomato sauce
4 teaspoons chili powder
1/4 teaspoon garlic powder
  or 1 garlic clove, minced

12 corn tortillas
8 ounces (2 cups) shredded part-skim mozzarella
  cheese

1. Pre-heat oven to 350 degrees.
2. Combine tomato sauce, chili powder, garlic powder in medium saucepan.
3. Spread 1/4 cup sauce in the bottom of a 9 inch square baking pan.
4. Top with 1 tortilla.
5. Top with 2 tablespoons sauce and 2 tablespoons of cheese.
6. Repeat layering of tortillas, sauce, cheese, ending with cheese.
7. Cover with aluminum foil. Bake until hot - about 25-30 minutes.
8. Meanwhile, heat remaining sauce until hot.
9. Remove tortilla stack from oven and transfer to serving platter. Cut into wedges and serve topped with hot sauce.

Yield: 6 servings

One serving =   290 calories, 9 grams fat, 400 milligrams calcium
            =   2 bread + 1 1/2 meat + 1 vegetables + fat

© 1993, *The Balancing Act Nutrition and Weight Guide*, G. Kostas, M.P.H., R.D., Dallas, Texas

Soups

Creamed Italian Tomato Soup

16 ounce jar spaghetti sauce
8 ounces part-skim ricotta cheese

Blend, heat and serve.

Yield: 4 servings

One serving =   150 calories, 8 grams fat
             =   1 meat + 2 vegetables + 1 fat

Potato-Vegetable Soup

1 cup frozen mixed vegetables
1 medium potato, sliced
2 cups skim milk

4 ounces part-skim mozzarella cheese, shredded
1 bouillon cube

Heat together the above ingredients until cheese melts.

Yield: 6 servings

One serving =   120 calories, 4 grams fat
             =   1 meat + 1/2 milk + 1 vegetable

Corn Chowder *

1/2 tablespoon margarine
1 cup onion, chopped
2 potatoes, peeled and diced into
        bite-size pieces
1 (12 oz.) can evaporated skim milk

1 (16 1/2 oz.) can cream-style corn
1 teaspoon salt
1/4 teaspoon pepper

1. Melt margarine; cook onion in margarine until tender and transparent.
2. In a soup pot, start potatoes in 4 cups water; cook potatoes until done. Do not drain.
3. Add all remaining ingredients including onion.
4. Cook over low to medium heat for 25 minutes, stirring occasionally.

Yield: 8 servings

One serving (1 cup) =   115 calories, 1 gram fat
             =   1 1/2 starches

* Source: <u>What's Cooking at the Cooper Clinic</u> cookbook. Reprinted with permission.

Low-Calorie Dressings

Dress Up Salads With Less Fat!

1. **Zero Salad Dressing**

   2 cups V-8 juice
   1/2 cup fresh lemon juice
   1 tablespoon chopped onion
   1 tablespoon chopped parsley

   Blend in blender.

   Yield: 2 cups
   1 tablespoon = 5 calories, 0 fat

2. **Mock Sour Cream**

   1 cup low-fat cottage cheese
   2 teaspoons lemon juice
   2 tablespoons chives

   Blend until smooth. May add skim milk to thin.

   Yield: 1 1/4 cups
   1 tablespoon = 10 calories, 0 fat

3. Mix 1/3 cup Blue Cheese dressing with 2/3 cup non-fat cottage cheese.
   1 tablespoon = 15 calories, 3 grams fat

4. Mexican hot sauce or Picante sauce
   1 tablespoon = 0 calories, 0 fat

5. Use 3-bean salad juice as dressing.
   1 tablespoon = 5 calories, 0 fat

6. Mix non-fat yogurt with cucumber bits, green onion bits, dill and mint.
   1 tablespoon = 10 calories, 0 fat

7. Mix 8 ounces non-fat yogurt and 1 packet Ranch style dry dressing mix.
   1 tablespoon = 10 calories, 0 grams fat

8. Mix 1 cup bottled Ranch style dressing and 1 cup non-fat yogurt.
   1 tablespoon = 30 calories, 3 grams fat

9. Flavored vinegars: wine vinegar, Tarragon vinegar, herb vinegars, balsamic
   1 tablespoon = 0 calories, 0 fat

10. Lemon juice
    1 tablespoon = 0 calories, 0 fat.

High-Fiber Recipes

Granola

4 cups dry oatmeal
1 cup bran flakes
2 cups All-Bran
1 cup raisins *
3/4 cup almonds
1/2 cup sunflower seeds
1 1/2 teaspoon cinnamon
1/2 teaspoon nutmeg
1 cup orange juice
1/2 cup wheat germ (optional)
2 tablespoons vanilla
1 small apple, peeled and chopped

Combine and bake 45 to 60 minutes at 250 degrees until browned.
* Add raisins during last 15 minutes only.

Yield: 10 cups (20 servings)

One serving (1/2 cup)   =   185 calories, 7 grams fat, 7 grams fiber
                        =   2 bread + 1 fat

Wholewheat Bran Muffins

2/3 cup all-purpose flour
1/2 cup wholewheat flour
1 tablespoon baking powder
1/2 teaspoon salt
1 cup All-Bran cereal
1 cup skim milk
1 egg

1. Stir together all-purpose flour, wholewheat flour, baking powder, and salt. Set aside.
2. Measure All-Bran cereal and milk into large mixing bowl. Stir to combine. Let stand about 2 minutes or until cereal is softened. Add egg. Beat well.
3. Add flour mixture, stirring only until combined. Portion batter into 12 greased muffin cups.
4. Bake at 400 degrees about 25 minutes or until lightly browned.

Yield: 12 muffins

1 muffin   =   70 calories, 1 gram fat, 3 grams fiber
           =   1 bread

Low-Sodium Recipes

Low-Sodium Vegetarian Pizza

Crust 3 cups flour
     1 1/2 tablespoons (2 envelopes) yeast
     1 cup lukewarm water
     2 tablespoons corn oil

Topping 2 tablespoons corn oil
     1 1/2 cups unsalted stewed tomatoes
     4 cups thinly sliced mushrooms *
     freshly ground black pepper to taste
     2 teaspoons dried oregano
     2 cups grated, part-skim mozzarella

  * May use 4 cups of any vegetable combination (broccoli, squash, carrots, mushrooms, onions, etc.)

1. Blend 1 cup of flour, yeast and 1/2 cup of lukewarm water in a mixing bowl or food processor. Blend well.
2. Add the oil and the remaining flour and water. Blend for about 1 minute. The dough will be a little sticky.
3. Scrape the dough onto a lightly floured board and knead briefly. Gather it into a ball, place in a bowl and cover with a cloth. Let stand for 30 minutes in a warm place.
4. Divide the dough in half. Pat out each piece of dough into a circle.
5. Add 1 tablespoon of oil to each of two 13 inch pizza pans. Place one circle of dough in the center of one pan. Press the dough with your knuckles all the way to the rim of the pans. Cover and let stand in a warm place for 30 minutes.
6. Pre-heat the oven to 400 degrees.
7. Spoon stewed tomatoes and mushrooms (or other vegetables) equally on top of each pizza. Sprinkle with pepper and equal amounts of remaining ingredients. Place in the oven and bake for 20 minutes.
8. Transfer the pizza to the lower rack and increase the oven temperature to 425 degrees. Bake for 5 minutes, or until browned on the bottom.

Yield: 2 pizzas, 16 slices (8 slices per pizza)

2 slices = 320 calories, 7 grams fat, 160 milligrams sodium
     = 2 bread + 1 meat + 2 vegetables + 2 fat

1 slice   = 160 calories, 3 grams fat, 80 milligrams sodium
     = 1 bread + 1/2 meat + 1 vegetable + 1 fat

Herb Blends (Salt-Free, Calorie-Free)

Prepare your own sodium-free herb blends to use in cooking and in the salt shaker at the table.

1. **Season-All** (Mix for meats and vegetables)

    1 teaspoon basil

    1 teaspoon marjoram

    1 teaspoon thyme

    1 teaspoon oregano

    1 teaspoon parsley

    1 teaspoon savory

    1 teaspoon mace

    1 teaspoon ground cloves

    1/4 teaspoon nutmeg

    1 teaspoon black pepper

    1/4 teaspoons cayenne

2. **All-Purpose Spice Blend**

    5 teaspoons onion powder

    2 1/2 teaspoons paprika

    1 1/4 teaspoons thyme

    1/4 teaspoon celery seed

    2 1/2 teaspoons garlic powder

    2 1/2 teaspoons mustard powder

    1/2 teaspoon ground white pepper

3. **Herb Seasoning Blend**

    2 tablespoons dill weed or basil

    1 teaspoon oregano
       leaves, crushed

    2 tablespoons onion powder

    1/4 teaspoon grated lemon peel (dried)

    1 teaspoon celery seed

    1/16 teaspoon black pepper

4. **Spicy Flavor Blend**

    2 tablespoons savory, crushed

    2 1/2 teaspoons onion powder

    1 3/8 teaspoons curry powder

    1 1/4 teaspoons cumin

    1 tablespoon powdered mustard

    1 1/4 teaspoons ground white pepper

    1/2 teaspoon garlic powder

Low-Sugar Desserts

No-Sugar Cookies

2 cups all-purpose flour
1/2 cup walnuts, chopped
1/2 cup dark seedless raisins
1/2 cup orange juice
1/2 cup margarine, softened

2 teaspoons double-acting baking powder
1 teaspoon grated orange peel
1/2 teaspoon salt
1/2 teaspoon ground cinnamon
1 egg

1. Pre-heat oven to 375 degrees.
2. In large bowl, with wooden spoon, stir all ingredients until well mixed.
3. Onto greased cookie sheets, drop dough by tablespoonfuls about 2 inches apart.
4. Bake about 20 minutes or until lightly browned.
5. With metal spatula, remove cookies to wire racks to cool. Store in tightly covered container.

Yield: 2 1/2 dozen cookies

One cookie = 80 calories, 5 grams fat
            = 1 bread

Peanut Butter Cookies

1/3 cup low-calorie mayonnaise
1/4 cup sugar
1 egg
1 cup peanut butter

1/2 teaspoon baking soda
1/4 teaspoon cinnamon
1 teaspoon vanilla
1 cup wholewheat flour

1. Cream together mayonnaise and sugar until well blended.
2. Beat in egg, peanut butter, baking soda, cinnamon and vanilla until smooth.
3. Add flour and beat until well blended.
4. Roll dough into balls about 3/4 inch in diameter and place on ungreased cookie sheets.
5. Bake at 375 degrees for 10-12 minutes or until browned.
6. Remove cookies from sheet and cool on wire racks.

Yield: 40 cookies

One cookie = 60 calories, 4 grams fat
            = 1 bread

© 1993, *The Balancing Act Nutrition and Weight Guide*, G. Kostas, M.P.H., R.D., Dallas, Texas

Apple Dessert

1/2 cup uncooked rolled oats
6 cups thinly sliced apples
1 cup unsweetened apple juice
1/2 cup raisins

1/2 cup finely chopped prunes
1/4 teaspoon cloves
1/4 teaspoon cinnamon
1/3 cup Grape Nut Flakes

1. Layer oats in bottom of 8 inch square baking pan, add apple slices.
2. Pour apple juice over and sprinkle with raisins, prunes, cinnamon and cloves.
3. Cover with foil.
4. Bake at 350 degrees for one hour.
5. Remove foil, sprinkle with Grape Nut Flakes and bake 15 minutes.

Yield: 6 servings

One serving = 180 calories, 1 gram fat
= 2 bread + 1/2 fruit

Hot Fudge Pudding Cake *

1 1/4 cup sugar, divided
1 cup flour
7 tablespoons cocoa powder, divided
2 teaspoons baking powder
1/4 teaspoon salt

1/2 cup skim milk
1/3 cup margarine, melted
1 1/2 teaspoon vanilla
1/2 cup brown sugar, firmly packed
1 1/4 cup hot water

1. In a medium mixing bowl, combine 3/4 cup sugar, flour, 3 tablespoons cocoa powder, baking powder and salt.
2. Blend in milk, melted margarine and vanilla; beat until smooth.
3. Pour batter into 8 or 9-inch square pan.
4. In a small bowl, combine remaining 1/2 cup sugar, brown sugar and remaining 4 tablespoons cocoa powder.
5. Sprinkle mixture evenly over batter.
6. Pour hot water over top; do not stir.
7. Bake at 350 degrees for 40 minutes or until center is almost set.
8. Let stand 15 minutes.
9. Spoon into dessert dishes, spooning sauce from bottom of pan over top.
10. Garnish with light Cool Whip (Optional).

Yield: 9 servings

One serving = 275 calories, 7 grams fat
= 3 bread + 1 fat

* Source: <u>What's Cooking at the Cooper Clinic</u> cookbook. Reprinted with permission.

Brownies De-light

With this recipe, you omit 1060 calories and 130 grams fat per batch.

1 box brownie mix, any brand
4 oz. non-fat plain yogurt

amount of water as shown on box
chocolate packet, if included

1. Omit 2 eggs and 1/2 cup oil from recipe directions on box of brownies. Instead, add yogurt to brownie mix and blend together in a mixing bowl.
2. Pre-heat oven to 350 degrees.
3. Pour mixture into pan sprayed with non-stick cooking spray; bake about 30 minutes, as directed on the brownie package.

Yield: 24 brownies (2" x 2")

One serving =   120 calories, 3 grams fat
            =   1 bread + 1 fat

Lucious Layer Cake

1 box yellow or white or lemon cake mix
1/3 cup applesauce (to replace 1/3 cup
    oil in directions)
Optional: low-fat vanilla frosting (i.e., Pillsbury's Lovin' Lites)

3 egg whites or 3/4 cup egg substitute
1 1/4 cups water

1. Pre-heat oven to 350 degrees. Spray 2 9-inch round cake pans with non-stick spray.
2. Mix all ingredients listed above with an electric mixer at low speed until moistened. Then beat at high speed for 2 minutes.
3. Pour half the batter in each pan. Bake 30-40 minutes, or until done. Cool. Remove from pans; may layer and frost cake.

Yield: 12 servings

	Without Frosting		With Frosting
One serving =	200 calories, 4 grams fat	=	330 calories, 6 grams fat
=	2 bread + 1 fat	=	3 1/2 bread + 1 fat

APPENDIX E

Meal Comparisons

- P-C-F Balance
- Fats and Cholesterol
- Fiber
- Sodium

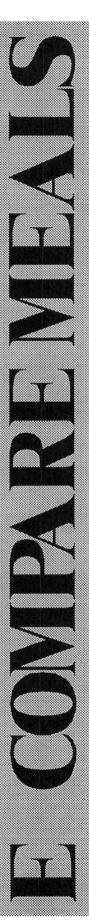

MEAL COMPARISON - P-C-F BALANCE

IMBALANCED
3000 Calories
10% Protein, 30% Carbohydrate, 60 % Fat

	*CAL	P (gm)	C (gm)	F (gm)
BREAKFAST				
1 fried egg	100	7	0	10
1 white toast	70	2	15	0
+ 1 tsp butter	35	0	0	5
+ 1 tbsp jam	50	0	12	0
2 strips bacon	100	0	0	10
8 ounces whole milk	150	8	12	10
LUNCH				
hamburger on bun with 3-ounce meat patty	390	29	32	20
20 french fries	280	4	40	20
12-ounce coke	150	0	40	0
1.2 ounce chocolate candy bar	190	0	11	20
SUPPER				
6 ounce ribeye steak	750	35	0	66
1 medium baked potato	140	4	30	0
+ 1 tbsp butter	100	0	0	12
+ 1 tbsp sour cream	30	0	0	3
2 rolls	140	4	30	0
+ 2 tsp butter	70	0	0	8
salad	25	2	5	0
+ 2 tbsp blue cheese	160	0	0	18
1/2 cup broccoli	25	2	4	0
+ 1 tsp butter	35	0	0	4
water	0	0	0	0
TOTALS:	**3000**	**97**	**231**	**206**

BALANCED
3000 Calories
16% Protein, 56% Carbohydrate, 28% Fat

	*CAL	P (gm)	C (gm)	F (gm)
BREAKFAST				
6 ounces orange juice	80	0	10	0
1 cup shredded wheat	140	4	30	0
8 ounces skim milk	80	8	12	0
1 banana	80	0	20	0
2 wholewheat toast	140	4	30	0
+ 2 tsp margarine	70	0	0	8
+ 1 tbsp jam	50	0	12	0
1 cup coffee	0	0	0	0
LUNCH				
turkey sandwich: 2 wholewheat bread	140	4	30	0
3 ounces turkey	150	24	0	6
1 ounce mozzarella cheese	80	7	0	5
lettuce/tomato/mustard	10	0	2	0
1 cup coleslaw	160	2	6	18
1/2 cup potato salad	180	0	9	17
1 medium apple	100	0	25	0
8 ounces iced tea	0	0	0	0
SNACK				
12 ounces apple juice	120	0	30	0
1 wholewheat bagel	170	4	32	2
SUPPER				
4 ounce lean steak filet	240	32	0	12
1 medium baked potato	140	4	30	0
+ 2 tsp margarine	70	0	0	8
2 wholewheat rolls	140	4	30	0
+ 1 tsp margarine	35	0	0	4
salad	25	2	5	0
+ 1 tbsp Italian dressing	80	0	0	9
1 cup broccoli	50	4	10	0
1 piece angel food cake	140	4	30	0
3/4 cup strawberries	40	0	10	0
8 ounces skim milk	80	8	12	0
SNACK				
4 cups air-popped popcorn	100	3	22	0
12 ounces pineapple juice	120	0	30	0
TOTALS:	**3000**	**118**	**400**	**90**

*Cal = Calcium, P = Protein, C = Carbohydrates, F = Fats

MEAL COMPARISON - FATS AND CHOLESTEROL

HIGH FAT MEAL PLAN
1700 Calories
20% Protein, 27% Carbohydrate, 53% Fat

	*CAL	Chol (mg)	Total Fat (gm)	Sat Fat (gm)
BREAKFAST				
1 orange	60	0	0	0
cheese omelet				
1 egg	80	250	6	2
1 ounce cheddar cheese	100	30	8	6
2 strips bacon	90	10	10	5
1 white toast	70	0	0	0
+ 2 tsp butter	70	25	8	4
LUNCH				
hamburger:				
3 ounce patty	240	80	20	9
1 bun	140	0	0	0
mustard	0	0	0	0
lettuce/tomato	10	0	0	0
10 french fries	140	10	10	2
1/2 cup coleslaw	120	4	10	0
1 chocolate chip cookie	70	6	5	1
SUPPER				
4 ounce sirloin steak	280	100	16	15
1 small baked potato	70	0	0	0
+ 1 tbsp butter	100	35	12	
+ 1 tbsp sour cream		30	5	3
1/2 cup broccoli	25	0	0	0
+ 2 tbsp cheese sauce	65	65	5	5
TOTALS:	**1730**	**645**	**115**	**52**

LOW FAT MEAL PLAN
1700 Calories
25% Protein, 57% Carbohydrate, 18% Fat

	*CAL	Chol (mg)	Total Fat (gm)	Sat Fat (gm)
BREAKFAST				
4 ounces orange juice	60	0	0	0
1 large banana	100	0	0	0
1 cup bran flakes	140	0	0	0
1 cup skim milk	90	5	0	0
2 wholewheat toast	140	0	0	0
1 ounce ricotta skim cheese	60	10	3	1
LUNCH				
tuna sandwich:				
1/2 cup tuna in water	120	60	0	0
1 tbsp diet mayonnaise	50	5	5	1
2 wholewheat bread	140	0	0	0
lettuce/tomato	10	0	0	0
carrot/celery sticks	25	0	0	0
1 large apple	100	0	0	0
1 cup skim milk	90	5	0	0
1 fat-free cookie	70	0	0	0
SUPPER				
4 ounce chicken breast				
(baked without skin)	200	80	6	2
1 medium baked potato	140	0	0	0
+ 1 tbsp diet margarine	50	0	6	0
+ 1 tbsp parmesan cheese	25	8	2	2
+ 2 tbsp non-fat yogurt	10	0	0	0
+ chives	0	0	0	0
1/2 cup broccoli	25	0	0	0
tossed salad	25	0	0	0
+ 1 tbsp ranch dressing	55	0	6	2
TOTALS:	**1725**	**173**	**28**	**8**

*Cal = Calcium, Chol = Cholesterol

   © 1993, *The Balancing Act Nutrition and Weight Guide*, G. Kostas, M.P.H., R.D., Dallas, Texas

MEAL COMPARISON - FIBER

Both meals contain approximately 1700 Calories, 20% Protein, 30% Fat, 50% Carbohydrates.

LOW FIBER MEAL PLAN

	Dietary Fiber (gm)	Calories
BREAKFAST		
orange juice, 1/2 cup	0.0	60
white toast, 1 slice	0.8	70
margarine, 1 tsp	0.0	35
poached egg, 1	0.0	80
skim milk, 1 cup	0.0	90
water, 1 cup	0.0	0
LUNCH		
tuna sandwich:		
1/2 cup tuna in water	0.0	120
2 tsp mayonnaise	0.0	90
2 slices white bread	1.6	140
banana, 1/2 6" medium	3.2	60
yogurt, 1 cup nonfat	0.0	100
water, 1 cup	0.0	0
SUPPER		
chicken 1/2 breast		
(3 ounces, no skin)	0.0	150
rice, white 1/2 cup	0.8	110
asparagus, 4 med spears	0.9	10
carrots, steamed, 1/2 cup	2.3	25
coleslaw, 1/2 cup	1.7	120
dinner roll, 1 small	0.8	80
margarine, 1 tsp	0.0	35
cantaloupe, 1/3	1.6	60
water, 1 cup	0.0	0
SNACK		
cupcake, 1 frosted		
(2-1/2 inches)	0.9	130
skim milk	0.0	90
TOTALS:	**14.6**	**1,700**

HIGH FIBER MEAL PLAN

	Dietary Fiber (gm)	Calories
BREAKFAST		
stewed prunes, 3 medium	3.9	60
All Bran cereal, 1/3 cup	9.0	80
poached egg, 1	0.0	80
wholewheat toast, 1	2.1	80
margarine, 1 tsp	0.0	35
water, 1 cup	0.0	0
LUNCH		
tuna sandwich:		
1/2 cup tuna in water	0.0	120
2 tsp mayonnaise	0.0	90
2 slices wholewheat bread	4.2	140
tomato slices and lettuce	1.0	10
carrots, 6 strips raw	0.8	5
apple, 1 medium w/skin	3.3	60
water, 1 cup	0.0	0
SUPPER		
chicken 1/2 breast		
(3 ounces, no skin)	0.0	150
baked potato, med w/skin	3.0	130
margarine, 1 tsp	0.0	35
spinach, 1/2 cup steamed	5.7	25
lettuce, 1 cup w/ 1/2 cup		
raw celery and	1.1	5
2 rings green pepper	0.2	5
1 tbsp french low-cal drsg	0.0	15
bran muffin, 1 large	3.2	150
skim milk, 1 cup	0.0	90
mixed fruit cup, 1 cup	3.2	120
water, 1 cup	0.0	0
SNACK		
popcorn, 3 C (no butter)	1.2	75
apple juice, 1 cup	0.0	120
TOTALS:	**42.6**	**1,700**

MEAL COMPARISON - SODIUM

Both meals contain approximately 1700 Calories, 20% Protein, 30% Fat, 50% Carbohydrates.

HIGH SODIUM MEAL PLAN

	Amount	Sodium (mg)	Calories
BREAKFAST			
cornflakes	1/2 cup	200	80
milk, 2%	1/2 cup	60	60
cantaloupe	1/3 melon	0	80
LUNCH			
tuna sandwich:			
wholewheat bread	2 slices	240	140
white tuna, canned in			
water	1/4 cup	200	60
mayonnaise	2 tsp	50	90
dill pickle	1/2 large	700	5
potato chips	10 chips	200	150
SNACK			
cheddar cheese	1 ounce	200	100
saltines	6	240	80
DINNER			
ham, cured	4 ounces	1,600	240
corn, canned	1/3 cup	100	80
green beans, canned	1/2 cup	270	25
biscuit, canned	1	300	115
margarine	2 tsp	100	70
lettuce / tomato salad	1 cup	5	50
bottled Italian dressing	1 tbsp	300	80
angel food cake	1 small slice	10	100
SNACK			
salted pretzels	38 sticks	100	80
TOTALS:		**4,875**	**1,700**

LOW SODIUM MEAL PLAN

	Amount	Sodium (mg)	Calories
BREAKFAST			
shredded wheat	3/4 cup	2	80
milk, 2%	1/2 cup	60	60
orange juice	1/2 cup	2	60
LUNCH			
tuna sandwich:			
wholewheat bread	2 slices	240	140
white tuna, canned in			
water, low sodium	1/4 cup	2	60
mayonnaise	2 tsp	50	90
celery, diced	1/4 cup	20	5
carrot sticks	1/2 cup	50	25
pear	1 medium	10	80
SNACK			
raisin bread	1 slice	120	80
milk, 2%	1 cup	120	120
margarine	1 tsp	50	35
DINNER			
ham, fresh	4 ounces	70	240
corn on the cob	1 small ear	0	80
green beans, frozen	1/2 cup	1	25
homemade biscuit	1	5	115
margarine	2 tsp	100	70
lettuce / tomato salad	1 cup	5	50
oil and vinegar	1 tbsp	1	80
baked apple			
with cinnamon	1 large	1	100
SNACK			
unsalted pretzels	38 sticks	5	80
TOTALS:		**935**	**1,700**

    © 1993, *The Balancing Act Nutrition and Weight Guide*, G. Kostas, M.P.H., R.D., Dallas, Texas

BOOK ORDER FORM
CLIP AND MAIL TODAY!

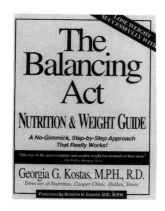 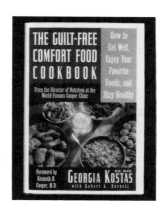 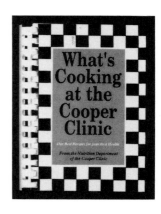

The Balancing Act Nutrition and Weight Guide
P.O. Box 671281, Dallas, Texas 75367-8281

Please send me _____ copies of **THE BALANCING ACT NUTRITION AND WEIGHT GUIDE** —
a step-by-step, no-gimmick approach to weight loss reflecting the Cooper Clinic philosophy of
health and fitness. Cost: $29.95 plus $4.50 shipping for each book. Texas residents add $2.47 tax.
Enclosed is my check for $ _____. Make checks payable to "The Balancing Act".
Mail to:

Name _____
Address _____
City _____State _____Zip _____

Visa, MasterCard and American Express accepted.
For phone orders, call the Cooper Clinic Nutrition Department at (214) 239-7223, ext. 161

The Guilt-Free Comfort Food Cookbook
P.O. Box 671281, Dallas, Texas 75367-8281

Please send me _____ copies of **THE GUILT-FREE COMFORT FOOD COOKBOOK** by Georgia
Kostas & Bob Barnett — a collection of American favorite "comfort foods" made healthy and guilt-free.
Nutrient Analysis included. Cost: $19.99 plus $4.00 shipping for each book. Texas residents add
$1.98 tax. Enclosed is my check for $ _____. Make checks payable to "Georgia Kostas &
Associates, Inc." Mail to:

Name _____
Address _____
City _____State _____Zip _____

Visa, MasterCard and American Express accepted.
For phone orders, call the Cooper Clinic Nutrition Department at (214) 239-7223, ext. 161

FOR OTHER PRODUCTS & SERVICES
FROM THE COOPER CLINIC

RECIPE ANALYSIS

Enclosed are _____ recipes that I would like analyzed by the Cooper Clinic at $15 each.
My check for $_____ is attached. (Make checks payable to "Cooper Clinic".)
Mail to: Nutrition Department-Cooper Clinic, 12200 Preston Road, Dallas, Texas 75230.

Name _____
Address _____
City _____State _____Zip _____

COMPUTERIZED DIET ANALYSIS

I would like to have my diet analyzed for 26 nutrients and receive nutritional
recommendations. Please send me the Nutrient Analysis for to record my intake. I will
return the form with $37 payment. (Make checks payable to "Cooper Clinic".)
Mail to: Nutrition Department-Cooper Clinic, 12200 Preston Road, Dallas, Texas 75230.

Name _____
Address _____
City _____State _____Zip _____

WHAT'S COOKING AT THE COOPER CLINIC - COOKBOOK

Please send me ___ copies of WHAT'S COOKING AT THE COOPER CLINIC at $14.95
plus $3.75 shipping for each book. Texas residents add $1.24 tax. Enclosed is my check
for $_____. (Make checks payable to "It's Cooking".) Mail to: Nutrition Department-
Cooper Clinic, 12200 Preston Road, Dallas, Texas 75230.

Name _____
Address _____
City _____State _____Zip _____

Visa, MasterCard and American Express accepted.
For phone orders, call the Nutrition Department at (214) 239-7223, ext. 161

© 1993, *The Balancing Act Nutrition and Weight Guide*, G. Kostas, M.P.H., R.D., Dallas, Texas

NUTRITION & WEIGHT LOSS HANDOUTS

REPRODUCIBLE MASTERS from
The Balancing Act Nutrition & Weight Guide

🍎 MENU MASTERS..$75

20 Pages: 71-91

PEOPLE LOVE THESE MEALS ! TRULY AN INNOVATIVE IDEA AND A GREAT TIME SAVER !

(1) 14 Days of delicious, healthy *Menus* at 1,000, 1,200, and 1,500 calories. All *Meals* are "quick-fix", "recipe-free," and very easy to assemble;

plus —

(2) 75 Quick and Easy "Mix-and-Match" meals: for *breakfast*, brown-bag *lunches*, and *suppers*... perfect for those who want pre-planned, easy, flexible meal choices. Any 3 meals add up to approximately 1,500 calories per day ... and 20-30 grams of fat per 1,000 calories.

🍎 OPTIMAL NUTRITION SERIES $50

10 Pages: 8-11, 17, 21, 41-44

SIMPLIFY BASIC NUTRITION WITH THESE CONCEPTS:

- *Optimal Nutrition* Guidelines
- *P-F-C Balance* Concept
- *Eating Plan Basics* — a teaching guide
- Helpful *Habits*
- Nutrition IQ *Quiz*

🍎 WEIGHT MANAGEMENT BASICS $65

16 Pages: 8, 9, 11, 12, 14, 15, 17, 27-29, 41-44, 94, and 95

KNOW WHERE TO BEGIN !

- *Eating* — Precise guidelines anyone can follow
- *Exercise* — Choose your own action plan
- *Body Composition* — "Rev up" your metabolism
- *Habits* — Your key to permanent weight loss
- Calorie and Fat *Comparisons* in Foods

🍎 HABITS: MAKING WEIGHT LOSS WORK.......................$65

16 Pages: 17, 37, 57, 135-137, 149-151, 153, 154, 203, and 220-223

THE RIGHT STRATEGIES AND SKILLS FOR YOU!

- *Planning, Portions, Pace*
- Recognizing Food *Cues*
- Identifying Your Best *Strategies*

🍎 FACTS ON FAT $65

16 Pages: 45, 67, 94, 95, 100-102, 108-110, 138-143

WAYS TO CUT BACK ON HIDDEN FAT!

- Fat in Foods and Quick Fat Gram Counter
- Cholesterol Update
- 15 Painless Way to Eat Less Fat

🍎 EATING OUT SERIES $60

13 Pages: 169-180, 183

HERE'S HOW TO EAT OUT ANYTIME, ANYWHERE:

- Ordering Tips
- Fast Foods
- Alcohol
- Restaurant Meal Comparisons
- Holidays

🍎 KEY NUTRIENTS $50

9 Pages: 141, 205-212

LEARN THE "WHY'S" AND "HOW'S" OF:

- Fiber
- Calcium
- Cholesterol
- Caffeine
- Water

🍎 TOP CHOICES: SNACKS & FUN FOODS $50

10 Pages: 69, 97-99, 129, 130, 144, 145, 161

CHOOSE THE BEST:

- Healthy Snacks
- Top Cereals
- Chocolate and Ice Cream Treats
- Cheeses

🍎 COOKING TIPS $50

9 Pages: 100, 163, 164, 127-132

TASTY TIPS TO LIGHTEN YOUR FAVORITE RECIPES!

- Cooking Tips to Cut Fat and Add Flavor
- Fun Foods: *Nachos, Pizza, Chips, Shakes, French Fries, Potatoes*
- 23 Easy *Vegetable Ideas* to "Veg'Out"
- Savory Seasonings without Sodium

🍎 SUGAR AND SODIUM $50

10 Pages: 155-160, 162-165

WHY AND WAYS TO LIMIT THEM:

- Hidden Sources
- Food Comparisons
- Savvy Seasonings
- Cooking Tips

------------------------------✂------------------ ORDER FORM ------------------✂------------------------------

REPRODUCIBLE MASTERS

Please send me the following Reproducible Masters:

____ set(s) of **Menu Masters**	$75 ea.
____ set(s) of **Optimal Nutrition Series**	$50 ea.
____ set(s) of **Weight Management Basics**	$65 ea.
____ set(s) of **Habits: Making Weight Loss Work**	$65 ea.
____ set(s) of **Facts on Fats**	$65 ea.
____ set(s) of **Eating Out Series**	$60 ea.
____ set(s) of **Key Nutrients**	$50 ea.
____ set(s) of **Top Choices: Snacks & Fun Foods**	$50 ea.
____ set(s) of **Cooking Tips**	$50 ea.
____ set(s) of **Sugar and Sodium**	$50 ea.

____ Total sets..................................... Sub-Total $_____

Please add $3.00 shipping per set X _____ sets = ... $_____

Texas residents add 8.25% tax. .... $_____

Reproducible Masters Total Amount.................. $_____

BOOKS *(Call for volume discounts.)*

Please send me _____ copies of *The Balancing Act Nutrition and Weight Guide* @ $29.95 ea...............................$_____

Please add $4.50 shipping per book X _____ books = ...$_____
Texas residents add $2.47 tax per book X _____ books = ...$_____

Total Book Amount...$_____

Reproducible Masters Total Amount (from previous column) ......$_____

TOTAL ORDER AMOUNT ....$_____

☐ Enclosed is my check to *"The Balancing Act"* for $_____.

Name _____

Address _____

City/State_____ Zip _____

Phone (   ) _____

For more information, please ☎ : (214) 239-7223.

✉ **Mail this order form to:** The Balancing Act, PO Box 671281, Dallas, Texas 75367-8281

SUGGESTIONS

    We would like to hear from you on how to improve the next edition of *The Balancing Act Nutrition & Weight Guide*. Give us your comments, corrections, criticisms, compliments, and suggestions; please send them to us at the address as shown below:

_____

_____

_____

_____

_____

_____

_____

_____

_____

_____

_____

_____

_____

_____

Thank you!

Send suggestions to: The Balancing Act
                                 P.O. Box 671281
                                 Dallas, TX 75367-8281